Clinical Pr KV-418-821

OBSTETRICS AND GYNECOLOGY

Clinical Progress in
OBSTETRICS AND GYNECOLOGY

Editor
Duru Shah
MD FRCOG FCPS FICS FICOG FICMCH DGO DFP
Scientific Director
Gynaecworld and Gynaecworld Assisted Fertility Center
Consultant Obstetrician and Gynecologist
Breach Candy Hospital/Jaslok Hospital/Sir Hurkisondas Hospital
Mumbai, Maharashtra, India

Associate Editor
Sudeshna Ray
MD MRCOG (London)
Consultant Obstetrician and Gynecologist
Jaslok Hospital and Research Center/Saifee Hospital
Mumbai, Maharashtra, India

JAYPEE BROTHERS MEDICAL PUBLISHERS (P) LTD

New Delhi • London • Philadelphia • Panama

Jaypee Brothers Medical Publishers (P) Ltd

Headquarters

Jaypee Brothers Medical Publishers (P) Ltd
4838/24, Ansari Road, Daryaganj
New Delhi 110 002, India
Phone: +91-11-43574357
Fax: +91-11-43574314
Email: jaypee@jaypeebrothers.com

Overseas Offices

J.P. Medical Ltd
83, Victoria Street, London
SW1H 0HW (UK)
Phone: +44-2031708910
Fax: +02-03-0086180
Email: info@jpmedpub.com

Jaypee Brothers Medical Publishers Ltd
The Bourse
111 South Independence Mall East
Suite 835, Philadelphia, PA 19106, USA
Phone: + 267-519-9789
Email: joe.rusko@jaypeebrothers.com

Jaypee Brothers Medical Publishers (P) Ltd
Shorakhute, Kathmandu
Nepal
Phone: +00977-9841528578
Email: jaypee.nepal@gmail.com

Jaypee-Highlights Medical Publishers Inc.
City of Knowledge, Bld. 237, Clayton
Panama City, Panama
Phone: +507-301-0496
Fax: +507-301-0499
Email: cservice@jphmedical.com

Jaypee Brothers Medical Publishers (P) Ltd
17/1-B Babar Road, Block-B, Shaymali
Mohammadpur, Dhaka-1207
Bangladesh
Mobile: +08801912003485
Email: jaypeedhaka@gmail.com

Website: www.jaypeebrothers.com
Website: www.jaypeedigital.com

Inquiries for bulk sales may be solicited at: jaypee@jaypeebrothers.com

This book has been published in good faith that the contents provided by the contributors contained herein are original, and is intended for educational purposes only. While every effort is made to ensure accuracy of information, the publisher and the editors specifically disclaim any damage, liability, or loss incurred, directly or indirectly, from the use or application of any of the contents of this work. If not specifically stated, all figures and tables are courtesy of the editors. Where appropriate, the readers should consult with a specialist or contact the manufacturer of the drug or device.

Clinical Progress in Obstetrics and Gynecology

First Edition: 2013

ISBN   978-93-5090-444-2

Printed at : Ajanta Offset & Packagings Ltd., New Delhi

Contributors

Ajay Rane
MBBS MD FRCOG FRCS FRANZCOG CU
FICOG (Hon) PhD
Consultant Urogynecologist
The Townsville and Mater Hospitals
Professor and Head
Department of Obstetrics and Gynecology
James Cook University
Townsville, Queensland, Australia

Anita Soni
MBBS MD DNB DGD
Consultant Obstetrician and Gynecologist
Dr LH Hiranandani Hospital
Mumbai, Maharashtra, India

Asha Kapadia
MBBS MD DABP
Head
Department of Medical Oncology
PD Hinduja National Hospital and Medical
Research Center
Mumbai, Maharashtra, India

Duru Shah
MD FRCOG FICS FICOG FICMCH DGO DFP
Consultant Obstetrician and Gynecologist
Breach Candy Hospital, Jaslok Hospital and
Sir Hurkisondas Hospital
Mumbai, Maharashtra, India

Isaac Manyonda
BSc MBBS PhD MRCOG
Professor and Consultant
Department of Obstetrics and Gynecology
St George's Hospital and University of London
London, UK

Jay Iyer
MBBS MD DNB MRCOG FRANZCOG
Consultant Obstetrics and Gynecology and
Pelvic Floor Surgeon
The Townsville and Mater Hospitals
Senior Lecturer
Department of Obstetrics and Gynecology
James Cook University
Townsville, Queensland, Australia

Latika Narang MRCOG
Specialist Registrar
Department of Obstetrics and Gynecology
St George's Hospital and St George's
University of London
London, UK

Madhuri Patil
MD DGO FCPS DFP FICOG (Mum)
Clinical Director
Dr Patil's Fertility and Endoscopy Clinic
Bengaluru, Karnataka, India

Mary Ann Lumsden
MRCOG FRCOG
Department of Obstetrics and Gynecology
School of Medicine
University of Glasgow
Scotland, UK

Muzammil Shaikh
MBBS MD
Junior Consultant
Department of Medical Oncology
PD Hinduja National Hospital and Medical
Research Center
Mumbai, Maharashtra, India

Neha Gupta MD
Senior Resident
Department of Obstetrics and Gynecology
Maulana Azad Medical College
New Delhi, India

Niraj Yanamandra MD
Consultant Obstetrics and Gynecology
Fernandez Hospital
Hyderabad, Andhra Pradesh, India

Rucha S Dagaonkar
DNB (Pulmonary Medicine)
Pulmonary Fellow
Department of Pulmonary Medicine
PD Hinduja National Hospital and Medical
Research Center
Mumbai, Maharashtra, India

Sabaratnam Arulkumaran
MD PhD
Professor and Head
Obstetrics and Gynecology
St George's University of London
London, UK

Seeru Garg
Clinical Associate
Department of Obstetrics and Gynecology
Dr LH Hiranandani Hospital
Mumbai, Maharashtra, India

Shantanu Abhayankar
MD FICOG
Modern Clinic
Wai, Maharashtra, India

Sigal Klipstein MD FACOG
In Via Fertility Specialists
Hoffman Estates, Illinoisis
Department of Obstetrics and Gynecology
University of Chicago
Chicago, USA

Stamatina Iliodromiti MD MRCOG
Department of Obstetrics and Gynecology
School of Medicine, University of Glasgow
Scotland, UK

Suchitra Dalvie MD MRCOG
Coordinator
Asia Safe Abortion Partenership
Mumbai, Maharashtra, India

Sujata Mishra
MD FICOG
Associate Professor
SCB Medical College, Cuttack
Chairperson, Medical Disorders in
Pregnancy Committee FOGSI
Academic Counselor
PGDMCH Course IGNOU
Member, Asia Pacific Society for Infections
in Gynecology and Obstetrics
Cuttack, Odisha, India

Suneeta Mittal
MD FAFM
Professor and Head
Department of Obstetrics and Gynecology
All India Institute of Medical Sciences
New Delhi, India

Vishwanath Karande
MD
InVia Fertility Specialists
Hoffman Estates
Illinois, USA

Zarir Udwadia
MD DNB FRCP FCCP
Consultant Chest Physician
Department of Pulmonary Medicine
PD Hinduja National Hospital and Medical
Research Center
Mumbai, Maharashtra, India

Preface

Newer research and newer therapies are emerging globally at a very rapid pace. During this period of engulfing time-crunch that every clinician and postgraduate faces, scanning indexed journals, attending regular continuing medical educations and conferences becomes a challenge that is largely unmet.

During the last 3 decades, we have had the most amazing investigational and therapeutic modalities that have emanated from extensive research being carried out all around the world! Bringing this research from the bench in the laboratory to the clinical setting, is the most meaningful of all advances that assist us in optimal management of our patients.

The present book on *Clinical Progress in Obstetrics and Gynecology* provides a ready resource of a review of subjects related to gynecology and obstetrics. The aim is to keep the reader abreast with the existing knowledge and future trends in the most notable and worked upon areas in our field.

To achieve the justified standard, we have selected subjects that are currently being researched, identified the experts with clinical experiences both nationally and internationally, to throw adequate light on the various subjects. We have expressed theory and practice, based on evidences, to ensure a refreshing revision and read. With emerging refurbishments, changing trends and continuous amendments, we would strive to bring similar updates on a regular basis.

We thank our authors for their well-explored contributions. We also thank Shri Jitendar P Vij (Group Chairman), Mr Ankit Vij (Managing Director) and Mr Tarun Duneja (Director-Publishing) of M/s Jaypee Brothers Medical Publishers (P) Ltd, New Delhi, India, for their excellent support.

We are quite hopeful that our readers would benefit adequately through our endeavor.

Duru Shah
Sudeshna Ray

Contents

Current Approaches to the Management of Fibroids

Chapter

Isaac Manyonda, Latika Narang

Introduction

Uterine leiomyomas are the most common benign pelvic tumors in women of reproductive age.[1] They are symptomatic in approximately 50% of cases, with the peak incidence of symptoms occurring among women in their 30s and 40s.[2] Uterine fibroids are estrogen dependent and are most often seen after the menarche, and tend to shrink after the menopause.[3] They are more commonly seen in women of African ancestry and afflicted women tend to be nulliparous or of low parity. Common symptoms include menorrhagia (that can lead to anemia and related symptoms), dysmenorrhea, pressure symptoms, abdominal distension, and sub-fertility. Where sub-fertility is an issue, it should always be borne in mind that the fibroid(s) may be incidental rather than the cause, except in cases where the fibroids are sub-mucosal.[4,5] Complications of fibroids include degeneration, prolapse of a submuous fibroid, ureteric obstruction, venous thromboembolism, intestinal obstruction (pressure effect from large fibroids) and rarely malignant transformation (indeed there is debate as to whether sarcomatous transformation does occur in a benign fibroid, or the fibroids are incidental in a uterus where a sarcoma develops). Traditional management is surgical, with hysterectomy being offered where the woman has completed her family or where fertility potential is deemed irrecoverable, and myomectomy where fertility is desired. Conventional open myomectomy is most commonly practiced, while the laparoscopic approach is argued by some to provide best prospects for fertility outcomes.[6] In more recent years the radiological interventions uterine artery embolization (UAE) and magnetic-resonance-guided focused ultrasound surgery (MRgFUS) have emerged as viable minimally invasive options.[7] The unmet need has remained effective medical therapies. While GnRH analogs once held promise, they are not suitable stand-alone or long-term treatments. Selective Progesterone Receptor Modulators are emerging as potential effective medical therapies, and ulipristal acetate has recently secured a European license as the first-in-class drug therapy that has completed Phase III clinical trials.

The positive news regarding this very common tumor is that 50% of afflicted women remain asymptomatic, so that no intervention is required. For the symptomatic 50%, the Holy Grail remains arguably a tablet that is taken orally, once a day or even better still once a week, with minimal or no side effects, and no negative impact on fertility. Such an ideal therapy remains elusive.

Expectant Management

It is estimated that 50% of women with uterine fibroids are without symptoms. With increasing use of ultrasound and more frequent clinical examinations during cervical screening, an increasing number of women will be diagnosed with asymptomatic fibroids. Such women warrant simple explanations of what fibroids are, what symptoms they may cause, and reassurance that as long as they remain asymptomatic no intervention is required.[8] In particular women will need reassurance that these benign tumors have minimal, if any, malignant potential. The practical reality is that once they know they have fibroids, many women inevitably become anxious and become aware of symptoms that they might have previously ignored, and therefore seek intervention. The proportion of women with fibroids who are symptomatic is, therefore, likely to increase over the years.

Surgical Management

Hysterectomy

Hysterectomy is the most common treatment for symptomatic fibroids, and it is considered definitive or curative, since there is no possibility of recurrence of the fibroids. Hysterectomy is particularly suited to women who have completed their families. It is associated with high patient satisfaction scores, with up to 90% of patients reporting at least moderate satisfaction at 2 years after the procedure.[9] However, many women later regret the loss of fertility or have concerns regarding their femininity.[10] Moreover, hysterectomy has an approximately 3% incidence of major complications.[11] While most hysterectomies the world-over are performed by the abdominal route, alternative approaches to hysterectomy include subtotal (open or laparoscopic), when the cervix is conserved, laparoscopic total hysterectomy and vaginal hysterectomy. A recent Cochrane review concluded that subtotal hysterectomy did not offer improved outcomes for sexual, urinary or bowel function when compared with total abdominal hysterectomy. However, women are more likely to experience ongoing cyclical bleeding up to a year after surgery with subtotal hysterectomy compared to total hysterectomy.[12]

In general, women with a uterus greater than 16 weeks gestational size are not suitable candidates for a laparoscopic hysterectomy, although some gifted surgeons may well have no difficulty with uteruses larger than this, and therefore, each surgeon should place an upper limit on uterine size based on their preference and expertise.[13] Vaginal hysterectomy in the presence of fibroids and/or absence of prolapse also requires expertise that may not be common-place. Allowing for the availability of expertise, the vaginal route does have advantages over the abdominal route. It has been reported that the duration of the procedure and hospital stay were longer after hysterectomy by the abdominal route. Perioperative complications were observed in 17% of patients after abdominal hysterectomy versus 7.69% after vaginal hysterectomy.[14] However, the operation becomes more challenging as the size and number of fibroids increases: the very large uterus is generally not compatible with removal via the vaginal route, even when the surgeon uses techniques to divide the uterus or morcellate the segments.[14]

Hysterectomy has been compared to the relatively newer radiological treatment uterine artery embolization (UAE), and to date, there have been three prospective, randomized trials comparing. These include the "REST" (Randomized Trial of Embolization versus Surgical Treatment for Fibroids) trial, the EMMY (EMbolization versus hysterectoMY) trial and the HOPEFUL study.[9,10,15,16] All three studies have shown both treatments to have very high clinical success rates and very high rates of patient satisfaction.

Myomectomy

For women with symptomatic fibroids desiring uterine conservation, the primary surgical treatment is myomectomy, most procedures being performed via the abdominal route (conventional abdominal myomectomy).

Conventional Abdominal Myomectomy

The time-honored conventional (open) abdominal myomectomy probably remains the most commonly performed uterus-preservation surgical procedure. When the fibroids are large, it can be technically challenging. It is an operation associated with considerable blood loss, potentially long hospital stay and recovery, and while evidence has shown improvement in fertility prospects, the risks of adhesion may compromise the very same fertility that the operation is performed to preserve. To optimize outcomes following conventional myomectomy, the authors would suggest the following measures or maneuvers:

- *Intraoperative blood loss reduction:* Administer 1g tranexmic acid by slow IV infusion at the time of induction of anesthesia. The authors dilute 20 units vasopressin in 100 mL normal saline, and inject this liberally into the myometrium surrounding the fibroids. The combination of the two creates a very dry operative field that lasts for about 45 minutes.[17]
- *Uterine incision:* In an attempt to minimize the risk of adhesion formation, and based on minimal research evidence available,[18] the authors prefer a single, midline, vertical incision to remove as many fibroids as possible.
- *Closure:* Following closure of dead space and prior to closure of serosal layer, the authors roll out surgical (oxidized regenerated cellulose hemostatic agent) into a ribbon and place it along the entire length of uterine incision, in the space between the myometrium and the serosa.

A major disadvantage of myomectomy is that 50–60% of patients will present with new myomas detected by ultrasound within 5 years following the procedure.[19,20] It has also been reported that more than one-third of these women will require additional surgical intervention for the leiomyomas within 5 years.[21]

Laparoscopic Myomectomy

Some consider laparoscopic myomectomy, the best treatment option for symptomatic women with uterine fibroids who wish to maintain their fertility.[6] Tulandi et al recommend laparoscopic myomectomy for fibroids of < 15 cm in size, and no more than three fibroids with a size of 5 cm.[6] Compared with laparotomy, laparoscopic myomectomy has the advantages of small incisions, decreased intraoperative bleeding, short hospital stay, less postoperative pain, rapid recovery and good assessment of other abdominal organs. No significant differences were found in terms of fertility and obstetrical outcome between the two groups.[22,23] Patient selection and the expertise of the surgeon, especially in laparoscopic suturing, play important role in the success and outcome of the procedure.[24]

Another advance in the field of laparoscopic surgery is the development of robotic-assisted laparoscopic surgery (RAS). RAS allows the surgeon to be seated comfortably while visualizing the abdominal and pelvic cavities in a three-dimensional view and the procedure can be more precise and accurate. [25] Much of this experience incorporated the "da Vinci surgical system" that was approved in April 2005 by the Food and Drug Administration (FDA) for gynecologic applications.[26]

However, due to recurrent symptoms, about 25% of women undergoing myomectomy will require further surgery.[27]

Laparoscopic-assisted Myomectomy

This procedure is similar to that of laparoscopic myomectomy, except the suturing and removal of fibroid is performed through a laparotomy incision. There have been no randomized studies so far comparing laparoscopic myomectomy and laparoscopic-assisted myomectomy.[28,29]

Vaginal Myomectomy

Davies et al demonstrated the feasibility of performing myomectomy via the vaginal route in a prospective study published in 1999.[30] It was carried out in 35 women with symptomatic fibroids requiring myomectomy, and was completed vaginally in 32 (91.4%) women. None of these women required a hysterectomy.

Hysteroscopic Myomectomy

It is an established surgical procedure for women with excessive uterine bleeding, infertility or repeated miscarriages. There is debate as to whether treatment with GnRH agonist before myomectomy offers any significant advantages.[31, 32] However, a recent review reports that preoperative GnRH agonist use in patients with submucous fibroids appears to be the most clinically relevant indication for their use.[33]

The choice of the technique for the hysteroscopic removal of submucous fibroids mostly depends on their type and location within the endometrial cavity. The operator has the possibility to choose among several alternative procedures, which are as follows:

- Resectoscopic excision by slicing
- Cutting of the base of fibroid and its extraction
- Ablation by Nd: yAG laser
- Vaporization of the fibroid using spherical or cylindrical electrodes.[34] The main disadvantage of vaporizing electrodes is the lack of tissue sample for pathology.
- Intrauterine morcellation, the main advantage with this approach being that it preserves tissue for histological examination.[35]
- *Office hysteroscopic myomectomy:* With the development of smaller diameter hysteroscopes (< 5 mm) with working channels and continuous flow systems, it is possible to treat several uterine pathologies in outpatient settings without cervical dilatation.[36]

Most studies have shown that hysteroscopic myomectomy is safe and effective in the control of menstrual disorders with a success rate ranging from 70 to 99%. Hysteroscopic myomectomy combined with endometrial ablation has been shown to provide good long-term results and has been shown to lead to an amenorrhic state in up to 95.5% of patients.[37,38]

Reproductive outcome in infertile women following hysteroscopic myomectomy have been investigated by several authors, but unfortunately the evidence thus far is not of the highest quality. Reported postsurgical pregnancy rates vary from 16.7 to 76.9% with a mean of 45%. This large variation reflects the difficulty in controlling for multiple infertility factors, small sample size, follow-up discrepancies and wide variations in patients' characteristics (i.e. age, primary or secondary infertility) as well as fibroid characteristics (i.e. number, size, intramural portion and presence of concomitant intramural fibroids).[39,40]

Laparoscopic Thermomyolysis or Cryomyolysis

These procedures are associated with side effects such as severe adhesion formation, fever, blood transfusion and conversion to hysterectomy.[41] Data on the safety and efficacy of these procedures are still insufficient.[42-44]

Laparoscopic Uterine Artery Occlusion

There is limited published data on laparoscopic uterine artery occlusion (LUAO). In a small retrospective study, 9% of women developed leiomyoma recurrence at a median follow-up of 23.6 months.[45] There are at least two studies comparing LUAO to UAE. In a small randomized controlled trial, LUAO achieved shorter hospital stays and reduced procedural pain compared to UAE, while achieving similar 3-month clinical success rates.[46] In another study, there was a similar degree of bleeding reduction between the two procedures.[47]

Temporary Transvaginal Uterine Artery Occlusion

In this procedure, the uterine arteries are noninvasively identified through the vagina, guided by audible Doppler ultrasound, when a clamp is then applied to occlude both arteries for 6 hours. This is sufficient time to induce fibroid ischemia and death without affecting the myometrium. Blood flow through the uterine arteries returns immediately following removal of the clamp.[48] While theoretically attractive, these techniques require complex facilities and considerable skills and there is limited data on their true efficacy in clinical settings.

Radiological Treatments

Uterine Artery Embolization (UAE)

It is a percutaneous transcatheter embolization technique using embolization material to occlude the uterine arteries. The rapidly growing fibroids are sensitive to the ischemia induced, and undergo infarction and involution, while the normal myometrium derives alternative blood supply from collaterals from the vaginal and ovarian arteries.

The UAE has become widely accepted because of the advantage of its minimal invasiveness. A number of large series have compared embolization with hysterectomy favoring embolization[49-54] as it leads to 80–90% symptom improvement for menorrhagia, pain and bulk-related symptoms. A register of 1387 patients reported that 84% and 83% of patients had an improvement in their symptoms after UAE at 6 and 24 months respectively. It also reported an improvement in mean health-related quality of life scores (on a scale from 0 to 100) from 44.1 at baseline to 79.5 after UAE at a maximum 3-year follow-up ($p < 0.001$).[55]

A randomized controlled trial (RCT) of 157 patients treated by UAE or surgery (hysterectomy or myomectomy) reported symptom improvement in both groups, but this improvement was significantly greater among patients treated by surgery than by UAE ($p = 0.004$ at 1 month, $p = 0.03$ at 12 months).[56]

A major side effect of UAE is severe pain after the procedure.[57-60] Rare but serious complications include severe infection leading to hysterectomy (1.5%) and ovarian failure (5%).[50,59,60] Another RCT reported that 28% (23/81) of UAE-treated patients had required hysterectomy at 5-year follow-up.[61,62] Some recent reviews have suggested that UAE may have a negative impact on reproduction, increasing subfertility, miscarriage rates and associated with poor obstetric outcomes, but the evidence is of poor quality, and challenging this are growing number of reported series of successful pregnancy outcomes following UAE. A head-to-head RCT of UAE versus myomectomy is clearly required to resolve these issues.

MR Guided Focused Ultrasound (MRgFUS)

Focused US (FUS) is the therapeutic use of US waves to induce focal thermal effects, ablation, or thermocoagulation in vivo.

The efficacy of magnetic resonance image (MRI)-guided transcutaneous focused ultrasound for treatment of uterine fibroids has been shown to be adequate, although further treatment may be required and the effect on subsequent pregnancy is uncertain. The side-effects are generally mild and the evidence on safety is adequate to support the use of this procedure provided.[63] Transient adverse effects include mild skin burn, nausea, short-term buttock or leg pain, and transient sciatic nerve palsy.[64-66]

A nonrandomized comparative study of 192 patients treated by MRI-guided transcutaneous focused ultrasound or abdominal hysterectomy reported improvements in all Short Form-36 quality of life domains for both treatment groups, although scores at 6 months were better in patients treated by hysterectomy.[63]

It has recently been demonstrated that the pretreatment of patients who have fibroids measuring 10 cm or greater with GnRHa, before MRgFUS, has a beneficial effect, enhancing the tissue response to high intensity focused ultrasound.[67]

Another advantage is that it can be used as an outpatient-based treatment and significantly reduces symptoms in more than 75% of women treated with fibroids. Another ongoing evaluation of the clinical application of MRgFUS is its impact on fertility. Rabinovici et al have reported on safe and successful outcomes of pregnancies after MRgFUS.[68]

Medical Management

Most of the current medical therapeutic approaches exploit the observations that uterine fibroids have significantly increased concentrations of estrogen (and more recently progesterone) receptors compared with normal myometrium[69,70] and that ovarian steroids influence fibroid growth. Most available therapies are therefore hormonal, or act on the relevant hormones or their receptors to interfere with fibroid growth.

GnRH Agonists

In the management of women with fibroid disease, GnRH agonists (GnRHa) are frequently used to reduce volume and vascularity prior to myomectomy[71,72] apparently to render the operation easier and reduce operative blood loss, and to enable a transverse suprapubic incision instead of a midline vertical one. They induce amenorrhea and thus aid in the correction of preoperative anemia.[73] Other gynecologists use GnRHa to shrink submucous fibroids greater than 5 cm in diameter to facilitate access and reduce blood loss and operating time at transcervical resection.[74] GnRHa are also occasionally used as a temporizing measure in women with symptomatic fibroids within the climacteric.[75]

The authors here argue that GnRHa have a limited, if any, role in the management of fibroid disease because they are not cost-effective,[76] render myomectomy more difficult because they destroy tissue planes, the more difficult enucleation in fact increasing rather than reducing perioperative blood loss and operating time.[77] When used prior to myomectomy, they increase the risk of "recurrence" because they obscure smaller fibroids that "recur" when the effects of the GnRHa wear off[78] and are associated with side effects in situations where they confer no benefits, or where alternative cheaper drugs with fewer side effects are available.

Progesterone, the Progesterone Receptor and Receptor Antagonists/Modulators

Progesterone plays a crucial part in human reproductive physiology. Its physiological effects impact the processes of endometrial differentiation, ovulation, implantation, successful development of the embryo, development of the mammary gland as well as regulation of central signals from the hypothalamic-pituitary (HP) axis. The effects of progesterone on target tissues are mediated via the progesterone receptor (PR), which belongs to the nuclear receptor family.[79] The PR exists as three separate isoforms (A, B and C) expressed from a single gene.[79] The PR functions as a ligand-activated transcription factor to regulate the expression of specific sets of target genes. PR antagonists oppose the biological actions of progesterone by inhibiting PR activation. Progesterone has dual actions on fibroid growth. It stimulates growth by up-regulating EGF and Bcl-2 and down-regulating tumor necrosis factor-alpha expression while it inhibits growth by down-regulating IGF-I expression.[80,81] While it has long been well established that estrogen promotes fibroid tumor growth, recent biochemical and clinical studies have suggested that progesterone and the progesterone receptors may also enhance proliferative activity in fibroids.[80,81] These observations have, therefore, raised the possibility that anti-progestins and agents or molecules that modulate the activity of the progesterone receptor could be useful in the medical management of uterine fibroids.

Levonorgesterol Intrauterine Device (LNG-IUS)

The LNG-IUS is effective in reducing menstrual blood loss and should be considered as an alternative to surgical treatment.[82] Levonorgestrel is released locally at a rate of 20 µg/day. At present there are no RCT's of use of LNG-IUS in treatment of menorrhagic women with uterine leiomyomas. There are of course, reports of its use in these women, with striking reduction in menorrhagia being reported, with consequent rise in hemoglobin.[82] However, it has not been shown to cause any significant reduction in leiomyoma volume or uterine volume, as assessed by MRI between pretreatment and 12 months of use.[83,84] A theoretical consideration is that while the LNG-IUS does indeed reduce menstrual loss (by inhibiting the proliferation of the endometrium) it could at the same time promote fibroid growth via its actions at the fibroid progesterone receptor. This would be an easy question to answer in any well-designed study of the impact of the LNG-IUS on fibroid disease.

Progesterone Receptor Modulators

Since the emergence of mifepristone (RU-486), the first progesterone receptor antagonist, more than 25 years ago hundreds of steroidal as well as nonsteroidal compounds displaying progesterone antagonist (PA) or mixed agonist/antagonist activity have been synthesized. Collectively, they are known as progesterone receptor modulators (PRMs). These compounds have a huge potential for use in the treatment of a number of pathological conditions of the female reproductive system including uterine fibroids, endometriosis, dysfunctional uterine bleeding

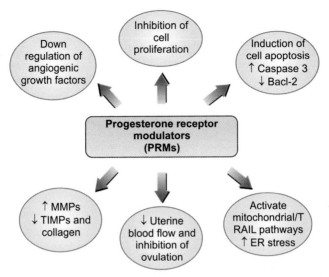

FIG. 1.1 Mechanisms of action of progesterone receptor modulators on uterine fibroids

and as potential contraceptives. Some of the PRMs that have been the subject of recent clinical trials/research studies in relation to fibroids treatment include mifepristone, CDB-4124 (telapristone), CP-8947 and J867 (asoprisnil) and CDB-2914 (ulipristal acetate). The potential mechanisms of action of PRMs on fibroids are depicted in Figure 1.1.

Evidence for Effectiveness of PRMs in Treatment of Uterine Fibroids

A number of clinical trials have established the potential of PRMs in the treatment of uterine fibroids. They are associated with a reduction in pain, bleeding, size of fibroids and overall improvement in quality of life. Unlike long-acting GnRH analogs, they do not have the drawbacks of the profound estrogen deficiency and decrease in bone mineral density.

Mifepristone (RU-486)

Early reports of the use of mifepristone for the treatment of fibroids date back to 2002, when De Leo et al used doses ranging from 12.5 to 50 mg daily and reported a reduction in uterine/fibroid volume of 40–50%, with amenorrhea in most subjects.[85] This report was corroborated by a paper a year later from a group who used mifepristone at a dose of 5 or 10 mg per day for one year, and found that it was effective in decreasing mean uterine volume by 50%, while amenorrhea occurred in 40–70% of the subjects.[86] Adverse effects included vasomotor symptoms, but no change in bone mineral density was noted. Hot flashes were increased over baseline in the 10 mg group, but 5 mg per day did not increase the incidence of vasomotor symptoms. Simple hyperplasia was noted in 28% of the women. This study therefore suggested that a dose as low as 5 mg per day of mifepristone may be efficacious for the treatment of uterine fibroids, with few side effects.[86] Antiglucocorticoid effects of long-term use of mifepristone are usually seen only with doses exceeding 200 mg daily.[87] The same group of researchers then followed up their preliminary findings with a randomized controlled trial (RCT) on the use of mifepristone for the treatment of uterine fibroids. This was a small study that included 42 women in a double-blind placebo controlled study design over a period of 6 months.[88] They reported that overall quality of life was improved significantly, while anemia rates and uterine volume were reduced significantly. The hyperplasia seen in some women may limit the use of this drug among those desiring a long-term medical therapeutic alternative. However, the apparent effectiveness of mifepristone in reducing myoma volume and improving fibroid-related symptoms and quality of life, and the minimal side-effects, all point to a need for a large RCT with sufficient power to define its true place in the medical management of uterine fibroids. A combination of mifepristone and the LNG-IUS could prove especially useful as the IUS would obviate the development of endometrial hyperplasia while also promoting a reduction in menstrual flow. In yet another recent randomised trial, 100 women were assigned to mifepristone 5 or 10 mg daily for 3 months without a placebo group. With both doses, there were equivalent reductions in fibroid and uterine volumes and symptomatic improvements.[89]

CDB-4124 (Telapristone)

A clinical trial (phase I/II) evaluated the efficacy of telapristone in symptomatic fibroids. This small 3-month study comprising 30 women, compared oral doses of 12.5, 25 and 50 mg telapristone with the GnRH analog Lupron and a placebo.[90] There was a significant reduction in tumor size and reduced bleeding with telapristone treatment.

J-867 (Asoprisnil)

Asoprisnil has high tissue selectivity and binds to progesterone receptors with a 3-fold greater binding affinity than progesterone.[91] The initial phase I studies established that asoprisnil induced a reversible suppression of menstruation, while having variable effects on ovulation.[92] The phase II multi-center double-blind placebo controlled studies by the same group of researchers compared the efficacy and safety of 3 doses (5, 10 and 25 mg and placebo) in 129 women over 12 weeks.[93,94] Asoprisnil reduced the uterine and fibroid volumes in a dose dependent manner. There was a dose dependent decrease in menorrhagia scores in women with menorrhagia at baseline, while amenorrhea rates increased as the dose increased (28.1% with 5 mg, 64.3% with 10 mg and 83.3% with 25 mg), but with no increase in the rates of unscheduled bleeding in all 3 asoprisnil groups. Compared to placebo, hemoglobin levels were improved in all three treatment groups, while adverse effects were evenly distributed. The initial clinical trials of asoprisnil suggested endometrial thickening to be one of the important side effects of the drug. However, overall safety data available so far have been reassuring and its impact on bone mineral density, fertility, recurrence rates of fibroids and endometrial hyperplasia are still under evaluation.

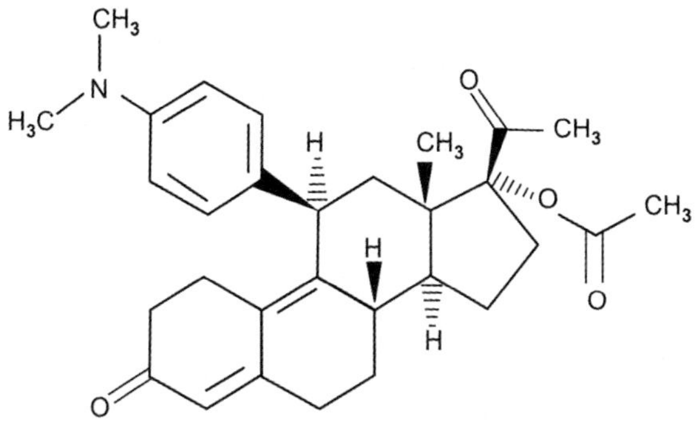

FIG. 1.2 Chemical structure of ulipristal acetate (17-acetoxy-11b-[4-N,N-dimethylaminophenyl]-19-norpregna-4,9-diene-3,20-dione)

CDB-2914 (Ulipristal Acetate or UA) (Fig. 1.2)

In Phase II and III clinical trials, a number of issues have been addressed using UA. In the first trial[95] in which UA was given at 10 mg or 20 mg in comparison against placebo for 3 cycles, UA showed a 92% reduction in bleeding versus 19% with placebo. Leiomyoma volume was significantly reduced with UA (29% versus 6%; p = 0.01). UA eliminated menstrual bleeding and inhibited ovulation (% ovulatory cycles 20% on UA versus 83% with placebo; p = 0.001). UA also improved the concern scores of the uterine leiomyoma symptom quality of life subscale (p = 0.04). One woman on UA developed endometrial cystic hyperplasia without evidence of atypia. No serious adverse events were reported. UA did not suppress estradiol and there were no differences in serum estradiol levels between the treatment and placebo groups (median estradiol was greater than 50 pg/ml in all groups). However, the numbers studied were small, with 22 patients being allocated and 18 completing the 3 cycles or 90–120 day trial.[95] An even more recent randomized, double blind, placebo controlled trial of efficacy and tolerability has also demonstrated positive results when UA was administered for 3–6 months, showing good control of bleeding, reduction in fibroid size, and improvement in quality of life in the treatment group.[96] UA has recently successfully completed two Phase III clinical trials (PEARL I and II) in Europe demonstrating its efficacy and safety for the treatment of symptomatic uterine fibroids in patients eligible for surgery.[97,98] PEARL I compared treatment with oral UA for up to 13 weeks at a dose of 5 mg per day (96 women) or 10 mg per day (98 women) with placebo (48 women) in patients with fibroids, menorrhagia and anemia. All patients received iron supplementation. The co-primary efficacy end points were control of uterine bleeding and reduction of fibroid volume at week 13, after that patients could undergo surgery. At 13 weeks, uterine bleeding was controlled in 91% of the women receiving 5 mg of UA, 92% of those receiving 10 mg of UA, and 19% of those receiving placebo (p < 0.001 for the comparison of each dose of UA with placebo). Treatment with UA for 13 weeks effectively controlled excessive bleeding due to uterine fibroids and reduced the size of the fibroids. PEARL II was a double-blind non-inferiority trial, which randomly assigned 307 patients with symptomatic fibroids and excessive uterine bleeding to receive 3 months of daily therapy with oral UA (at a dose of either 5 mg or 10 mg) or once-monthly intramuscular injections of the GnRH analog leuprolide acetate (at a dose of 3.75 mg). The primary outcome was the proportion of patients with controlled bleeding at week 13, with a pre-specified non-inferiority margin of –20%.Uterine bleeding was controlled in 90% of patients receiving 5 mg of UA, in 98% of those receiving 10 mg, while the figure for leuprolide acetate was 89%. Both UA doses were non-inferior to once monthly leuprolide acetate in controlling uterine bleeding and were significantly less likely to cause hot flashes.[98]

Adverse Effects and Limitations Associated with Long-term Use of PRMs

Endometrial Hyperplasia and Thickening
A National Institute of Health (NIH) sponsored workshop evaluated endometrial specimens from women receiving mifepristone, asoprisnil and UA.[80,99,100] Pathologists were blinded to agent, dose and exposure interval. It was concluded that there was little evidence of mitosis consistent with the anti-proliferative effect of PRMs. No biopsy demonstrated atypical hyperplasia. There was asymmetry of stromal and epithelial growth and prominent cystically dilated glands with both admixed estrogen (mitotic) and progestin (secretory) epithelial effects. This histology has not previously been encountered in clinical practice. The panel designated these changes as PRM associated endometrial changes (PAECs).[80,99,100] Despite the paucity of mitoses, pathologists may associate the cystic glandular dilatation observed with PRMs with simple hyperplasia and should be aware of the potential diagnostic pitfalls of misdiagnosing hyperplasia in women receiving PRMs.[80,101] In another study, biopsies were obtained from 58 premenopausal women participating in clinical trials of the telapristone. Biopsies were obtained at 3 and 6 months, and women were receiving daily doses of oral therapy that ranged from 12.5–50 mg. Out of 174 samples 103 contained histologic changes not seen in the normal menstrual cycle.[102] Whereas the majority of the histology was atrophic, novel cystic changes were seen with increasing doses. Cystically dilated glands with mixed secretory and mitotic features were noted.[102] These lesions are not considered to be premalignant and no malignancies were found.

A few studies have reported endometrial thickening detected on ultrasound after use of high or low dose Mifepristone.[103, 104] During 3 months treatment with ulipristal in normal women, no thickening was observed and examination of hysterectomy specimens after 3 months of asoprisnil (10 or 25 mg) showed that when compared with placebo, there was a trend for decreased endometrial thickness.[80, 105] With use of telapristone in the treatment of fibroids, there was a minimum increase in endometrial thickness of 3.3 and 4.2 mm with the 12.5 and 25 mg doses, respectively, after 3 months of treatment.[80] It has been suggested that, unlike in the situation where there is unopposed estrogen effect, the endometrial thickening in women on PRMs is related to cystic glandular dilation and not endometrial hyperplasia. The overall evidence emerging from the recent clinical trials regarding the safety of PRMs appears to be reassuring. Clinicians detecting endometrial thickening in women treated with PRMs need to be aware that administration of PRMs for longer than 3 months may lead to endometrial thickening. This is related to cystic glandular dilation, not endometrial hyperplasia and pathologists need to be aware of PAEC and avoid misclassifying the appearance as hyperplasia. It is also important to consider the limitations of the current data while describing the effects of PRMs on the endometrium. Most existing studies have described the endometrial changes over short periods (months) of follow-up; however, atypical hyperplasia and possibly malignant changes take years to develop and long-term studies are, therefore, necessary to evaluate such outcomes.

Although breakthrough bleeding has been reported as one of the side effects of PRMs, sufficient data assessing their long term use are not available. It is also argued that PRMs are not useful for treatment of large fibroids as they cause a modest decrease in their size; however, larger clinical trials with varying doses and duration of therapy of PRMs in future will be able to provide a definite answer to this question.

Gestrinone

It is a steroid that possesses antiestrogen receptor and antiprogesterone receptor properties in the endometrium. A report from Italy evaluated the use of gestrinone in the treatment of premenopausal women with uterine leiomyomas at a dose of 2.5 mg twice per week over a 6-month period.[106] The authors reported a 32–42% reduction in uterine volume. A subsequent study reported up to 60% leiomyoma shrinkage in size.[107] However, gestrinone acts as a contraceptive agent and also has several unfavorable side effects, such as mild androgenicity, weight gain, seborrhea, acne, hirsutism and occasional hoarseness.

Other Treatment Modalities

Endometrial Ablation

Selected women with submucous fibroids, who have completed their families, can be treated by endometrial ablation.[108,109] Conventional endometrial ablation techniques cannot be used when the uterine cavity is remarkably enlarged (>12 cm) and distorted as result of submucous or intramural myomas.

Hydrothermal ablation has already been demonstrated to be safe and effective in treating women with menorrhagia and submucous fibroids up to 4 cm in diameter.[110]

Microwave endometrial ablation (MEA) has also been used for treating menorrhagia effectively. It is now possible to treat even enlarged (12–16 cm in length) and distorted uterine cavity as a result of large submucous fibroids, with the advent of a thinner (4 mm) curved microwave probe.[111,112] Available data about the outcome of MEA in patients with menorrhagia caused by submucous myomas are few but encouraging.

Image Guided Thermal Therapy

This can be achieved by using either magnetic resonance thermometry or laser ablation. The laser ablation of fibroids was first described in 1989 as a procedure performed via laparoscopic (intramural or subserosal fibroids) or hysteroscopic route (submucosal fibroids).[113] It was found to decrease fibroid volume by 50% to 70% in symptomatic women. In 1999, Law et al first reported percutaneous treatment of uterine fibroids by neodymium: yttrium-aluminum-garnet (Nd: YAG) laser under MR guidance.[114]

The reduction in mean fibroid volume was 31% at 3 months follow-up, and 41% at the one year follow-up, in the follow-up series study.[115]

Cryotherapy

Cryoablation is the thermal ablation method that causes cell death by rapid freezing followed by rapid thawing.[116] The temperature must be lower than –20~50°C to completely destroy tissue. Like laser ablation this was also initially introduced using either laparoscopic or hysteroscopic route.[117, 118] Reduction of fibroid volume ranged widely from 31% to about 80% in the follow-up studies.[119,120]

Radiofrequency Ablation

Ablation of solid tumors with radiofrequency energy results from heating that is produced when ions follow the oscillations of a high-frequency alternating electric field.[121]

It was first used in 2005 in the management of uterine fibroids via a surgical laparoscopic approach[122, 123] and subsequently with US guidance.[124-126] A large area of necrosis (up to 6 cm in diameter) can be achieved in a single access with RFA, and, therefore, compared to cryotherapy it is relatively time efficient.

Acupuncture

The effectiveness of acupuncture for the management of uterine fibroids remains uncertain.[127] More evidence is required to establish the efficacy and safety of acupuncture for uterine fibroids. There is a continued need for well-designed RCTs with long-term follow-up.

Concluding Remarks

As recently as 20 years ago the choices for the woman with symptomatic fibroids were confined to abdominal hysterectomy and conventional abdominal myomectomy. Now, there is a multitude of additional choices, including laparoscopic and vaginal myomectomy, uterine artery embolization (UAE) and more recently magnetic resonance-guided focused ultrasound surgery (MRgFUS). Developments in purely medical therapies had, until recently, been singularly disappointing, but the emergence of ulipristal acetate as the first-in-class progesterone receptor modulator licensed for clinical use in Western Europe renders it highly likely that a definitive and effective stand-alone medical therapy will soon be developed. As yet, however, there is no panacea. UAE and MRgFUS are yet to be subjected to the rigorous evaluation demanded by the modern concept of evidence-based medical care. There are limitations on the size and number of fibroids that can be treated with laparoscopic or vaginal myomectomy. The license for ulipristal acetate dictates that it is used for no more than 3 months preceding surgery and this treatment is therefore not stand-alone, and further clinical trials of its efficacy are urgently required. Fibroid disease is essentially benign and treatment modalities aim not to save lives, but to improve its quality. Therefore, any evaluation and research on these new treatments must include as the main outcomes health-related quality of life, functional clinical outcomes such as symptom relief and impact on fertility, and a cost-effectiveness analysis as dictated by the finite resources for health care.

References

1. Stewart EA. Uterine fibroids. Lancet. 2001;357(9252):293–8.
2. Wise LA, Palmer JR, Stewart EA, et al. Age specific incidence rates for self-reported uterine leiomyomata in Black Women's Health Study. Obstet Gynecol. 2005;105:563–68
3. Simms-Stewart D, Fletcher H. Counselling patients with uterine fibroids: a review of the management and complications. Obstet Gynecol Int. 2012;2012:539365. Epub 2012 Jan 9.
4. Pritts EA. Fibroids and infertility: a systematic review of the evidence. Obstetrical and Gynecological Survey. 2001;56(8):483–91.
5. Poncelet C, Benifla JL, Batallan A, Daraï E, Madelenat P. Myoma and infertility: analysis of the literature. Gynecol Obstet Fertil. 2001;29(6):413–21.
6. Agdi M, Tulandi T. Endoscopic management of uterine fibroids. Best Practice & Research Clinical Obstetrics and Gynaecology. 2008;22(4):707–6.
7. Magnetic resonance image-guided transcutaneous focused ultrasound for uterine fibroids. National Institute of Clinical Excellence; IPG413. 2011.
8. Divakar H, Manyonda I. Asymptomatic uterine fibroids. Clinical Obstetrics and Gynaecology. 2008; 22(4): 643–54
9. Hehenkamp WJ, Volkers NA, Birnie E, Reekers JA, Ankum WM. Symptomatic uterine fibroids: treatment with uterine artery embolization or hysterectomy--results from the randomized clinical Embolisation versus Hysterectomy (EMMY) Trial. Radiology. 2008; 246(3):823–32.
10. A Hirst, S Dutton, O Wu, A Briggs, C Edwards, L Waldenmaier, et al. A multi-centre retrospective cohort study comparing the efficacy, safety and cost-effectiveness of hysterectomy and uterine artery embolisation for the treatment of symptomatic uterine fibroids. The HOPEFUL study. Health Technol Assess. 2008;12(5):1–248.
11. Garry R, Fountain J, Mason S, Hawe J, Napp V, Abbott J, et al. The eVALuate study: two parallel randomised trials, one comparing laparoscopic with abdominal hysterectomy, the other comparing laparoscopic with vaginal hysterectomy. BMJ. 2004;328(7432):129.
12. Lethaby A, Mukhopadhyay A, Naik R. Total versus subtotal hysterectomy for benign gynaecological conditions. Cochrane Database Syst Rev. 2012;18(4):CD004993.
13. Agdi M, Tulandi T. Endoscopic management of uterine fibroids. Best Practice and Research Clinical Obstetrics and Gynaecology. 2008;22(4):707–16.
14. Traoré M, Togo A, Traoré Y, Dembélé BT, Diakité I, Traoré SO, et al. Hysterectomy: indications and advantages of the vaginal route in Mali. Med Trop (Mars). 2011;71(6):636–7.

15. Edwards RD, Moss JG, Lumsden MA, Wu O, Murray LS, Twaddle S, et al. Uterine artery embolization versus surgery for symptomatic uterine fibroids. N Engl J Med. 2007;356:360–70.
16. Pinto I, Chimeno P, Romo A, et al. Uterine fibroids: uterine artery embolization versus abdominal hysterectomy for treatment—a prospective, randomized, and controlled clinical trial. Radiology. 2003;226(2):425–31.
17. Frederick J, Fletcher H, Simeon D, et al. Intramyometrial vasopressin as a haemostatic agent during Myomectomy. Br J Obstet Gynaecol. 1994;101:435–7.
18. Tulandi T, Murray C, Guralnick M. Adhesion formation and reproductive outcome after myomectomy and second look laparoscopy. Obstet Gynecol. 1993;82:213–5.
19. Fedele L, Parazzini F, Luchini L, Mezzopane R, Tozzi L, Villa L. Recurrence of fibroids after myomectomy: a transvaginal ultrasonographic study. Hum Reprod. 1995;10(7):1795–6.
20. Hanafi M. Predictors of leiomyoma recurrence after myomectomy. Obstet Gynecol. 2005;105(4):877–81.
21. Stewart EA, Faur AV, Wise LA, Reilly RJ, Harlow BL. Predictors of subsequent surgery for uterine leiomyomata after abdominal myomectomy. Obstet Gynecol. 2002;99(3):426–32.
22. Seracchioli R, Rossi S, Govoni F et al. Fertility and obstetric outcome after laparoscopic myomectomy of large fibroid: a randomized comparison with abdominal myomectomy. Hum Reprod. 2000;15:2663–8.
23. Rosetti A, Sizzi O, SOranna L et al. Long-term results of laparoscopic myomectomy: recurrence rate in comparison with abdominal myomectomy. Hum Reprod. 2001; 16:770–4.
24. Milad MP, Sankpal RS. Laparoscopic approaches to uterine fibroids. Clin Obstet Gynecol. 2001;44:401–11.
25. Advincula AP, Xu X, Goudeau S 4th, et al. Robot-assisted laparoscopic myomectomy versus abdominal myomectomy: a comparison of short-term surgical outcomes and immediate costs. J minim invasive gynecol. 2007;14(6):698–705.
26. Advincula AP, Song A. The role of robotic surgery in gynecology. Curr Opin Obstet Gynecol. 2007;19(4):331–6.
27. Candiani GB, Fedele L, Parazzini F. Risk of recurrence after myomectomy. Br J Obstet Gynaecol. 1991;98:385–9.
28. Nezhat C, Nezhat F, Bess O. et al. laparoscopically assisted Myomectomy- a report of a new technique in 57 cases. Int J Fertil. 1994;39:34–44.
29. Pelosi III MA, Pelosi MA. Laparoscopic assissted transvaginal myomectomy. J Am Assos Gynecol Laparosc. 1997;4:241–6.
30. Davies A, Hart R, Magos AL. The excision of uterine fibroids by vaginal Myomectomy: a prospective study. Fertil Steril. 1999;71:961–4.
31. Lethaby A, Vollenhoven B, Sowter M. Preoperative GnRH analogue therapy before hysterectomy or myomectomy for uterine fibroids. Cochrane Database Syst Rev. 2001;2:CD000547.
32. Lethaby A, Vollenhoven B, Sowter M. Efficacy of pre-operative gonadotrophin hormone releasing analogues for women with uterine fibroids undergoing hysterectomy or myomectomy: a systematic review. BJOG. 2002;109:1097–1108.
33. Gutmann JN,Corson SL. GnRH agonist therapy before myomectomy or hysterectomy. J Minim Invasive Gynecol. 2005;12:529–37.
34. Glasser MH. Endometrial ablation and hysteroscopic myomectomy by electrosurgical vaporization. J Am Assoc Gynecol Laparosc. 1997;4:369–74.
35. Emanuel MH, Wamsteker K. The intra uterine morcellator: a new hysteroscopic operating technique to remove intrauterine polyps and fibroids. J Minim Invasive Gynecol. 2005;12:62–6.

36. Bettocchi S, Ceci O, Di Venere R et al. Advanced operative office hysteroscopy without anaesthesia: analysis of 501 cases treated with a 5 Fr. bipolar electrode. Hum Reprod. 2002;17:2435–8.
37. Loffer FD. Preliminary experience with the VersaPoint bipolar resectoscope using a vaporizing electrode in a saline distending medium. J Am Assoc Gynecol Laparosc. 2000;7:498–502.
38. Polena V, Mergui JL, Perrot N et al. Long-term results of hysteroscopic myomectomy in 235 patients. Eur J Obstet Gynecol Reprod Biol. 2007;130:232–7.
39. Cheong Y, Ledger WL. Hysteroscopy and hysteroscopic surgery. Obstet Gynecol Reprod Med. 2007;17:99–104.
40. Somigliana E, Vercellini P, Daguati R, Pasin R, DeGiorgi O, Crosignani PG. Fibroids and female reproduction: a critical analysis of the evidence. Hum Reprod Update. 2007;13:465–76.
41. Aubuchon M, Pinto AB, Williams DB. Treatment of uterine fibroids. Prim Care Update Ob Gyns. 2002;9:231–7.
42. Zreik TG, Rutherford TJ, Palter SF, et al. Cryomyolysis, a new procedure for the conservative treatment of uterine fibroids. J Am Assoc Gynecol Laparosc. 1998;5:33–8.
43. Odnusi KO, Rutherford TJ, Olive DL, et al. Cryomyolysis in the management of uterine fibroids: technique and complications. Surg Technol Int. 2000;VIII:173–8.
44. Ciavattini A, Tsiroglou D, Litta P et al. Pregnancy outcome after laparoscopic cryomyolysis of uterine fibroids: report of nine caese. J Minim Invasive Gynecol. 2006;13:141–4.
45. Holub Z, Eim J, Jabor A, Hendl A, Lukac J, Kliment L.Complications and myoma recurrence after laparoscopic uterine artery occlusion for symptomatic myomas. J Obstet Gynaecol Res. 2006;32(1):55–62.
46. Cunningham E, Barreda L, Ngo M, Terasaki K, Munro MG. Uterine artery embolization versus occlusion for uterine leiomyomas: a pilot randomized clinical trial. J Minim Invasive Gynecol. 2008;15(3):301–7.
47. Hald K, Klow NE, Qvigstad E, Istre O. Laparoscopic occlusion compared with embolization of uterine vessels: a randomized controlled trial. Obstet Gynecol. 2007; 109(1):20–7.
48. Istre O, Hald K, Qvigstad E. Multiple myomas treated with a non-invasive, Doppler-directed, transvaginal uterine artery clamp. J Am Assoc Gynecol Laparosc. 2004;11: 273–6.
49. Walker WJ, Pelage JP. Uterine artery embolization for symptomatic fibroids: Clinical results in 400 women with imaging follow up. Br J Obstet Gynaecol. 2002;109:1262–72.
50. Pron G, Bennett J, Common A, et al. The Ontario uterine fibroid embolization trial: Uterine fibroid reduction and symptom relief after uterine artery embolization for fibroids. Fertil Steril. 2003;79:120–7.
51. Pinto I, Chimeno P, Romo A, et al. Uterine fibroids: Uterine artery embolization versus abdominal hysterectomy for treatment. A prospective, randomized, and controlled clinical trial. Radiology. 2003;226:425–531.
52. Spies JB, Cooper JM, Worthington-Kirsch R, et al. Outcome of uterine embolization and hysterectomy for leiomyomas: Results of a multicenter study. Am J Obstet Gynecol. 2004;191:22–31.
53. Spies JB, Spector A, Roth AR, et al. Complications of uterine artery embolization for leiomyomata. Obstet Gynecol. 2002;100:873–80.
54. Pron G, Mocarski E, Cohen M, et al. Hysterectomy for complications after uterine artery embolization for leiomyoma: Results of a Canadian multicenter clinical trial. J Am Assoc Gynecol Laparosc. 2003;10:99–106.

55. O'Grady EA, Moss JG, Belli AM, et al. UK uterine artery embolisation for fibroids registry 2003–2008. The British Society of Interventional Radiology. 2009.
56. Edwards RD, Moss JG, Lumsden MA, et al. Uterine-artery embolization versus surgery for symptomatic uterine fibroids. New England Journal of Medicine. 2007;356:360–70.
57. Goodwin S, Walker W. Uterine artery embolisation for the treatment of uterine fibroids. Curr Opin Obstet Gynaecol. 1998;10:315–20.
58. Worthington-Kirsch RL, Popky GL, Hutchins FL. Uterine arterial embolization for leiomyomas: Quality-of-life assessment and clinical response. Radiology. 1998;208:625–9.
59. Roth AR, Spies JB, Walsh S, et al. Pain after uterine fibroid embolization for leiomyomata: Can its severity be predicted and dose the severity predict outcome? J Vasc Interv Radiol. 2000;11:1047–52.
60. Spies JB, Roth A, Jha RC, et al. Leiomyomata treated with uterine fibroid embolization: Factors associated with successful symptom and imaging outcome. Radiology. 2002;222:45–52
61. Hehenkamp WJ, Volkers NA, Birnie E, Reekers JA, Ankum WM. Symptomatic uterine fibroids: treatment with uterine artery embolization or hysterectomy--results from the randomized clinical Embolisation versus Hysterectomy (EMMY) Trial. Radiology. 2008;246(3):823–32.
62. Volkers NA, Hehenkamp WJK, Birnie E, et al. Uterine artery embolization versus hysterectomy in the treatment of symptomatic uterine fibroids: 2 years' outcome from the randomized EMMY trial. American Journal of Obstetrics and Gynecology. 2007; 196:519e1–519e11.
63. Magnetic resonance image-guided transcutaneous focused ultrasound for uterine fibroids. National Institute of Clinical Excellence; IPG413, 2011.
64. Hindley J, Gedroyc W, Regan L, et al. MRI guidance of focused ultrasound therapy of uterine fibroids: early results. AJR Am J Roentgenol. 2004;183:1713–9.
65. Stewart EA, Rabinovici J, Tempany CM, et al. Clinical outcomes of focused ultrasound surgery for the treatment of uterine fibroids. Fertil Steril. 2006;85:22–9.
66. Fennessy F, Tempany CM, McDannold N, et al. MRI-guided focused ultrasound surgery of uterine leiomyomas: results of different treatment guideline protocols. Radiology. 2007;243:885–93.
67. Smart OC, Hindley JT, Regan L, et al. Gonadotrophin-releasing hormone and magnetic-resonance–guided ultrasound surgery for uterine leiomyomata. Obstetrics and Gynecology. 2006;108(1):49–54
68. Rabinovici J, David M, Fukunishi M, et al. MR guided focused ultrasound pregnancies: pregnancy outcome following magnetic resonance guided focused ultrasound surgery (MRgFUS) for conservative treatment of uterine fibroids. Fertil Steril. In Press.
69. Wilson EA, Yang F, Rees ED. Estradiol and progesterone binding in uterine leiomyomata and in normal uterine tissue. Obstet Gynecol. 1980;55: 20–4.
70. Tamaya T, Fujimoto J, Okada H. Comparison of cellular levels of steroid receptors in uterine leiomyomas and myometrium. Acta Gynaecol Scand. 1985;64:307–9.
71. Maheux R, Guilloteau C, Lemay A, Bastide A, Fazekas AT. Regression of leiomyomata uteri following hypoestrogenism induced by repetitive LHRH agonist treatment: preliminary report. Fertil Steril. 1984;42:644–6.
72. Friedman AJ, Barbieri RL, Benacerraf BR. Treatment of leiomyomata with intranasal or subcutaneous leuprolide, a gonadotropin-releasing hormone agonist. Fertil Steril. 1987; 48: 560–4.
73. Friedman AJ, Barbieri RL, Doubilet PM, Fine C, Schiff I. A randomized, double-blind trial of a gonadotropin releasing-hormone agonist (leuprolide) with or without medroxyprogesterone acetate in the treatment of leiomyomata uteri. Fertil Steril. 1988; 49(3):404–9.

74. Campo S, Campo V, Gambadauro P. Short-term and long-term results of resectoscopic myomectomy with and without pretreatment with GnRH analogs in premenopausal women. Acta Obstet Gynecol Scand. 2005;84:756–60.

75. Lethaby A, Vollenhoven B, Sowter M. Pre-operative GnRH analogue therapy before hysterectomy or myomectomy for uterine fibroids. Cochrane Database Syst Rev. 2001;(2):CD000547.

76. Lethaby AE, Vollenhoven BJ. An evidence-based approach to hormonal therapies for premenopausal women with fibroids. Best Practice and Research Clinical Obstetrics and Gynaecology. 2008;22(2):307–31.

77. Mukhopadhaya N, De Silva C, Manyonda IT. Conventional myomectomy. Best Practice and Research Clinical Obstetrics and Gynaecology. 2008;22(4):677–705.

78. Candiani GB, Fedele L, Parazzini F, Villa L. Risk of recurrence after myomectomy. Br J Obstet Gynaecol. 1991;98(4):385–9.

79. Giangrande PH, McDonnell DP. The A and B isoforms of the human progesterone receptor: two functionally different transcription factors encoded by a single gene. Recent Prog Horm Res. 1999;54:291–313.

80. Spitz IM. Clinical utility of progesterone receptor modulators and their effect on the endometrium. Current Opinion in Obstetrics and Gynecology. 2009;21:318–24.

81. Maruo T, Matsuo H, Samoto T, Shimomura Y, Kurachi O, Gao Z et al. Effects of progesterone on uterine leiomyoma growth and apoptosis. Steroids. 2000;65:585–92.

82. The management of menorrhagia in secondary care. Evidence based clinical guideline No. 5. London: Royal College of Obstetricians and Gynaecologists. 1999.

83. Maruo T, Laoag-fernandez JB, Pakarinen P, et al. Effects of the levonorgesterone-releasing intrauterine system on proliferation and apoptosis in the endometrium. Hum Reprod. 2001;16:2103–8.

84. Maruo T, Ohara N, Matsuo H et al. Effects of levonorgesterone-releasing IUS and progesterone receptor modulator PRM CDB-2914 on uterine leiomyomas. Contraception. 2007;75:S99–S103.

85. De Leo V, Morgante G, La Marca A, Musacchio MC, Sorace M, Cavicchioli C, et al. A benefit-risk assessment of medical treatment for uterine leiomyomas. Drug Saf. 2002;25:759–79.

86. Eisinger SH, Meldrum S, Fiscella K, le Roux HD, Guzick DS. Low-dose mifepristone for uterine leiomyomata. Obstet Gynecol. 2003;101:243–50.

87. Spitz IM, Grunberg S, Chabbert-Buffet N, Lindenberg T, Gelber H, Sitruk-Ware R. Management of patients receiving long term treatment with mifepristone. Fertil Steril. 2005;84:1719–26.

88. Fiscella K, Eisinger SH, Meldrum S. Effect of Mifepristone for symptomatic leiomyomata on quality of life and uterine size. Obstet Gynecol. 2006;108:1381–87.

89. Carbonell Esteve JL, Acosta R, Heredia B, Pérez Y, Castañeda MC, Hernández AV. Mifepristone for the treatment of uterine leiomyomas: a randomized controlled trial. Obstet Gynecol. 2008;112:1029–36.

90. Wiehle RD, Goldberg J, Brodniewicz T, Jarus-Dziedzic K, Jabiry-Zieniewicz Z. Effects of a new progesterone receptor modulator, CDB-4124, on fibroid size and uterine bleeding. US Obstetr Gynaecol, Touch briefings. 2008;1–4.

91. Brahma PK, Martel KM, Christman GM. Future directions in myoma research. Obstet Gynecol Clin North Am. 2006;33:199–224.

92. Chwalisz K, Elger W, Stickler T, Mattia-Goldberg C, Larsen L. The effects of one-month administration of asoprisnil (J867), a selective progesterone receptor modulator, in normal women. Hum Reprod. 2005;20:1090–99.

93. Chwalisz K, Lamar Parker R, Williamson S, Larsen L, McCrary K, Elger W. Treatment of uterine leiomyomas with the novel selective progesterone receptor modulator (SPRM) J867. J Soc Gynecol Inves. 2003;10(2) abstract 636.

94. Chwalisz K, Larsen L, McCrary K, Edmonds A. Effects of the novel selective progesterone receptor modulator (SPRM) asoprisnil on bleeding patterns in subjects with leiomyomata. J Soc Gynecol Invest. 2004;11:320A–21A.

95. Levens ED, Potlog-Nahari C, Armstrong AY, Wesley R, Premkumar A, Blithe DL, et al. CDB-2914 for uterine leiomyomata treatment: a randomized controlled trial. Obstetr Gynecol. 2008;111:1129–36.

96. Nieman LK, Blocker W, Nansel T, Mahoney S, Reynolds J, Blithe D, et al. Efficacy and tolerability of CDB-2914 treatment for symptomatic uterine fibroids: a randomized, double-blind, placebo-controlled, phase IIb study. Fertil Steril. 2011;95(2):767–72.e1-2.

97. Donnez J, Tatarchuk TF, Bouchard P, Puscasiu L, Zakharenko NF, Ivanova T, et al; PEARL I Study Group. Ulipristal acetate versus placebo for fibroid treatment before surgery. N Engl J Med. 2012;366(5):409–20.

98. Donnez J, Tomaszewski J, Vázquez F, Bouchard P, Lemieszczuk B, Baró F, et al; PEARL II Study Group. Ulipristal acetate versus leuprolide acetate for uterine fibroids. N Engl J Med. 2012;366(5):421–32.

99. Horne FM, Blithe DL. Progesterone receptor modulators and the endometrium: changes and consequences. Hum Reprod Update. 2007;13:567–80.

100. Mutter GL, Bergeron C, Deligdisch L, Ferenczy A, Glant M, Merino M, et al. The spectrum of endometrial pathology induced by progesterone receptor modulators. Mod Pathol. 2008;21(5):591–8.

101. Williams AR, Critchley HO, Osei J, Ingamells S, Cameron IT, Han C, et al. The effects of the selective progesterone receptor modulator asoprisnil on the morphology of uterine tissues after 3 months treatment in patients with symptomatic uterine leiomyomata. Hum Reprod. 2007;22:1696–704.

102. Ioffe OB, Zaino RJ, Mutter GL. Endometrial changes from short-term therapy with CDB-4124, a selective progesterone receptor modulator. Mod Pathol. 2009;22:450–9.

103. Lakha F, Ho PC, Van der Spuy ZM, Dada K, Elton R, Glasier AF, et al. A novel estrogen-free oral contraceptive pill for women: multicentre, double-blind, randomized controlled trial of mifepristone and progestogen-only pill (levonorgestrel). Hum Reprod. 2007;22:2428–36.

104. 104.Baird DT, Brown A, Critchley HO, Williams AR, Lin S, Cheng L. Effect of long-term treatment with low-dose mifepristone on the endometrium. Hum Reprod. 2003;18:61–8.

105. Chabbert-Buffet N, Pintiaux-Kairis A, Bouchard P. Effects of the progesterone receptor modulator VA2914 in a continuous low dose on the hypothalamicpituitary-ovarian axis and endometrium in normal women: a prospective, randomized, placebo-controlled trial. J Clin Endocrinol Metab. 2007;92:3582–9.

106. La Marca A, Giulini S, Vito G, Orvieto R, Volpe A, Jasonni VM. Gestrinone in the treatment of uterine leiomyomata: effects on uterine blood supply. Fertil Steril. 2004;82(6):1694–6.

107. Coutinho EM. Treatment of large fibroids with high doses of gestrinone. Gynecol Obstet Invest. 1990;30(1):44–7.

108. Hickey M, Farquhar CM. Update on treatment of menstrual disorders. Med J Aust. 2003;178:625–9.

109. Loffer FD. Endometrial ablation in patients with fibroids. Curr Opin Obstet Gynecol. 2006;18:391–3.

110. Glasser MH, Zimmerman JD. The HydroThermAblator system for management of menorrhagia in women with submucous fibroids: 12- to 20-month follow-up. J Am Assoc Gynecol Laparosc. 2003;10:521–7.

111. Kanaoka Y, Hirai K, Ishiko O Microwave endometrial ablation for an enlarged uterus. Arch Gynecol Obstet. 2003;269:30–2.
112. Kanaoka Y, Hirai K, Ishiko O. Microwave endometrial ablation for menorrhagia caused by large submucous fibroids. J Obstet Gynaecol Res. 2005;31:565–70.
113. Nisolle M, Smets M, et al. Laparoscopic myolysis with the neodymium-Ytrium Aluminium Garnet Laser. J Gynaecol Surg. 1993;9:95–9.
114. Law PA, Gedroyc WM, Regan L. Magnetic resonance guided percutaneous laser ablation of uterine fibroids. Lancet. 1999;354:2049–50
115. Hindley JT, Law PA, Hickey M, et al. Clinical outcomes following percutaneous magnetic resonance image guided laser ablation of symptomatic uterine fibroids. Human Reproduction. 2002;17(10):2737–41.
116. Rubinsky B, Lee CY, Bastacky J, et al. The process of freezing and the mechanism of damage during hepatic cryosurgery. Cryobiology. 1990;27:85–97.
117. Olive DL, Rutherford T, Zreik T, et al. Cryomyolysis in the conservative treatment of uterine fibroids. J Am Assoc Gynecol Laparosc. 1996;3(suppl):S36.
118. Zupi E, Piredda A, Marconi D, et al. Directed laparoscopic cryomyolysis: a possible alternative to myomectomy and/or hysterectomy for symptomatic leiomyomas. Am J Obstet Gynecol. 2004;190:639–43.
119. Cowan BD. Myomectomy and MRI-directed cryotherapy. Semin Reprod Med. 2004;22(2):143–8.
120. Sakuhara Y, Shimizu T, Kodama Y, et al. Magnetic resonance-guided percutaneous cryoablation of uterine fibroids: early clinical experiences. Cardiovasc Intervent Radiol. 2006;29(4):552–8.
121. Organ LW. Electrophysiologic principles of radiofrequency lesion making. Appl Neurophysiol. 1976;39:69–76.
122. Bergamini V, Ghezzi F, Cromi A, et al. Laparoscopic radiofrequency thermal ablation: a new approah to symptomatic uterine myomas. Am J Obstet Gynecol. 2005;192:768–73.
123. Milic A, Asch MR, Hawrylyshyn PA, et al. Laparoscopic ultrasound-guided radiofrequency ablation of uterine fibroids. Cardiovasc Intervent Radiol. 2006;29:694–8.
124. Kim HS, Tsai J, Jacobs MA, et al. Percutaneous image-guided radiofrequency thermal ablation for large symptomatic uterine leiomyomata after uterine artery embolization: a feasibility and safety study. J Vasc Interv Radiol. 2007;18:41–8.
125. Recaldini C, Carrafiello G, Lagana D, et al. Percutaneous Sonographically Guided Radiofrequency Ablation of Medium-Sized Fibroids: Feasibility Study. AJR Am J Roentgenol. 2007;189:1303–6
126. Cho HH, Kim JH, Kim MR. Transvaginal radiofrequency thermal ablation: A day-care approach to symptomatic uterine myomas. Australian and New Zealand Journal of Obstetrics and Gynaecology. 2008;48:296–301.
127. Acupuncture for uterine fibroids. Zhang Y, Peng W, Clarke J, Liu Z. Cochrane Database Syst Rev. 2010;(1):CD007221.

Tumor Markers in Gynecological Cancers

Chapter

2

Asha Kapadia, Muzammil Shaikh

Tumor markers indicate biological changes that signal the existence of malignancy in a host organism. Tumor markers are produced by the tumor itself or by the body in response to the presence of cancer or certain benign conditions. A tumor marker is a molecular or tissue based process requiring a special assay that is beyond routine clinical, radiographic, or pathologic examination that provides information on future behavior of a cancer.[1] These substances can usually be detected in elevated quantities in the blood, urine, or body tissues of patients with certain types of cancer. Following the development of monoclonal antibodies, an array of new tumor markers has been discovered during the past 2 decades.

Tumor markers are not elevated in all cancer patients, particularly patients with early-stage cancer. The various tumor markers differ in their usefulness for screening, diagnosis, prognosis, assessing therapeutic response and detecting recurrence.[2]

Endometrial, cervical and ovarian cancers are the three most common malignancies of the female reproductive tract presenting in advanced stage with poor outcome and it is critical to detect the disease at the earliest possible stage. The discovery of useful serum biomarkers for the early detection of gynecologic cancers has thus been a high priority.

Serum Markers for Ovarian Cancer

The overall mortality of ovarian cancer has remained unchanged despite new chemotherapeutic agents, which have significantly improved the five-year survival rate.[3] The main reason is lack of success in diagnosing ovarian cancer at an early stage, as the great majority of patients with advanced stage of ovarian carcinoma, die of the disease. In contrast, if ovarian cancer is detected early, 90% of those with well-differentiated disease confined to the ovary survive. Symptoms that are associated with ovarian cancer are typically nonspecific and the association is often not recognized until the disease is advanced.[4] Previous studies showed that ultrasonography (USG), with or without color Doppler, provided high sensitivity. However, ultrasonography's specificity and positive predictive values were unsatisfactory.[5,6] The search for tumor markers for the early detection and outcome prediction of ovarian carcinoma represents one of the critical subjects in the study of ovarian cancer.

Serum Markers in Epithelial Ovarian Cancer

Ovarian cancer is composed of several related but distinct tumor categories including surface epithelial tumors, sex-cord stromal tumors, germ cell tumors and metastatic tumors.[7] The serous carcinoma is the most important, representing the majority of all primary ovarian carcinomas with a dismal clinical outcome.[8] Therefore, unless otherwise specified, serous carcinoma is what is generally thought of as "ovarian cancer".

The most widely studied ovarian cancer body fluid and tissue-based tumor markers are listed in Table 2.1, which also summarizes the phase of development of each marker and the level of evidence (LOE) for its clinical use. The LOE grading system is based on a previous report describing the framework to evaluate clinical utility of tumor markers.[1]

Serum CA 125

In 1981, Bast et al identified the CA125 antigen.[9]

Uses of CA 125

Screening/Early Detection

Elevated serum CA 125 levels have been detected in 50% and 92% of ovarian cancers in early and late stages, respectively.[10] The positive predictive value of the CA 125 assay for the early detection of ovarian cancer is 57%.[11] Elevated CA 125 occurs in other cancers, such as in endometrial, breast, pancreatic, gastrointestinal, and lung cancers. Raised CA 125 levels are sometimes found in patients with benign gynecologic conditions, such as menstruation, pregnancy, endometriosis, and pelvic inflammatory disease, and even in non-gynecologic conditions, such as hepatitis and pancreatitis.[12] The predictive value of pre-treatment CA 125 levels for prognosis is controversial; however, changes in CA 125 levels correlate with the regression, stability and progression of the disease in 87–94% of instances.[12] A National Cancer Institute (NCI) consensus development panel concluded that neither CA125 nor transvaginal ultrasonography effectively reduces mortality from ovarian cancer.[13] The same panel did recommend annual CA125 determinations, in addition to pelvic and ultrasound examinations, in women with a history of hereditary ovarian cancer who have an estimated lifetime risk of 40%.

Discrimination of Pelvic Masses

In contrast to its use in early detection, CA125 is more widely accepted as an adjunct in distinguishing benign from malignant disease in women, particularly in postmenopausal women presenting with ovarian masses.[13,14]

Postoperative Use

Elevations of CA125 greater than 35 U/mL after debulking surgery and chemotherapy indicate that residual disease is likely (> 95% accuracy) and that chemotherapy will be required. Monitoring with CA 125 testing in women with

TABLE 2.1 Currently available serum markers for ovarian cancer

Cancer Marker	Year Discovered	Proposed Uses	Phase of Development	LOE
CA125	1981	Tumor monitoring	Accepted clinical use	I, II
Osteopontin	2002	Tumor monitoring	Research/Discovery	III, IV
Carcinoembryonic antigen (CEA)	1995	Tumor monitoring	Research/Discovery	IV
Tumor-associated trypsin inhibitor (TATI)	1991	Tumor monitoring	Research/Discovery	IV, V
Kallikreins 5,6, 7,8, 9,10, 11,13,14,15	1996	Differential diagnosis, tumor monitoring, prognosis prediction	Research/Discovery	IV, V
Lysophosphatidic acid (LPA)	1995	Detection	Evaluation	IV, V
Tissue polypeptide antigen (TPA)	1994	Tumor monitoring	Research/Discovery	IV
Cancer-associated serum antigen (CASA)	1991	Tumor monitoring, prognosis prediction	Research/Discovery	IV
Plasminogen activator inhibitor-1 (PAI-1)	1995	Prognosis prediction	Research/Discovery	V
Interleukin-6 (IL-6)	1995	Prognosis prediction	Research/Discovery	IV
Prostasin	2001	Differential diagnosis	Research/Discovery	IV
Urinary β-core hCG (hCGβcf)	2000	Prognosis prediction	Evaluation	III, IV
Insulin-like growth factor binding protein-2 (IGFBP-2)	2004	Prognosis prediction	Research/Discovery	IV
Tumor released DNA	2002	Detection	Research/Discovery	IV
Human leukocyte antigen-G (HLA-G)	1990	Differential diagnosis	Research/Discovery	V
Her-2/neu	1985	Tissue marker for prognosis prediction and treatment outcome prediction of Herceptin	Evaluation	IV
Akt-2	1987	Tissue marker for prognosis prediction	Research/Discovery	V
Mitogen-activated protein kinase (MAPK)	2003	Tissue marker for prognosis prediction	Research/Discovery	V

elevated preoperative CA125 concentrations, along with a routine history and physical, and rectovaginal pelvic examination, has been advocated instead of surgery for asymptomatic women after primary therapy.[13]

Monitoring Treatment

Serial measurement of CA125 may also play a role in monitoring response to chemotherapy. Declining CA125 concentrations appear to correlate with treatment response even when disease is not detectable by either palpation or imaging.

Prognosis

The CA125 is recommended during primary therapy as a potential prognostic marker since CA125 concentrations, both preoperative and postoperative, may be of prognostic significance.[15-17] After primary surgery and chemotherapy, declines in CA125 concentrations during chemotherapy have generally been observed to be independent prognostic factors and in some studies the most important indicator. Persistent elevations indicate a poor prognosis.

Other Markers for Ovarian Cancer

Several other potential tumor-associated markers have been reported in body fluid and tissue of ovarian cancer patients. Although these experimental markers could represent promising new biomarkers and their clinical usefulness need to be validated by assessing the sensitivity and specificity in larger groups of patients with stage I disease.

The Kallikrein Family

Kallikreins are a subgroup of the serine protease enzyme family that play an important role in the progression and metastasis of human cancers.[18]

Osteopontin

It has been found as a potential diagnostic biomarker for ovarian cancer. Osteopontin expression has been found to be higher in invasive ovarian cancer than in borderline ovarian tumors, benign ovarian tumors and normal ovarian surface epithelium.[20] Osteopontin increased earlier than CA125 in 90% of the study patients who developed recurrent disease, indicating that osteopontin may be a clinically useful adjunct to CA125 in detecting recurrent ovarian cancer.

Lysophosphatidic Acid (LPA)

It was first identified in ascites of ovarian cancer patients and has since been demonstrated to play a biological role in ovarian cancer cell growth.[20-23]

Carcinoembryonic Antigen (CEA)

It is an oncofetal antigen and elevated serum levels of CEA are frequently found in a variety of benign diseases and cancers, including ovarian carcinoma. The sensitivity of CEA as a marker to detect ovarian cancer is approximately 25%, and the positive predictive value is only 14%.[24] Although CEA is not a marker for early diagnosis because of its low sensitivity, CEA can be useful in determining treatment response in ovarian cancer patients.

Plasminogen Activator Inhibitor-1 and -2 (PAI-1 and -2)

Fibrinolytic markers include PAI-1 and PAI-2, for which diagnostic and prognostic values havebeen reported in ovarian cancer. Whether PAI-1 can be used clinically for screening and/or monitoring ovarian cancer awaits further studies, including correlation with clinical treatment events and comparison with CA125. In contrast, expression of PAI-2 in tumors has been shown to be a favorable prognostic factor in ovarian cancer patients.[25]

Interleukin-6 (IL-6)

High levels of IL-6 have been detected in the serum and ascites of ovarian cancer patients.[26] IL-6 correlates with tumor burden, clinical disease status, and survival time of patients with ovarian cancer.

Her-2/neu

The c-erbB-2 oncogene expresses a transmembrane protein known as Her-2/neu. Amplification of Her-2/neu has been found in several human cancers, including ovarian carcinoma. In ovarian cancer, 9% to 38% of patients have elevated levels of the HER-2/neu protein.[27-29] Elevation of p105 in serum or the over-expression immunohistochemically of Her2/neu in tumors has correlated with an aggressive tumor type, advanced clinical stages and poor clinical outcome.[30] Furthermore, the test could be potentially useful for detecting recurrent disease.

The National Academy of Clinical Biochemistry (NACB) Panel recommends CA125 as the only marker for clinical use in ovarian cancer for the following indications: early detection in combination with transvaginal ultrasound (TVUS) in hereditary syndromes, differential diagnosis in suspicious pelvic mass, detection of recurrence, monitoring of therapy and prognosis. The NACB Panel does not recommend CA125 for screening of ovarian cancer. All other markers are either in the evaluation phase or in the research/discovery phase. Therefore, the NACB Panel does not recommend these biomarkers for clinical use in ovarian cancer.

Serum Tumor Markers in Non-epithelial Ovarian Cancer

Ovarian Germ Cell Tumors (OGCN)

These tumors arise primarily in young women between 10 and 30 years of age; they represent 70% of ovarian neoplasms in this age group.[29] OGCNs are often associated with hormonal or enzymatic activity. Some of these proteins can be measured in the serum, providing a highly sensitive and variably specific marker for the presence of certain histologic components. Some tumor markers are present in some, but not all tumors of a specific histology. Tumor markers produced by tumor's types are as follows:

Human Chorionic Gonadotropin (hCG)

Elevated in embryonal cell carcinomas, and ovarian choriocarcinomas, mixed germ cell tumors and some dysgerminomas

Alpha Feto Protein (AFP)

Elevated inendodermal sinus tumors, embryonal cell carcinomas and polyembryoma carcinomas, mixed germ cell tumors and some immature teratomas[31-33] most dysgerminomas are associated with a normal AFP.

Lactate Dehydrogenase (LDH)

Elevated in dysgerminomas.

Sex Cord Stromal Tumors

Ovarian sex cord-stromal tumors are a heterogeneous group of benign or malignant tumors that develop from the cells surrounding the oocytes, are rare, comprising only 1.2% of all primary ovarian cancers.[34] Hormonal activity of granulosa cell tumors permits the use of a variety of serum tumor markers in the diagnostic evaluation.

Inhibin

It is a peptide that produced by the ovaries in response to follicle stimulating hormone and luteinizing hormone. Inhibin usually becomes undetectable after menopause, unless produced by certain ovarian tumors, mostly mucinous epithelial ovarian carcinomas and granulosa cell tumors.[35-40] An elevated inhibin level in a postmenopausal woman or a premenopausal woman presenting with amenorrhea and infertility is suggestive of the presence of a granulosa cell tumor, but not specific. Although most commercial laboratories only provide assays for inhibin A, serum levels of inhibin B seem to be more frequently elevated.[41]

Estradiol

It was one of the first markers identified in the serum of patients with granulosa cell tumors. In general, however, estradiol is not a sensitive marker for the presence of a granulosa cell tumor. Approximately 30% of tumors do not produce estradiol, perhaps related to the lack of theca cells that produce androstenedione, a necessary precursor for estradiol synthesis.

Mullerian Inhibiting Substance (MIS)

It is produced by granulosa cells in the developing follicles, has emerged as a potential tumor marker for granulosa cell tumors. As with inhibin, MIS is typically undetectable in postmenopausal women. Although an elevated MIS level appears to be highly specific for ovarian granulosa cell tumors,[42-44] this test is not available for clinical use.

Serum Markers for Other Gynecological Cancers

Gestational Trophoblastic Disease (GTD)

The GTD is a proliferative disorder of trophoblastic cells. It defines a heterogeneous group of interrelated lesions arising from the trophoblastic epithelium of the placenta. All forms of GTD are characterized by a distinct tumor marker, the beta subunit of human chorionic gonadotropin (hCG). There are several histologically distinct types of GTD:
- Hydatidiform mole (complete or partial)
- Persistent/invasive gestational trophoblastic neoplasia (GTN)

- Choriocarcinoma
- Placental site trophoblastic tumors.

The tumor marker for GTD is human chorionic gonadotropin (hCG). It is a family of pituitary and placental glycoprotein hormones that share the same alpha subunit and differs in the beta subunit from follicle stimulating hormone, luteinizing hormone, and thyroid stimulating hormone. Different assays detect intact or fragments of beta-hCG by enzyme linked sandwich assays (radioimmunoassay). The serum hCG concentration is always elevated in women with GTD and is usually higher than that observed with intrauterine or ectopic pregnancies of the same gestational age. About 40% of complete moles are associated with hCG levels >100,000 mIU/mL (normal nonpregnant < 5 mIU/mL and peak normal pregnancy level typically < 100,000 mIU/mL). Compared to other types of GTD, PSTT is associated with lower levels of hCG relative to tumor size because of the lack of syncytiotrophoblastic proliferation.[45,46]

Serum Markers for Cervical Cancer

Screening for cervical cancer with cervical cytology reduced the incidence of cervical cancer by more than 50% over the past 30 years in the United States.[47] However, it is estimated that 50% of the women in whom cervical cancer is diagnosed each year will have never had cervical cytology testing.[47] One approach for further reducing the incidence and the mortality of cervical cancer would be to increase the screening rates among groups of women at highest risk, who currently are not being screened. Another would be the establishment of appropriate serum testing for the early detection of cervical cancer. The squamous cell carcinoma antigen, SCC, is the most commonly used serum marker for squamous cell cervical carcinoma, that makes up 85–90% of all cervical carcinomas. Elevated serum SCC levels have been detected in 28–88% of cervical squamous cell carcinomas (Table 2.2).[48-56] Pre-treatment levels of SCC have been shown to be related to the stage of the disease, size of the tumor, depth of the stromal invasion, the lymph-vascular space involvement and lymph node metastasis.[48,50,52,53,55-58] Elevated SCC levels were also demonstrated to have predictive value for prognosis in some studies.

TABLE 2.2 Diagnostic serum markers for cervical cancer in clinical use

Serum markers	SCC	CYFRA21-1	CA 125	CA 19-9	CEA	IAP
Positive rates	Squamous 28–85%	Squamous 42–52%	Adeno 27–75%	Adeno 35–42%	Adeno 26–48%	43–51%

Positive rates (elevated serum levels) detected for the indicated serum markers, in cases of squamous cell carcinoma (Squamous), adenocarcinoma (Adeno), or for all histological types

TABLE 2.3 Diagnostic serum markers for endometrial cancer in clinical use

Serum markers	CA 125	CA 19-9	CA 15-3	CA 72-4	CEA	IAP
Positive rates	11–43%	22–24%	24–32%	22–32%	14–22%	55–76%

Positive rates (elevated serum levels) detected for the indicated serum markers, in cases of endometrial cancer are shown

The serum SCC level also proved to be an independent predictor of response to neoadjuvant chemotherapy in locally advanced cervical cancer patients who received neoadjuvant chemotherapy and radical surgery.[58] SCC has also been used in the follow-up examination of cervical cancer patients. Increased serum SCC was shown to precede the clinical detection of recurrence of the disease.[51,52,59]

Other Tumour Markers in Carcinoma Cervix

Serum markers for endometrial cancer: In current practice, screening for endometrial cancer is not undertaken because of the lack of an appropriate, cost-effective and acceptable test that actually reduces mortality (Table 2.3).[60]

Conclusion

For gynecologic cervical, endometrial, and ovarian cancers only a small handful of tumor-associated antigens, such as SCC and CA 125, have been routinely used as tumor markers. Some markers are useful, not only as diagnostic tools, but also as a predictive marker for the prognosis and the clinical course after treatment. Recent breakthroughs in proteomics and bioinformatics technology will expand our understanding of tumor-specific biomarkers. Such investigations will establish newer and more useful biomarkers for the more accurate detection and management of ovarian, endometrial and cervical cancers.

References

1. Hayes DF, Bast R, Desch CE, et al. A tumour marker utility grading system (TMUGS): a framework to evaluate clinical utility of tumour markers. J Natl cancer Inst. 1996;88:1456.
2. Tchagang AB, Tewfik AH, DeRycke MS, Skubitz KM, Skubitz AP. Early detection of ovarian cancer using group biomarkers. Mol Cancer Ther. 2008;7(1):27–37.
3. Jemal A, Tiwari RC, Murray T, Ghafoor A, Samuels A, Ward E, et al. Cancer Statistics, 2004. CA Cancer J Clin. 2004;54:8–29.
4. Clarke-Pearson, Daniel L. Clinical practice: screening for ovarian cancer. N Engl. 2009;361:170–7.
5. Lerner JP, Timor-Tritsch IE, Federman A, Abramovich G. Transvaginal ultrasonographic characterization of ovarian masses with an improved, weighted scoring system. Am. J. Obstet. Gynecol, 1994;170:81–5.
6. Kupesic S, Plavsic BM. Early ovarian cancer: 3-D power Doppler. Abdom. Imaging. 2006;31:613–9
7. Young RH, Clement PB, Scully RE. The Ovary. In: Sternberg SS, ed. Diagnostic Surgical Pathology. 3rd ed. Philadelphia: Lippincott Williams and Wilkins. 1999:2307–94.
8. Seidman JD, Horkayne-Szakaly I, Haiba M, Boice CR, Kurman RJ, Ronnett BM. The histologic type and stage distribution of ovarian carcinomas of surface epithelial origin. Int J Gynecol Pathol. 2004;23:41–4.
9. Bast RC Jr, Feeney M, Lazarus H, Nadler LM, Colvin RB, Knapp RC. Reactivity of a monoclonal antibody with human ovarian carcinoma. J Clin Invest. 1981;68:1331–7.
10. Jacobs I, Bast RC Jr. The CA 125 tumour-associated antigen: a review of the literature. Hum. Reprod. 1989;4:1–12.

11. Nossov V, Amneus M, Su F, Lang J, Janco JM, Reddy ST. The early detection of ovarian cancer: from traditional methods to proteomics. Can we really do better than serum CA-125Am. J. Obstet. Gynecol. 2008;199:215–23.
12. Gadducci A. Cosio S, Carpi A, Nicolini A, Genazzani AR. Serum tumor markers in the management of ovarian, endometrial and cervical cancer. Biomed Pharmacother. 2004;58:24–38.
13. NIH consensus conference. Ovarian cancer. Screening, treatment, and follow-up. NIH consensus development conference. JAMA. 1995;273:491–7.
14. Ovarian Cancer. NCCN clinical practice guidelines in oncology v1. 2005.
15. Cooper BC, Sood AK, Davis CS, Ritchie JM, Sorosky JI, Anderson B, et al. Preoperative CA125 levels: an independent prognostic factor for epithelial ovarian Cancer. Obstet Gynecol. 2002;100:59–64.
16. Gadducci A, Cosio S, Fanucchi A, Negri S, Cristofani R, Genazzani AR. The predictive and prognostic value of serum CA125 half-life during paclitaxel/platinum-based chemotherapy in patients with advanced ovarian carcinoma. Gynecologic Oncology. 2004;93:131–6.
17. Rustin GJ. The clinical value of tumour markers in the management of ovarian cancer. Ann Clin Biochem. 1996;33:284–9.
18. Diamandis EP, Yousef GM. Human tissue kallikreins: a family of new cancer biomarkers. Clin Chem. 2002;48:1198–205.
19. Kim JH, Skates SJ, Uede T, Wong KK, Schorge JO, Feltmate CM, et al. Osteopontin as a potential diagnostic biomarker for ovarian cancer. JAMA. 2002;287:1671–9.
20. Xu Y, Shen Z, Wiper DW, Wu M, Morton RE, Elson P, et al. Lysophosphatidic acid as a potential biomarker for ovarian and other gynecologic cancers. JAMA. 1998;280:719–23.
21. Pustilnik TB, Estrella V, Wiener JR, Mao M, Eder A, Watt MA, et al. Lysophosphatidic acid induces urokinase secretion by ovarian cancer cells. Clin Cancer Res. 1999;5:3704–10.
22. Hu YL, Albanese C, Pestell RG, Jaffe RB. Dual mechanisms for lysophosphatidic acid stimulation of human ovarian carcinoma cells. J Natl Cancer Inst. 2003;95:733–40.
23. Fang X, Yu S, Bast RC, Liu S, Xu HJ, Hu SX, et al. Mechanisms for lysophosphatidic acid-induced cytokine production in ovarian cancer cells. J Biol Chem. 2004;279:9653–61.
24. Tuxen MK, Soletormos G, Dombernowsky P. Tumor markers in the management of patients with ovarian cancer. Cancer Treat Rev. 1995;21:215–45.
25. Chambers SK, Ivins CM, Carcangiu ML. Expression of plasminogen activator inhibitor-2 in epithelial ovarian cancer: a favorable prognostic factor related to the actions of CSF-1. Int J Cancer. 1997;74:571–5.
26. Gastl G, Plante M. Bioactive interleukin-6 levels in serum and ascites as a prognostic factor in patients with epithelial ovarian cancer. In: Bartlett JMS, ed. Methods in Molecular Medicine- Ovarian Cancer. Totowa: Humana press Inc. 2000:121–3.
27. Meden H, Fattahi-Meibodi A, Marx D. ELISA-based quantification of p105 (c-erbB-2, HER2/neu) in serum of ovarian carcinoma. In: Bartlett JMS, ed. Methods in molecular medicine- ovarian cancer. Totowa: Humana press, Inc. 2000:125–33.
28. Meden H, Kuhn W. Overexpression of the oncogene c-erbB-2 (HER2/neu) in ovarian cancer: a new prognostic factor. Eur J Obstet Gynecol Reprod Biol. 1997;71:173–9.
29. Cheung TH, Wong YF, Chung TK, Maimonis P, Chang AM. Clinical use of serum c-erbB-2 in patients with ovarian masses. Gynecol Obstet Invest. 1999;48:133–7.
30. Hellstrom I, Goodman G, Pullman J, Yang Y, Hellstrom KE. Overexpression of HER-2 in ovarian carcinomas. Cancer Res. 2001;61:2420–3.
31. Zalel Y, Piura B, Elchalal U, et al. Diagnosis and management of malignant germ cell ovarian tumors in young females. Int J Gynaecol Obstet. 1996;55:1.

32. Ihara T, Ohama K, Satoh H, et al. Histologic grade and karyotype of immature teratoma of the ovary. Cancer. 1984;54:2988.
33. Mann JR, Raafat F, Robinson K, et al. The United Kingdom Children's Cancer Study Group's second germ cell tumor study: carboplatin, etoposide and bleomycin are effective treatment for children with malignant extracranial germ cell tumors, with acceptable toxicity. J Clin Oncol. 2000;18:3809.
34. Quirk JT, Natarajan N. Ovarian cancer incidence in the United States, 1992–1999. Gynecol Oncol. 2005;97:519.
35. Lappöhn RE, Burger HG, Bouma J, et al. Inhibin as a marker for granulosa-cell tumors. N Engl J Med. 1989;321:790.
36. Jobling T, Mamers P, Healy DL, et al. A prospective study of inhibin in granulosa cell tumors of the ovary. Gynecol Oncol. 1994;55:285.
37. Boggess JF, Soules MR, Goff BA, et al. Serum inhibin and disease status in women with ovarian granulosa cell tumors. Gynecol Oncol. 1997;64:64.
38. Healy DL, Burger HG, Mamers P, et al. Elevated serum inhibin concentrations in postmenopausal women with ovarian tumors. N Engl J Med. 1993;329:1539.
39. Gustafson ML, Lee MM, Scully RE, et al. Müllerian inhibiting substance as a marker for ovarian sex-cord tumor. N Engl J Med. 1992;326:466.
40. Robertson DM, Stephenson T, Pruysers E, et al. Characterization of inhibin forms and their measurement by an inhibin alpha-subunit ELISA in serum from postmenopausal women with ovarian cancer. J Clin Endocrinol Metab. 2002;87:816.
41. Mom CH, Engelen MJ, Willemse PH, et al. Granulosa cell tumors of the ovary: the clinical value of serum inhibin A and B levels in a large single center cohort. Gynecol Oncol. 2007;105:365.
42. Rey RA, Lhommé C, Marcillac I, et al. Antimüllerian hormone as a serum marker of granulosa cell tumorsof the ovary: comparative study with serum alpha-inhibin and estradiol. Am J Obstet Gynecol. 1996;174:958.
43. Lane AH, Lee MM, Fuller AF Jr, et al. Diagnostic utility of Müllerian inhibiting substance determination in patients with primary and recurrent granulosa cell tumors. Gynecol Oncol. 1999;73:51.
44. Chang HL, Pahlavan N, Halpern EF, MacLaughlin DT. Serum Müllerian inhibiting substance/anti-Müllerian hormone levels in patients with adult granulosa cell tumors directly correlate with aggregate tumor mass as determined by pathology or radiology. Gynecol Oncol. 2009;114:57.
45. Schmid P, Nagai Y, Agarwal R, et al. Prognostic markers and long-term outcome of placental-site trophoblastic tumours: a retrospective observational study. Lancet. 2009;374:48.
46. Hoekstra AV, Keh P, Lurain JR. Placental site trophoblastic tumor: a review of 7 cases and their implications for prognosis and treatment. J Reprod Med. 2004;49:447.
47. The American College of Obstetricians and Gynecologists (ACOG). ACOG Practice Bulletin No. 109. Clinical Management Guidelines for Obstetricians and Gynecologists. Cervical Cytology Screening. Obstet. Gynecol. 2009;114:1409–20.
48. Massuger LF, Koper NP, Thomas CM, Dom KE, Schijf CP. Improvement of clinical staging in cervical cancer with serum squamous cell carcinoma antigen and CA 125 determinations. Gynecol. Oncol. 1997;64:473–6.
49. Lehtovirta P, Viinikka L, Ylikorkala O. Comparison between squamous cell carcinoma-associated antigen and CA-125 in patients with carcinoma of the cervix. Gynecol. Oncol. 1990;37:276–8.
50. Gadducci A, Ferdeghini M, Caenaro GF, Prontera C, Malagnino G, Annichiarico C, et al. Immunoacid protein (IAP) as marker for cervical and endometrial carcinoma: alone and in comparison with CA 125 and SCC. Cancer J. 1992;5:272–8.

51. Kainz C, Sliutz G, Mustafa G, Bieglmayr C, Koelbl H, Reinthaller A, Gitsch G. Cytokeratin subunit 19 measured by CYFRA 21-1 assay in follow-up of cervical cancer. Gynecol. Oncol. 1995;56:402–25.
52. Micke O, Prott FJ, Schäfer U, Tangerding S, Pötter R, Willich N. The impact of squamous cell carcinoma (SCC) antigen in the follow-up after radiotherapy in patients with cervical cancer. Anticancer Res. 2000;20:5113–5.
53. Takeda M Sakuragi N, Okamoto K, Todo Y, Minobe S, Nomura E, et al. Preoperative serum SCC, CA125, and CA19-9 levels and lymphnode status in squamous cell carcinoma of the uterine cervix. Acta Obstet Gynecol Scand. 2002;81:451–7.
54. Ohara K, Tanaka Y, Tsunoda H, Nishida M, Sugahara S, Itai Y. Assessment of cervical cancer radioresponse by serum squamous cell carcinoma antigen and magnetic resonance imaging. Obstet Gynecol. 2002;100:781–7.
55. Duk JM, Groenier KH, de Bruijn HW, Hollema H, ten Hoor KA, van der Zee AG. Pretreatment serum squamous cell carcinoma antigen: a newly identified prognostic factor in early-stage cervical carcinoma. J Clin. Oncol. 1996;14:111–8. 17.
56. Gadducci A, Scambia G, Benedetti-Panici P, Ferdeghini M, Battaglia F, Caenaro GF, et al. The prognostic relevance of pretreatment serum immunosuppressive acidic protein (IAP) in patients with squamous cell carcinoma of the uterine cervix: a comparison with squamous cell carcinoma antigen (SCC). Cancer J. 1994;7:241–7.
57. Gaarenstroom KN, Kenter GG, Bonfrer JM, Korse CM, Van de Vijver MJ, Fleuren GJ, et al. Can initial serum cyfra 21-1, SCC antigen, and TPA levels in squamous cell cervical cancer predict lymph node metastases or prognosis? Gynecol Oncol. 2000;77:164–70.
58. Scambia G, Benedetti P, Foti E, Ferrandina G, Leone FP, Marciano M, et al. Multiple tumour marker assays in advanced cervical cancer: relationship to chemotherapy response and clinical outcome. Eur J Cancer. 1996;32A:259–63.
59. Ngan HY, Cheng GT, Yeung WS, Wong LC, Ma HK. The prognostic value of TPA and SCC in squamous cell carcinoma of the cervix. Gynecol Oncol. 1994;52:63–8.
60. Berek JS, Ed. Novak's Gynecology, 13th ed.; Lippincott Williams and Wilkins: Philadelphia, PA, USA. 2002;1143-1398.

Emergency Contraception– Rational Use for Women's Health

Chapter 3

Suneeta Mittal, Neha Gupta

Emergency Contraception (EC) is a method of contraception that can be used to prevent pregnancy after an act of unprotected sexual intercourse. It is also called 'morning after' or post-coital method, although the time frame for EC use extends beyond the morning after. Thus, the term Emergency Contraception (EC) encompasses methods that are for one time use following a contraceptive accident and are effective if used within a short time frame after sexual exposure. As the name signifies, it is meant only for contraceptive emergency situations and not for routine or repeated use.

Emergency contraception is effective only in the first few days following intercourse before the ovum is released from the ovary and before the sperm fertilizes the ovum. Emergency contraceptive pills cannot interrupt an established pregnancy or harm a developing embryo.

History

Dr Ary Haspels, a Dutch family planning pioneer, in mid-1960s, first administered high doses of estrogen to a 13-year-old rape victim. This became the first standard regimen for emergency use of steroidal hormones to prevent pregnancy.[1] Research on other regimens soon followed. In mid-1970s, Canadian physician Albert Yuzpe used high doses of combined oral contraceptive pills which soon became the preferred regimen for emergency contraception.[2] This combination regimen containing 100 µg ethinyl estradiol and 0.5 mg levonorgestrel (LNG) taken twice at 12-hour-interval within 72 hours of exposure is commonly known as Yuzpe Regimen. Further research revealed that a single dose of 0.75 mg of LNG within 72 hours of unprotected intercourse was effective in preventing pregnancy but resulted in a higher incidence of menstrual disturbances. These earlier studies, however, suggested that LNG might prove useful in emergency post-coital contraception.[3] During this period, post-coital insertion of intrauterine device was also shown to be effective in preventing pregnancy.[4]

The first WHO sponsored comparative study of 834 women in Hong Kong, suggested that LNG alone used within 48 hours of unprotected intercourse was as effective as the Yuzpe regimen and caused fewer side effects.[5] The subsequent multicenter study conducted by WHO at 21 centers in 14 countries and involving

1998 women confirmed these results. This study in which India also participated, revealed that LNG regimen (0.75 mg dose repeated 12 hours later) was more effective than Yuzpe regimen up to 72 hours and was much better tolerated. WHO study also found that the sooner the drug is taken after unprotected intercourse, more effective it is.[6]

In 1995, the Rockefeller Foundation convened a meeting in Bellagio, Italy to discuss emergency contraception and expand its access and use in developing countries. Due to the Consortium's effort, EC formulation of combined estrogen-progestin regimen was added to the WHO Model List of Essential Drugs in 1995 and the levonorgestrel-only regimen was added in 1997. The Consortium identified a stepwise strategic approach for introduction of EC in four countries—Indonesia, Kenya, Mexico and Sri Lanka. The other countries where EC is approved and registered are Bangladesh, Brazil, Canada, China, Czech Republic, Egypt, Ghana, Jamaica, Mexico, Nigeria, South Africa, Venezuela, Vietnam, Yemen, USA, UK, France and most European countries.

In the light of these facts, a landmark step was taken in India in January 2001. A consortium on national consensus for EC was organized to provide recommendations and guidelines for appropriate use and follow-up of EC in India. It was organized by WHO-CCR in Human Reproduction, AIIMS, New Delhi and the expert group consisted of national and international technical experts, policy makers, representatives from NGOs, media and pharmaceutical companies and legal and ethical experts. Following this, the Government of India approved manufacturing and marketing of LNG EC as a dedicated product to be available on prescription (Pill 72 and Ecee 2). GOI also introduced 'E Pill' in its National Family Welfare Program in 2002. Finally, the much debated 'over the counter (OTC) availability of EC' came in to being in 2005, a year before OTC availability in US[7] following another consortium meet organized by AIIMS for expanding access to emergency contraception.

Need for Emergency Contraception in India

The relevance of EC can be derived from the fact that attempts to stabilize the population have not met success yet. While every unwanted pregnancy is a burden on maternal physical and mental health, it is also a contributor to infant morbidity and mortality. NFHS III figures reveal the couple protection rate to be 56% and unmet need to be 12.8%. A significant percentage of maternal mortality arises out of unsafe abortions taking place in women with unwanted pregnancies. The desire to limit family size and to space the next birth are the main reasons given by the majority of those who seek an abortion. Rational use of emergency contraception in India can play a very important role in reducing maternal mortality and morbidity, and women's health. It can also indirectly contribute towards reduction of perinatal mortality and morbidity by preventing unwanted births.

In India, knowledge about various temporary and permanent methods among men and women ranges between 45% and 97%, knowledge about EC is only 20% in men and 11% in women (NFHS III).[8]

Indications of Use of Emergency Contraception

- Unanticipated sexual intercourse
- Teenage sex
- Unprotected exposure (sexual assault, rape, sexual coercion)
- Contraceptive accidents with natural and regular methods
- Miscalculation of safe period
- Failed coitus interruptus
- Condom rupture or slippage
- Late insertion of spermicide
- Pill forgotten for 2 consecutive days or pill free interval of 9 or more days between packets
- More than 12 hours delay in taking progesterone only pill
- Delay of progestin injectable contraceptive injection by 2 weeks
- Delay of combined estrogen and progestin injectable contraceptive injection by 3 days
- Expelled or misplaced IUD.

Contraindications of Use of Emergency Contraception

The only situation in which a copper-bearing IUD should never be used as emergency contraception is if a woman is already pregnant. There are other contraindications to using a copper-bearing IUD as ongoing contraception that also should be considered before its use as emergency contraception.

Pregnancy is the only contraindication of EC pill use. The WHO medical eligibility criteria for EC use is given in Table 3.1.[9]

The ECPs do not protect against STI/HIV. If there is risk of STI/HIV (including during pregnancy or postpartum), the correct and consistent use of condoms is recommended, either alone or with another contraceptive method. Male latex condoms are proven to protect against STI/HIV.

Current Methods of Emergency Contraception

Table 3.2 gives a summary of the various methods of emergency contraception.

High dose estrogen was the first scientific method introduced in 1960s. Association of diethylstilbestrol (DES) with potential side effects on female offspring resulted in discontinuation of diethylstilbetrol (DES). High dose estrogen is associated with significant nausea and vomiting and causes disruption of menstrual pattern as well. 10% of pregnancies are likely to be ectopic pregnancies after treatment failure. Thus, estrogens are no longer used as emergency contraception.

Yuzpe Regimen

It is a combined ethinyl estradiol and norgestrel pill each containing 100 µg ethinyl estradiol and 0.5 mg norgestrel, 2 tablets given twice, 12 hours apart within 72 hours of unprotected intercourse. Combined pills are universally available and

TABLE 3.1 The WHO medical eligibility criteria for EC use

Condition	Yuzpe Regime Category	LNG EC Category	Clarification/Evidence
Pregnancy	NA	NA	NA = not applicable Clarification: Although this method is not indicated for a woman with a known or suspected pregnancy, there is no known harm to the woman, the course of her pregnancy, or the fetus if ECPs are accidentally used
Breastfeeding	1	1	
Past ectopic pregnancy	1	1	
History of severe cardiovascular complications (ischemic heart disease, cerebrovascular attack, or other thromboembolic conditions	2	1	
Angina pectoris	2	1	
Migraine	2	1	
Severe liver disease	2	1	
Repeated EC use	1	1	Clarification: Recurrent ECP use is an indication that the woman requires further counseling on other contraceptive options. Frequently repeated ECP use may be harmful for women with conditions classified as 2, 3 or 4 for CHC or POC use
Rape	1	1	

Category 1: A condition for that there is no restriction for the use of contraceptive method
Category 2: A condition where the advantages of using the method generally outweigh the theoretical or proven risks
Category 3: A condition where the theoretical or proven risks usually outweigh the advantages of using the method
Category 4: A condition that represents an unacceptable health risk if the contraceptive method is used

women find them familiar to use but as there are many formulations available, there is confusion about doses to be used for emergency contraception. Table 3.3 summarizes the dose of different COC formulations to be used.

Intrauterine Contraceptive Device

A trained health care provider can insert a copper T within 5 days of unprotected intercourse. This is the most effective EC method but it is undesirable in young women or in women with multiple sexual partners, women with active STI or at high-risk of STI such as following sexual assault. Irregular bleeding associated

TABLE 3.2 Methods of emergency contraception

Method and Dose	Time after Intercourse	Failure Rate (%)	Comments
No contraceptive method	–	4–40 (overall 8)	Risk based on cycle day
Vaginal douching	immediately	15–20	Very low efficacy
High dose estrogen (DES 50 mg or Ethinyl Estradiol 5 mg × 5 days)	< 72 hours	0.3–1.6	Severe nausea, vomiting, headache and irregular bleeding. Failure to complete regimen. Ectopic pregnancy and fetal malformations reported
Yuzpe regimen (Ethinyl Estradiol 100 µg + LNG 0.5 mg)	<72 hours. Repeat after 12 hours	0.2–3.2	Nausea, vomiting, headache and irregular bleeding. Risk of estrogen use. Low efficacy
Danazol 800 mg × 3 doses, 1200 mg × 2 doses	72 hours	0.8–1.8	Androgenic side effects on repeated use, costly
IUD (copper bearing)	120 hours	0.1	Risk of PID. Unsuitable for nullipara, rape victims
Centchroman 50 mg 2 tablets	72–120 hours. Repeat after 12 hours	To be evaluated	Menstrual delay
LNG 0.75 mg × 2 or 1.5 mg × 1	120 hours	1.1	Cheap, safe and effective. Severity of nausea, vomiting much less
Anti-progestin RU-486 (Mifepristone) 10 mg single dose	120 hours	0.9–1.3	Menstrual delay. Risk of ectopic pregnancy

TABLE 3.3 Combined oral contraceptive as EC- how many pills to be taken

Brand Name	Estrogen	Progestogen	No. of Tablets to be Used
Ovral	EE 0.05 mg	Levonorgestrel 0.25 mg	2 + 2
Ovral G	EE 0.05 mg	Norgestrel 0.5 mg	2 + 2
Ovral L	EE 0.03 mg	Levonorgestrel 0.15 mg	4 + 4
Mala D	EE 0.03 mg	Norgestrel 0.30 mg	4 + 4
Mala N	EE 0.03 mg	Norgestrel 0.30 mg	4 + 4
Femilon	EE 0.02 mg	Desogestrel 0.15 mg	5 + 5
Pearl	EE 0.03 mg	Norgestrel 0.30 mg	4 + 4
Loette	EE 0.02 mg	Levonorgestrel 0.10 mg	5 + 5
Novelon	EE 0.03 mg	Desogestrel 0.15 mg	4 + 4

Note: a. Triphasic pills should not be used as EC to avoid miscalculation of dose.
   b. Only white colored tablets should be used while prescribing from the 28 pill packs where red pills are non-hormonal iron tablets.

with Copper T insertion may mark the diagnosis of early pregnancy. For the suitable clients it has the advantage that there are no systemic side effects and can be used as an ongoing method of contraception. It can be used as a 'third chance', where EC pill has been vomited or the woman is unable to take the full dose due to intractable nausea or vomiting.

Mifepristone

It is an antiprogestogen that acts as anti-implantation agent when given post coitally, menses inducer when given in luteal phase and abortifacient when given in early pregnancy. It is effective as a single dose of 600 mg, 100 mg and 10 mg when used as emergency contraception. Current accepted dose for emergency contraception is 10 mg. In a comparative trial of mifepristone with Yuzpe regimen, side effects were less common with mifepristone but menstrual disturbances occurred more frequently.[10] Menstrual delay can add to the anxiety of women and breakthrough ovulation can occur resulting in failure if further sexual exposure occurs. There is also a higher risk of ectopic pregnancy. Currently, it is not licensed for use as EC in India.

Levonorgestrel—the Method of Choice

The progesterone only pill containing 0.75 mg LNG, 2 tablets taken 12 hours apart or a single tablet containing 1.5 mg LNG, taken within 72 hours of unprotected intercourse has shown to be more effective and with fewer side effects. Further studies have shown that the second pill could be delayed to 12–18 hours of the 1st one in case subsequent 12 hours fell at an inconvenient time, e.g. midnight. Current recommendations say that the regimen is efficacious up to 5 days, although the efficacy is higher, the earlier the pills are taken. Currently LNG is the most accepted and dedicated method for emergency contraception (a product that is specifically packaged and labeled for use as emergency contraception).

Ulipristal Acetate

Ulipristal acetate (UPA) is a selective progesterone receptor modulator approved for EC use in the United States in August 2010. UPA is administered as a one-time, 30-mg dose within 120 hours of intercourse. Based on clinical trials, UPA seems to be a reasonably tolerable and effective method of EC when used within 120 hours of intercourse. UPA is at least as effective as LNG when used within the first 72 hours after unprotected intercourse. However, UPA may be more effective than LNG when used between 72 to 120 hours after unprotected intercourse, extending the window of opportunity for EC. UPA may provide a new option for women who require EC up to 5 days after unprotected intercourse.[11] Side effects are mild and similar to those seen with levonorgestrel. Currently Ulipristal acetate has not been approved in India.

Mechanism of Action of Emergency Contraception[12]

Levonorgestrel-only emergency contraceptive pills:

- Inhibit or delay an egg from being released from the ovary when taken before ovulation; LNG ECPs inhibit the pre-ovulatory luteinizing hormone (LH) surge, impeding follicular development and maturation and/or the release of the egg itself. This is the primary and possibly the only mechanism of action for LNG ECPs.[13] It does not have any effect on histological or biochemical characteristics of endometrium and therefore does not prevent implantation.[14, 15]
- Possibly prevent the sperm and the egg from meeting by affecting the cervical mucus or the ability of sperm to bind to the egg.[16]

Emergency contraception is not the same as early medical abortion. EC is effective only in the first few days following intercourse before the ovum is released from the ovary and before the sperm fertilizes the ovum. This is also the basis for the window period of 5 days for use effectiveness of EC.

Medical abortion is an option for women in the early stage of an established pregnancy, but requires a different drug from levonorgestrel. EC cannot interrupt an established pregnancy or harm a developing embryo.[17]

Available data from the studies in humans indicate that the contraceptive effect of 10 mg mifepristone used as a single dose for EC is mainly because of impaired ovarian function, either by blocking the LH surge or by postponing the surge, rather than inhibiting implantation. In contrast, higher doses affect both ovulation and implantation. The drug can act as an abortifacient, if taken after implantation but here the dose and time frame are different and the two situations should not be confused in concept or practice.

Thus, Mifepristone and LNG seem to affect follicular development after selection of the dominant follicle but before the rise in LH have begun. The effect on follicular development and ovulation varies from delayed follicular development to arrested or persistent unruptured follicles. The LH peak is either blocked or delayed and blunted. Mifepristone is effective up to 5 days after intercourse and, in contrast to LNG and Yuzpe regimen, there appears to be no decrease in efficacy with time (Table 3.4).

There is some evidence that ulipristal acetate can produce changes in the uterine lining, but whether these changes would impair the implantation of a fertilized egg is unknown. If emergency contraceptive pills were effective at preventing implantation of a fertilized egg, their failure rates would surely be lower than they are. Levonorgestrel EC fails about 2.2% of the time, and the failure rate for

TABLE 3.4 Efficacy of different EC regimens[18]

	Crude Pregnancy Rate (%)	Prevented Fraction (%)
Yuzpe regimen	3.2	75
LNG pill	1.1	85
Mifepristone	0.9	85-90
CuT IUD	0.1	99–100

ulipristal acetate is around 1.4%. The copper IUD is the most effective emergency contraceptive method by far, with a failure rate of less than one per thousand; the extremely high efficacy of the IUD used as EC suggests that it does have the ability to inhibit implantation. IUD acts primarily through spermicidal and ovicidal mechanisms, and a possible harmful effect on embryo that has not yet implanted. Only copper bearing IUDs can be used as EC.

Effectiveness and Probability of Conception

Emergency contraceptive methods are less effective than regular methods. The efficacy of emergency contraception is influenced by the time elapsed since unprotected intercourse and the time in a women's cycle at which she had sex. The earlier the EC is taken after unprotected intercourse, the more effective it is. The closer a woman is to ovulation at the time of unprotected intercourse lower is the efficacy. As a woman is not capable of conceiving throughout cycle, EC effectiveness is better expressed in terms of 'prevented fraction' of pregnancies after calculating the probability of conception rather than the percentage failure.

The formula for calculating the prevented fraction of pregnancy is:
Observed pregnancies/expected pregnancies
For calculating the expected pregnancies, conception risk in menstrual cycle is calculated by probability of conception on that day of the cycle. The day of ovulation is calculated by subtracting 14 days from the expected date of next period and depending on the day of coitus in relation to this day, probability is estimated. Thus efficacy of EC is expressed either as overall pregnancy rate or the prevented fraction of pregnancies.

The probability of conception after single act of intercourse is around 8%. But the number of fertile days of a menstrual cycle is difficult to quantify. A normally sexually active couple not using contraception has an average 20–25% monthly chance of conception. Further 25% of zygotes do not implant and another 17% are lost before a pregnancy becomes clinically recognizable. About 8% of pregnancies are lost even after clinical confirmation. Therefore, in a vast majority of cases, EC addresses a theoretical or statistical risk, rather than an actual chance of fertilization having occurred and relieves the woman's apprehension of unwanted pregnancy considerably.

Prescribing the Pill

Emergency contraceptive can be prescribed at any time of the cycle following an act of unprotected intercourse as it allays the anxiety arising out of the possibility of an unwanted pregnancy, howsoever low the theoretical or statistical risk may be.
But before prescribing the following points should be noted:
- Counseling – it should be done using the 'GATHER' approach.
  - G-Greet the client and build a rapport
  - A-Ask questions effectively without being judgmental. Identify the client's needs

- T-Tell the relevant information about EC so that she can make an informed choice about the method of EC and ongoing contraception
- H-Help the client to reach the decision and give other related information
- E- Explain about the method in detail. That it protects a single act, its efficacy, side effects and the need to follow-up in case period is delayed by more than 7 days
- R-Return for follow-up if period is delayed beyond 7 days and for ongoing contraceptive methods.

- History—Date of last menstrual period and average cycle length, number of hours since the act of unprotected intercourse, any use of regular contraception, any history suggestive of STI and any relevant medical history.
- Examination—General and systemic examination is not essential. Pelvic examination is also not necessary except in cases of sexual assault, if there is a suspected pregnancy, for assessment of PID or there is consideration for IUD insertion or an overdue Pap smear.
- Laboratory Test—No specific test is required. Urine pregnancy test must be done if pregnancy is suspected. STI screening should be done in high-risk cases.
- Give clear instructions regarding the correct use of EC. The following points need to be emphasized:
  - EC should be taken as early as convenient after the act of unprotected intercourse to ensure better efficacy.
  - Failure rate is high if there are multiple unprotected sexual acts and the first act was more than 120 hours away from the date of prescription of EC.
  - The common side effects should be explained.
    - Nausea and vomiting—routine administration of antiemetics is not recommended with the LNG regimen. The dose of EC should be repeated if there is vomiting within two hours of EC intake.
    - Bleeding—any irregular bleeding or spotting after EC should not be misunderstood as periods. Next menstrual period may occur one week prior or later than the expected time. Women having excessive or prolonged bleeding should be evaluated for pregnancy (intrauterine or ectopic) and its complications.
    - Missed period— a urine pregnancy test may be done when delay is more than one week. If negative at this stage, wait for another one week. However pregnancy test is mandatory if periods are delayed by more than two weeks from the expected date.
    - Headache, mastalgia, dizziness, giddiness, abdominal cramps, etc. are minor side effects that are usually self-limiting.
  - EC does not prevent pregnancy from sexual acts after treatment. Client should be told to avoid exposure or use barrier method during further sexual acts, till the next period.
  - EC is a good back up method and not to be used as a regular method. EC pills are not intended for repeated use. Although they can be prescribed to a

woman who has used them before or within the same menstrual cycle, EC pill is less effective and has more side effects as compared to most modern methods over long-term use. A woman using it four times a month will be consuming same dose of hormone that is present in a monthly pill pack, that will have more side effects, thus will be better off using regular pills.

– The client should be explained about the small risk of failure of EC, but absent fetal risk if pregnancy occurs. Also EC does not increase the risk of ectopic pregnancy but chances of ectopic among failures are higher, therefore, it should be ruled out.

Important Tips for Prescription

- Tablets are to be swallowed with sips of water.
- There is no difference in side effects or efficacy whether the pills are taken on empty or full stomach.
- The treatment should not be delayed unnecessarily as the efficacy declines over time.
- The ideal interval between 2 doses of LNG EC is 12 hours. However, it is permissible to take the second dose between 10–24 hours of the first dose.
- Do not prescribe extra pills to women with undue anxiety. More pills will not make it more effective, but will increase the risk of nausea and vomiting.

Follow-up

- Woman experiences symptoms that suggest possible complications OR has any concerns
- Woman has not menstruated 7 days beyond expected period
- Visit to initiate a regular method of contraception
- Counseling about preventing pregnancy or HIV/STD infection.

Women are advised to come for follow-up if the periods are delayed for more than one week from the expected date or if she has lower abdominal pain or heavy bleeding. At the follow-up visit, details of post-treatment menstrual period should be recorded to ensure that the treatment was successful and the woman should be explained about all the methods of regular contraception available and a suitable method initiated.

Follow-up algorithm is mentioned in Figure 3.1.

Initiating Regular Contraception after Emergency Contraception

Currently available methods of contraceptives should be explained. The client should be given an opportunity to choose a specific method that can be started as per the following guidelines:

- Barrier methods and spermicides:
  – These can be initiated immediately following ECP use.
- Oral contraceptives:
  – The client may wait until the beginning of her menstrual cycle and then

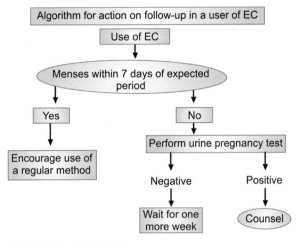

FIG. 3.1 Algorithm for follow-up

start a new pack according to the package instructions for the pill brand being used. She should be advised to use a barrier contraceptive method or abstain from intercourse for the remainder of the current cycle. Alternatively, the client may start oral contraceptives on the day after she takes the EC. She may begin a new pack of pills, or if she was using oral contraceptives before taking the EC (i.e. the EC was indicated because of missed pills), she may resume taking pills from the pack that she was previously using. She should use a barrier method for at least 7 days after starting or restarting the oral contraceptive pills. She may have some irregular bleeding until the onset of menses.

- Injectables:
  - Initiate progestin-only injectables within 7 days after the beginning of the next menstrual cycle. Initiate combined injectables within 5 days after the beginning of the next menstrual cycle. The client should use a barrier contraceptive or abstain from intercourse for up to 7 days after she receives the injection.
- Implants (Norplant):
  - Insert within 7 days after the beginning of next menstrual cycle. Use a back-up method or abstain from intercourse until the implants are inserted.
- Intrauterine device (IUD):
  - Insert during the next menstrual period. The client should use a barrier contraceptive or abstain from intercourse until the IUD is inserted. If the client intends to use an IUD as a long-term method and meets IUD screening criteria, emergency insertion of a copper-bearing IUD may be the EC prescribed.
- Natural family planning:
  - Natural family planning may be initiated after the normal menstrual period following ECP use. An alternative non-hormonal contraceptive method should be used in the interim period.

- Female or male sterilization:
  - Perform the operation only after informed consent can be ensured. It is not recommended that clients make this decision under the stressful conditions that often surround ECP use. Defer female sterilization until after the client's menstrual period, to ensure that she is not pregnant. Use a back-up method or abstain from intercourse until the sterilization procedure is performed.

Key Facts for Awareness

- Emergency contraception can prevent most pregnancies when taken after intercourse.
- Emergency contraception can be used following unprotected intercourse, contraceptive failure, incorrect use of contraceptives, or in cases of sexual assault.
- There are two methods of emergency contraception: emergency contraceptive pills (ECPs) and copper-bearing intrauterine devices (IUDs).
- When inserted within 5 days of unprotected intercourse, a copper-bearing IUD is the most effective form of emergency contraception available.
- The emergency contraceptive pill regimen recommended by WHO is one dose of levonorgestrel 1.5 mg, taken within 5 days (120 hours) of unprotected intercourse.

Warning and Precautions

- Pregnancy—No effect on fetal development
- Nursing mothers—No adverse effect
- Fertility following discontinuation—Rapid returns
- Drug interaction—No significant interaction.

Record Keeping for EC Use

1. Name (optional)
2. Age
3. Marital status
4. Date of LMP
5. Length of duration of coitus (in hour)
8. Past use of ECPs menstrual cycle
6. Number of unprotected acts in current cycle
7. Time since last act of unprotected
9. Past use of regular contraceptive
10. Method prescribed.

Management of Side Effects

- Advanced counseling leads to better tolerance
- Antiemetic 1 hour before Yuzpe reduces incidence of nausea to 30% and vomiting 10%

- No routine recommendation of antiemetic with LNG
- If vomiting within 2 hours—Dose can be repeated
- If pills are visible in emesis : Dose to be repeated.

How Frequently can One Take it?

- Should be used only once
- Repeated use in the same menstrual cycle will increase chance of pregnancy. It can result in menstrual irregularities
- However, if required it is permissible to use is repeatedly with side effects mentioned above that would in any case be milder than an unwanted pregnancy risk.

Social and Ethical Issues with Emergency Contraception Use

Emergency contraceptive pills (ECP) are effective, safe and cheap, with profound global health and economic benefits. Emergency contraception availability presents many opportunities for enhanced contraceptive care and evidence is lacking for contraindications to this expanded role. Issues related to morality, its perceived status as an abortifacient and harmful behavior should it be easily available, has limited the widespread use of ECP in many countries.

Increased access to emergency contraceptive pills enhances use but has not been shown to reduce unintended pregnancy rates.[19] Women's ability to benefit from emergency contraception is hampered by lack of knowledge and conservative cultural or social mores. Various Indian studies have shown the low level of awareness and knowledge about the correct use of EC among women as well as health care providers.[20] Low awareness of pharmacists' prescriptive authority has also created barriers to use. Opposition from activist groups also exists. Those opposed to EC, should know that biochemical evidence of pregnancy is possible only 6–9 days after fertilization. Thus, a physician prescribing EC within 120 hours of intercourse cannot intent pregnancy termination. Since, all methods of emergency contraception act either prior to implantation or prevent implantation, EC cannot be considered synonymous with termination of pregnancy or abortion.

There is need to popularize emergency contraception in India for its better usage among women to avoid unwanted pregnancies and abortions—with the help of media, government and health-management agencies and health care providers.

- Public awareness campaigns should be carried out to increase awareness and availability of EC. More emphasis is needed on the appropriate and effective use of EC, especially targeted to the 16–20-year-old age group.[21] Currently social marketing will not be a good option because of very low awareness about these methods. Overt publicity to increase awareness will also not be acceptable to authorities as well as society. Knowledge about these methods needs to be spread in the community in a subtle way. Getting the support and participation of community leaders, women's groups and non-government organizations will help. PHC staff and ASHA's need to be involved in counseling and dispensing.

- Both advocacy of EC and the awareness of the risk of unprotected sex should be improved through sex education programs in schools.
- Pharmacists, being the main EC providers in direct contact with sexually active adolescents, should receive systematic training and take the responsibility for offering information about the correct usage of EC and other, more reliable contraceptive methods.[22]
- Clinicians caring for women of reproductive age should also recognize the importance of ready access to this medication to help prevent unintended pregnancies.[23] It is very crucial that both health care providers and doctors should be fully aware of all aspects of EC for better delivery of EC-related services. People coming to family planning clinics should be told about rational use of EC pills. It is important to counsel women regarding the use of regular contraception and keep EC in reserve for emergency purpose. Dissemination of information to women visiting family planning clinics has been found to be effective in promoting better usage of emergency contraceptive pills.[24] Advance prescription will provide an opportunity to take the drug as soon as possible. This is especially useful for women using barrier or fertility awareness based methods. Advance prescription does not compromise the correct use of regular contraception.
- For effective and timely use of emergency contraception, there is a need to ensure availability at primary health care level. The training of health workers for proper counseling and follow-up of emergency contraception users and a distribution system for regular supply of drugs needs to be worked out.
- Facility for providing emergency contraception, counseling, back up abortion service and training of peripheral health care workers should be available at referral hospitals (secondary care level).
- The Medical Termination of Pregnancy Act (MTP Act) of India, 1971 creates no bar to the use of emergency contraception pills.

Future of Postcoital Contraceptives

There is enormous potential for EC in improving the reproductive health of the country. Research is ongoing. Mifepristone may follow the path of LNG and dedicated products in prescribed dosages that are currently not available may become approved and available. LHRH analogs, anti-hCG, ORF 13811 are some other products being tested for use as EC.

EC: Useful Information

- Emergency contraceptive is effective if taken within 120 hours after unprotected intercourse
- Sooner the ECPs are taken after unprotected intercourse more effective they are
- Repeated unprotected intercourse in the same cycle cannot be protected by single use of ECPs
- ECPs can prevent only 85% of pregnancies after unprotected intercourse

- Woman must be examined if period overdue by >1 week
- Initiate regular contraception soon after
- Emergency contraception (EC) offers women a last chance to prevent pregnancy after unprotected sex, whether a contraceptive method was not used (or was not used correctly), the method fails (such as a condom breaking or slipping), or in cases of sexual assault.

References

1. Haspels AA. Emergency contraception: a review. Contraception. 1994;50:101–8.
2. Trussell J, Ellertson C, Stewart F: The effectiveness of the Yuzpe regimen of post coital contraception. Family Planning Perspectives. 1996;28(2):58–64.
3. Landgren BM, Johannison E, Aedo AR, Kumar A, Yong-en S. The effect of levonorgestrel administered in large doses at different stages of the cycle on ovarian fuction and endometrial morphology. Contraception. 1989;39(3):275–87.
4. Lippes J, Malik T, Tatum HJ. The post coital copperT. Adv Plann Parenth. 1976;11: 24–9.
5. Ho PC, Kwan MS. A prospective randomised comparison of levonorgestrel with the Yuizpe regimen in post coital contraception. Human Reproduction. 1993;8:389–92.
6. Task force on postovulatory methods of fertility regulation. Randomized controlled trial of levonorgestrel versus the Yuzpe regimen of combined oral contraceptives for emergency contraception. The Lancet. 1998;352:428–33.
7. Consortium for National Consensus on Emergency Contraception in India. Published by WHO-CCR in Human Reproduction 2001. Available from URL: www.aiims.ac.in
8. http://www.nfhsindia.org/factsheet.html
9. Medical eligibility criteria for contraceptive use. 4th ed. World Health Organization, Geneva, Switzerland, 2009.
10. Webb AMC, Russell J, Elstein M. Comparison of the Yuzpe regimen, danazol and mifepristone (RU 486) in oral post coital contraception. BMJ. 1992;305:927–31.
11. Richardson AR, Maltz FN. Ulipristal acetate: review of the efficacy and safety of a newly approved agent for emergency contraception. Clin Ther. 2012;34(1):24–36. Epub 2011 Dec 9
12. International consortium for emergency contraception. Statement on mechanism of action, 2008.
13. Okewole IA, Arowojolu AO, Odusoga OL, Oloyede OA, Adeleye OA, Salu J, et. al. Effect of single administration of levonorgestrel on the menstrual cycle. Contraception. 2007;75:372–7.
14. Meng CX, Andersson KL, Bentin-Ley U, Gemzell-Danielsson K, Lalitkumar PG. Effect of levonorgestrel and mifepristone on endometrial receptivity markers in a three-dimensional human endometrial cell culture model. Fertility and Sterility. 2009;91(1):256-64. Epub 2008 Jan 18.
15. Durand M, Seppala M, Cravioto M del C, Koistinen H, Koistinen R, Gonzalez-Macedo J, et al. Late follicular phase administration of levonorgestrel as an emergency contraceptive changes the secretory pattern of glycodelin in serum and endometrium during the luteal phase of the menstrual cycle. Contraception. 2005;71:451–7.
16. Kesseru E, Camacho-Ortega P, Laudahn G, Schopflin G. In vitro action of progestogens on sperm migration in human cervical mucus. Fertility and Sterility. 1975;26(1):57–61.
17. De Santis M, Cavaliere AF, Straface G, Carducci F, Caruso A. Failure of the emergency contraceptive levonorgestrel and the risk of adverse effects in pregnancy and on fetal development: an observational cohort study. Fertility and Sterility. 2005;84(2):296–9.

18. Emergency contraception with update on regular contraception-Guidebook for health care providers. Mittal S. Published by WHO-CCR in human reproduction. 2006.
19. Raymond EG, Trussell J, Polis CB. Population Effect of Increased Access to Emergency Contraceptive Pills: A Systematic Review. Obstet Gynecol. 2007;109(1):181–8.
20. Puri S, Bhatia V, Swami HM, Singh A, Sehgal A, Kaur AP. Awareness of emergency contraception among female college students in Chandigarh, India. Indian J Med Sci. 2007;61(6):338–46.
21. Fitter M, Urquhart R. Awareness of emergency contraception: a follow-up report. J Fam Plann Reprod Health Care. 2008;34(2):111–3.
22. Xu J, Cheng L. Awareness and usage of emergency contraception among teenagers seeking abortion: a Shanghai survey. Eur J Obstet Gynecol Reprod Biol. 2008;141(2):143–6. Epub 2008 Oct 1.
23. Prine L. Emergency contraception, myths and facts. Obstet Gynecol Clin North Am. 2007;34(1):127–36, ix-x.
24. Tripathi R, Rathore AM, Sachdeva J. Emergency contraception: Knowledge, attitude and practices among health care providers in North India. J Obstet Gynaecol Res. 2003;29:142–6.

Current Management of Tubal Pregnancy

4

Chapter

Vishwanath Karande, Sigal Klipstein

An ectopic, or extra-uterine, pregnancy is defined as a pregnancy implanted outside of the uterine cavity. The most common location of an ectopic pregnancy is within the fallopian tube. This chapter will be limited to the medical and surgical management of tubal pregnancy. Discussions of extra-uterine pregnancies that occur in locations other than the fallopian tube (ovarian, abdominal, cervical, cesarean section scar) are beyond the scope of this chapter.

Incidence

Approximately 1–2% of all pregnancies in Europe and the USA are ectopic. In the Western world, tubal ectopic pregnancy (EP) remains the most common cause of maternal mortality in the first trimester of pregnancy. Ectopic pregnancy mortality rates in the United States steadily declined during the late 20th century, through 2007.[1] The decline in these deaths has been attributed to improvements in the sensitivity, accuracy, and use of pregnancy testing, ultrasound for diagnosis, and improvements in therapeutic modalities, including laparoscopic surgery and medical management of ectopic pregnancy. This success relies heavily on access to early care so that women who have signs and symptoms of ectopic pregnancy can be identified, diagnosed and treated. The contribution of any change in the incidence of ectopic pregnancy to the decline in mortality is unknown. Obtaining a reliable incidence rate for ectopic pregnancy in the United States is difficult. The latest estimate of 19.7 EPs per 1,000 pregnancies in the United States for 1990–1992 was reported using inpatient National Hospital Discharge Survey and outpatient National Hospital Ambulatory Medical Care Survey data. However, hospital discharge data are no longer considered an accurate surveillance data source for all ectopic pregnancies because more of these pregnancies are managed on an outpatient basis and with nonsurgical interventions. Other surveillance approaches suggest that the frequency of ectopic pregnancy in the United States has not changed substantially in the United States since the early 1990s.[2,3] The EP rate increases progressively with age and is three to four times higher for women ages 35–44 than for those ages 15–24.

Risk Factors for Tubal Ectopic Pregnancy

The major risk factors for tubal EP include: tubal damage as a result of surgery or infection (particularly *Chlamydia trachomatis*), smoking and in vitro fertilization.

Previous tubal surgery, and in particular tubal ligation, is a risk factor for tubal pregnancy (7.3/1000 procedures over a 10-year period). Of the tubal sterilization procedures, bipolar coagulation poses the highest risk of a subsequent ectopic pregnancy (17.1/1000 procedures) and postpartum salpingectomy poses the lowest risk (1.5/1000 procedures). Another risk factor for ectopic is a pregnancy that occurs in a woman with an intrauterine device (IUD). While the overall pregnancy rate in women with an IUD is exceedingly low, 50% of the pregnancies that occur will be extrauterine.[4]

The exact mechanism by which C. trachomatis infection leads to tubal EP remains relatively unknown. Lower genital tract chlamydial infection may ascend to the upper reproductive tract and result in salpingitis. Also, it is possible that an antibody response to chlamydial heat shock protein (HSP 60) may cause a tubal inflammatory response leading to tubal blockage or a predisposition to tubal implantation.[6] The risk for EP is increased 2-fold for women with circulating anti-chlamydial antibodies and the majority of women with EPs have high levels of these antibodies. Women with a previous documented chlamydial infection have a 2-fold increase in the incidence of hospitalization for EP. In women who have had three or more chlamydial infections, the risk of ectopic pregnancies is increased 4-fold. Overall, women with surgically documented salpingitis have a 4-fold increased risk of EP; the risk is approximately 10% after one episode of pelvic infection and this risk increases progressively with each subsequent infection.[4]

Cigarette smoking significantly increases the risk of tubal EP. Inhalation of cigarette smoke may alter embryo-tubal transport. Cigarette smoke may also affect ciliary beat frequency and smooth muscle contraction.[7]

The incidence of tubal EP after in vitro fertilization is relatively high at 2 – 5%. Several theories for this increase have been proposed. It has been suggested that high placement of embryos in the uterine cavity, higher volumes of transfer media and rapid plunging of the syringe attached to the embryo transfer catheter and transfer of may increase incidence of tubal pregnancy. Risk of tubal pregnancy increases with the number of embryos transferred during IVF treatment. Each of these embryos has a risk of implanting in the fallopian tube. Women undergoing IVF because of tubal factor (previous infection, surgery or tubal pregnancy) are at higher risk for tubal EP than women undergoing IVF for male factor.[8,9,10] It is also proposed that an 'embryo factor' may be present. This involves the cell adhesion protein, E-cadherin that is essential for blastocyst formation prior to implantation. In IVF, the embryos are exposed to a different growth factor and cytokine milieu during *in vitro* culture compared with naturally conceived embryos. This results in a difference in localization if E-cadherin making such embryos unable to implant within the uterus and instead migrate into the Fallopian tube and attach to the tubal epithelium.[6]

Risk for EP is increased as much as 10-fold for women with a previous EP, compared to the general population. The overall risk is 10% for women with one previous EP and at least 25% for women having two or more. The risk of recurrence is approximately 8% after medical treatment with methotrexate (single-dose regimen), 10% after salpingectomy and 15% after a linear salpingostomy.[11] Approximately 60% of women who have an EP will subsequently achieve a successful intrauterine pregnancy.

Pathogenesis

More than 98% of ectopic pregnancies occur in the Fallopian tubes. Of all ectopic pregnancies, 70% are located in the tubal ampulla, 12% in the isthmus, 11% in the fimbria and 2% in the interstitial (cornual) segment. The remaining 5% occur in the ovaries, cervix or abdomen.

A tubal pregnancy may be caused by a combination of 1) retention of the embryo within the Fallopian tube because to impaired embryo-tubal transport and 2) alterations in the tubal environment allowing early implantation to occur. In histopathologic studies, post-inflammatory changes (chronic salpingitis, salpingitis isthmica nodosa) are frequently seen. Other abnormalities observed include diverticuli and foci of persistent decidual transformation.

The histopathology of EPs varies with the site of implantation. In approximately 50% of ampullary EPs, trophoblastic proliferation occurs entirely within the tubal lumen and the muscularis remains intact. In these cases, the dilated appearing ampullary portion consists mainly of coagulated blood and not trophoblastic tissue. In the remainder, the trophoblast penetrates the tubal wall and proliferates in the loose connective tissue between the muscularis and the serosa. In contrast, ectopic implantation in the tubal isthmus typically penetrates the tubal wall relatively early, probably because the more muscular segment is less distensible. Not all EPs will rupture. Some may resolve without intervention, presumably by spontaneous regression in situ or tubal abortion (expulsion via the fimbria).[4]

The incidence of chromosomal abnormalities in ectopic pregnancies (approximately 5%) is similar to that expected when maternal age and gestational age are considered.[12]

Diagnosis of Tubal Ectopic Pregnancy

The three classic symptoms of EP are delayed menses, vaginal bleeding and lower abdominal pain. Other symptoms include shoulder pain (from irritation of the diaphragm by blood in the peritoneal cavity), lightheadedness and shock (from severe intra-abdominal hemorrhage). With the availability of highly sensitive and specific assays for the β-subunit of human chorionic gonadotropin (hCG) and transvaginal ultrasonography (TVU), and sometimes with a dilatation and curettage, it is now possible to diagnose or rule out an EP within a short time. Tubal pregnancies are now being diagnosed early, often before they become symptomatic. Treatment with methotrexate (MTX), a folic acid antagonist highly toxic to rapidly replicating tissues, achieves results comparable to surgery for the treatment of appropriately selected ectopic pregnancies and is used commonly.[13] An unruptured EP can be managed with either surgery or methotrexate. Surgery is specifically indicated in cases of suspected tubal rupture and when MTX is contraindicated.

Use of Transvaginal Ultrasonography and Serial Human Chorionic Gonadotropin Levels

A gestational sac (or sacs) should become visible by TVU between 5.5 and 6.0 weeks gestational age.[14,15] In sequence, structures such as a gestational sac ("double decidual sign"), yolk sac, and fetal pole with later cardiac motion become visible by TVU. When gestational age is not known, hCG levels can provide alternate criteria for timing and interpretation of TVU.[16,17]

It now is widely accepted that above the discriminatory zone of 1,500–2,500 IU/L, a normal intrauterine pregnancy (IUP) should be visible by TVU.[18] The absence of an intrauterine gestational sac when the hCG concentration is above the discriminatory zone implies an abnormal gestation. The specific cutoff value for hCG used at each institution will depend on clinical expertise and the specific characteristics of the hCG assay used. A more conservative discriminatory zone, that is, higher hCG level, may be used to minimize the risk of terminating a viable pregnancy.[19] In the case of multiple pregnancy, hCG levels are higher at an earlier stage of development than in singleton intrauterine gestations, but the rate of increase remains similar.[20]

If the initial hCG level is below the discriminatory zone, and TVU cannot definitively identify an intrauterine or extrauterine gestation, then serial hCG measurements are needed to document either a growing, potentially viable or a nonviable pregnancy. The minimum rise for a potentially viable pregnancy in women who present with symptoms of pain and/or vaginal bleeding is 53% per two days, based on the 99th percentile confidence interval (CI) around the mean of the curve for β-hCG rise (up to 5,000 IU/L) over time.[17] Intervention when the β-hCG level rises less than 66% over 2 days, a practice supported by previous data, may potentially result in the interruption of a viable pregnancy.[21] When the hCG levels have risen above the discriminatory zone, ultrasound should be used to document the presence, or absence, of an IUP.

A proportion of patients presenting with pain, bleeding, and a positive pregnancy test will have a pregnancy of unknown location (PUL). This term is applied to women without evidence of either an intrauterine pregnancy (IUP) or an EP on TVU. It can be clinically challenging to manage these patients. Generally, patients with PUL are reassessed within 48 hours from presentation to determine the change in hCG level and to aid the frequency and method of follow-up.

Morse et al[22] followed 1005 patients with PUL until diagnosed with EP (n = 179), IUP (n = 259), or miscarriage (n = 567). They then investigated the accuracy of serial hCG levels to predict the outcome in these patients. They determined that the optimal balance in sensitivity and specificity used with minimal expected 2-day increase in hCG of 35% and the minimal 2-day decrease in hCG level of 36–47% (depending on level) achieved 83.2% sensitivity, 70.8% specificity to predict EP.

However, 16.8% of EPs and 7.7% of IUPs would be misclassified solely using serial hCG levels. Consideration of a third hCG and early ultrasound decreased IUP misclassification to 2.7%. They suggest that solely using serial hCG values can result in misclassification. Clinical judgment should also come into play and not just "prediction rules".

Declining hCG values suggest a failing pregnancy. Serial hCG levels can be used to show that the gestation is regressing spontaneously. After a complete abortion, hCG levels decline at least 21–35% every 2 days, depending on the initial value.[23] However, a decline in hCG concentrations at this rate, or faster, does not exclude entirely the possibility of a resolving EP or its rupture.

The absence of a gestational sac with an hCG above the discriminatory zone, or an abnormally rising or declining hCG level, suggests an abnormal pregnancy but does not distinguish an EP from a failed intrauterine gestation. The presumption of an EP in such circumstances can be incorrect in up to 50% of cases. A uterine curettage and evaluation of uterine contents may be helpful to differentiate an abnormal IUP from an EP.[18] Also, if hCG levels continue to rise after curettage, the diagnosis of EP is established.

Medical Treatment of Tubal Pregnancy

Approximately 40% of women diagnosed with an EP are candidates for a trial of medical management, and 90% of those can be treated successfully without surgery.[18] Various treatments of tubal pregnancy have been reported including the local and systemic use of prostaglandin F2α[24] and local instillation of hyperosmolar glucose.[25] Other agents that have been locally instilled (ultrasound-guided or via laparoscopy) include MTX, potassium chloride, vasopressin, actinomycin and the progesterone receptor antagonist mifepristone.[26] However, over the years, systemically administered MTX has emerged as the most widely used drug for the medical treatment of tubal pregnancy.

Effort should be made to diagnose an EP definitively before medical treatment with MTX. Medical treatment for a suspected EP without a definitive diagnosis does not reduce complication rates or cost because many women with undiagnosed miscarriage would otherwise be exposed to MTX and its side effects unnecessarily. Exposure of a viable pregnancy to MTX may result in embryopathy, a very serious and avoidable complication that is being reported with increasing frequency.[27]

The use of MTX for the medical management of EP is now well established, widely accepted and has been used for more than 25 years.[28-32] MTX is a folic acid antagonist.[33] Folic acid normally is reduced to tetrahydrofolate by the enzyme dihydrofolate reductase (DHFR), a step in the synthesis of DNA and RNA precursors. MTX inhibits DHFR, causing depletion of cofactors required for DNA and RNA synthesis. Folinic acid (leucovorin) is an antagonist to MTX that can help reduce otherwise prohibitive side effects, particularly when higher doses of MTX are used.

Ideally, a candidate for medical management with MTX should meet the following criteria: i. hemodynamic stability, ii. no severe or persistent abdominal pain, iii. commitment to follow-up until the EP has resolved, and iv. normal baseline liver and renal function tests.

Contraindications to methotrexate therapy include:
- Absolute contraindications
- Intrauterine pregnancy
- Evidence of immunodeficiency
- Moderate to severe anemia, leukopenia or thrombocytopenia
- Sensitivity to methotrexate
- Active pulmonary disease
- Active peptic ulcer disease
- Clinically important hepatic dysfunction
- Clinically important renal dysfunction
- Breastfeeding

Relative contraindications:
- Embryonic cardiac activity detected by TVU
- High initial hCG concentration (> 5,000 mIU/mL)
- EP > 4 cm in size as imaged by TVU
- Refusal to accept blood transfusion
- Non-compliant or unable to participate in follow-up.

Prior to the first dose of MTX, women should be screened with a complete blood count; liver function tests, serum creatinine and blood type and Rh. Women with a history of pulmonary disease should be screened with a chest x-ray because of the risk of interstitial pneumonitis in patients with underlying lung disease.

There are two commonly used MTX treatment regimens: "multiple dose" and "single dose." Schema for treatment and follow-up for the two regimens are summarized in Tables 4.1 and 4.2, respectively. The multiple-dose protocol is a regimen adapted from early experience with MTX treatment for trophoblastic disease and was the regimen first used to treat EP. The multiple-dose protocol alternates MTX treatment with leucovorin therapy. MTX is continued until hCG falls by 15% from its peak concentration. Approximately 50% of patients so treated will not require the full 8-day regimen. The term "single dose" actually is

TABLE 4.1 Single-dose methotrexate (MTX) treatment protocol

Treatment day	Laboratory evaluation	Intervention
Pretreatment	hCG, CBC with differential, liver function tests, creatinine, blood type and antibody screen	Rule out spontaneous miscarriage. Rhogam if Rh negative
1	hCG	MTX 50 mg/m² IM
4	hCG	
7	hCG	MTX 50 mg/m² IM if β-hCG decreased <15% between day 4 and 7

Note: Surveillance every 7 days (until hCG < 5 mIU/mL). IM = intramuscularly
Reproduced by permission from reference 18.

TABLE 4.2 Multiple-dose methotrexate (MTX) treatment protocol

Treatment day	Laboratory evaluation	Intervention
Pretreatment	hCG, CBC with differential, liver function tests, creatinine, blood type and antibody screen	Rule out spontaneous miscarriage. Rhogam if Rh negative
1	hCG	MTX 1.0 mg/kg IM
2		LEU 0.1 mg/kg IM
3	hCG	MTX 1.0 mg/kg IM if < 15% decline day 1 – day 3 If > 15%, stop treatment and start surveillance
4		LEU 0.1 mg/kg IM
5	hCG	MTX 1.0 mg/kg IM if < 15% decline day 1 – day 3 If > 15%, stop treatment and start surveillance
6		LEU 0.1 mg/kg IM
7	hCG	MTX 1.0 mg/kg IM if < 15% decline day 1 – day 3 If > 15%, stop treatment and start surveillance
8		LEU 0.1 mg/kg IM

Note: Surveillance every 7 days (until hCG < 5 mIU/mL)
Screening laboratory studies should be repeated 1 week after last dose of MTX. LEU = leucovorin.
Reproduced by permission from reference 18

a misnomer.[34,35] Whereas it describes the number of MTX injections planned, the regimen includes provisions for additional doses of MTX when the response is inadequate.[18]

In both single- and multiple-dose MTX treatment protocols, once hCG levels have met the criteria for initial decline, hCG levels are followed serially at weekly intervals to ensure that concentrations decline steadily and become undetectable. Complete resolution of an EP usually takes between 2 and 3 weeks but can take as long as 6 to 8 weeks when pretreatment hCG levels are in higher ranges. When declining hCG levels again rise, the diagnosis of a persistent EP is made.

When the criteria described earlier are fulfilled, treatment with MTX yields treatment success rates comparable to those achieved with conservative surgery. Numerous open-label studies have been published demonstrating the efficacy of both MTX treatment regimens. One review concluded that MTX treatment was successful in 78–96% of selected patients. Post-treatment hysterosalpingography documented tubal patency in 78% of cases; 65% of patients who attempted subsequent pregnancies succeeded and the incidence of recurrent EP was a relatively low 13%.

There have been no randomized trials directly comparing the two different MTX treatment protocols.

A hybrid protocol, involving two equal doses of MTX (50 mg/m^2) administered on days 1 and 4 without leucovorin rescue and follow-up as described previously for the single-dose protocol, may offer a more optimal balance between convenience and efficacy.[36] The protocol also allows for more than 2 doses of MTX when hCG values do not decrease 15% between days 4 and 7.

Women undergoing treatment with methotrexate should avoid: intercourse, pelvic examinations, TVU, sun exposure (because of the risk of methotrexate dermatitis), foods and vitamins containing folic acid (including prenatal vitamins), and gas-forming foods.

Predictors of Methotrexate Failure

The most commonly identified predictors of MTX treatment failure are adnexal fetal cardiac activity, size and volume of the gestational mass (> 4 cm), high initial hCG concentration (> 5,000 mIU/mL), presence of free peritoneal blood, rapidly increasing hCG concentrations (>50%/ 48 hours) before MTX and continued rapid rise in hCG concentrations during MTX.

Dudley et al. in a retrospective case-control analysis, studied eighty-one women diagnosed with an ectopic pregnancy and treated with MTX. They proceeded to identify risk factors for tubal rupture in the 19 patients that experienced subsequent tubal rupture.[37] The hCG incremental rate both before and after MTX represented an independent risk factor for subsequent tubal rupture. hCG values prior to ectopic diagnosis that increased at least 66% over 48 hours and rising hCG values after treatment with MTX may be considered signs of impending rupture and as an indication for surgical intervention. The mean time to rupture in this series was 6.1 days (range 1 – 17 days).

Whereas the prognosis for successful medical treatment has been demonstrated repeatedly to correlate with the initial hCG level, no consensus on a threshold value that best predicts success or failure has been established. One study noted that the failure rate of single-dose treatment was 13% (6/45) for initial hCG values between 5,000 IU/L and 9,999 IU/L, 18% (4/22) for concentrations between 10,000 IU/L and 14,999 IU/L, and 32% (7/22) when hCG values exceeded 15,000 IU/L.[38] Analysis after combining all published data yields an OR for failure of 5.45 (95% CI, 3.04–9.78) when the initial hCG value above 5,000 IU/L compared with that observed when hCG concentrations are below that threshold. The failure rate for single-dose MTX treatment stratified by initial hCG level is illustrated in Figure 4.1.[18] Because the failure rate rises with the pretreatment hCG concentration, the single-dose MTX treatment regimen may be better reserved for patients with a relatively low initial hCG value.

Side Effects of Methotrexate

Overall, MTX is a safe and effective treatment for an unruptured EP. Very rarely, life-threatening complications have been reported with MTX. Rarely patients may complain of gastric distress, nausea and vomiting, stomatitis, dizziness, severe neutropenia (rare), reversible hair loss (rare) and pneumonitis (rare). Some patients

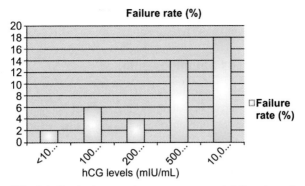

Failure rate (%)

hCG levels (mIU/mL)

☐ Failure rate (%)

FIG. 4.1 Single-dose methotrexate treatment failure based on hCG level

develop transient pain ("separation pain") between 3 and 7 days after treatment begins, but such pain normally resolves within 4 to 12 hours after onset. When pain is severe and persistent, it is prudent to evaluate the patient's vital signs and hematocrit and if rupture is suspected, surgery should be performed.[18]

Signs of treatment failure or suspected rupture are indications to abandon medical management and to proceed with surgical treatment. Signs suggesting treatment failure or possible rupture include: hemodynamic instability increasing abdominal pain regardless of trends in hCG levels, and rapidly increasing hCG concentrations (> 53% over 2 days) after four doses in the multi-dose regimen or after two doses in the single-dose regimen.[39]

Serial ultrasonographic examinations after MTX treatment may be considered unnecessary because ultrasonographic findings cannot demonstrate or predict treatment failure, unless evidence of recent tubal rupture is observed.[18]

Rh (D) immunoglobulin treatment (at least 50 μg) is recommended routinely for all Rh-negative women who have an ectopic pregnancy or early spontaneous abortion. The evidence to support this recommendation, however, is weak.

Heterophilic Antibodies

Heterophilic antibodies are important to recognize because persistent false positive tests may be interpreted as evidence of EP or gestational trophoblastic disease and lead to inappropriate evaluation and treatments having serious potential consequences. A false-positive hCG usually remains at the same level over time, neither increasing nor decreasing. When the clinical presentation is uncertain or inconsistent with the test result, a true-positive hCG can be confirmed by i. obtaining similar result with a different assay method; ii. demonstrating hCG in the urine; and iii. obtaining parallel results with serial dilutions of the hCG standard and the patient's serum.[40]

Surgical Treatment of Ectopic Pregnancy

Laparoscopy is the mainstay for the surgical management of tubal pregnancy. It has almost completely replaced laparotomy as the treatment of choice when surgery is indicated.[41] Surgery is indicated in patients where medical management is contraindicated (see above) or has failed.

Salpingectomy Versus Salpingostomy

Surgical treatment for EP can be radical (salpingectomy) or conservative (salpingostomy). There have been no randomized controlled trials comparing the two treatment modalities, though observational studies have found no difference in the chance of achieving an IUP with either surgical approach. The preferred approach when the contralateral tube is normal remains unresolved.[42]

Laparoscopic Salpingectomy

A salpingectomy involves the removal of a segment or the whole length of the Fallopian tube that contains the EP. Indications for salpingectomy include a severely damaged Fallopian tube, an ectopic in a woman who has undergone tubal ligation, in a previously reconstructed tube and recurrent ectopic pregnancy on the same side. Patients with uncontrolled bleeding after salpingostomy, a large tubal pregnancy, a heterotopic pregnancy and patients who have completed childbearing may also be offered this approach.[43]

Various techniques have been described for salpingectomy:
- Use of a pre-tied ligature loop to tie the damaged segment that can then be safely resected.
- Coagulation of the proximal and distal part of the Fallopian tube and the mesosalpinx with bipolar cautery, followed by excision of the segment with laparoscopic scissors.
- The same procedure can be done using a laser, a harmonic scalpel (Ethicon Endo Surgery, Cincinnati, OH) or a LigaSure device (Covidien, Mansfield, MA).
  The specimen can be removed with a grasper through one of the ports or using a specially designed pouch (Endobag, US Surgical Corporation, Norwalk, CT). If the contralateral tube is normal, salpingectomy does not compromise the subsequent pregnancy rate. It also avoids the complication of persistent or recurrent ectopic pregnancy on the ipsilateral tube.

Laparoscopic Linear Salpingostomy

A salpingostomy may be considered in women who wish to preserve their fertility.[44] The tube is immobilized with an atraumatic laparoscopic grasper and the tubal wall can be injected with a dilute vasopressin solution (0.2 IU/mL of normal saline) at the area of maximum distension to reduce bleeding. This step, however, is not mandatory and may cause a rise in the blood pressure. A 1–2 cm longitudinal incision is made on the antimesenteric side of the tube with a needlepoint monopolar cautery (or with a laser, scissors or Harmonic scalpel). The tubal pregnancy is then flushed out using a suction irrigator. It is important not to pull out the tissue as the resultant bleeding may require repeated cautery with subsequent damage to the tube. The

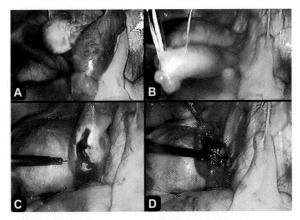

FIG. 4.2 Salpingostomy for a right ampullary tubal pregnancy. (A) Dilated ampullary portion with a tubal pregnancy; (B) A dilute vasopressin solution is injected in the anti-mesenteric part of the tube; (C) A linear incision is made with a monopolar needle cautery; (D) The tubal pregnancy is flushed out with a suction irrigator (hydro dissection) (*For color version see Plate 1*)

specimen can be delivered using a grasper or a bag (Fig. 4.2). If the pregnancy is close to the fimbrial end, it can be expressed ('milked out') without tubal injury. The laparoscopic approach may be more complicated in patients with a cornual or interstitial pregnancy. In most cases, laparoscopic excision can be performed successfully.[45] Diluted vasopressin should be used to facilitate hemostasis. Sometimes, laparoscopic suturing may be required to control blood loss. Cornual resection or hysterectomy is seldom required today.

Adjunctive Use of MTX

A persistent EP can develop after salpingostomy or medical management. Consequently, it is important to monitor hCG levels until they fall to below 5 mIU/mL. When hCG levels rise or plateau, persistent trophoblastic tissue can be treated successfully with a single dose of MTX. MTX also can be given immediately after a salpingostomy as a prophylactic measure, especially in circumstances where incomplete resection is more likely.[46,47] Risk for persistent EP is increased in very early gestations, those measuring less than 2 cm in diameter, and when initial hCG concentrations are relatively high.[47]

Conclusion

- 1–2% of pregnancies in the US are tubal pregnancies. The exact incidence is difficult to compute as an increasing number of patients are being treated medically on an outpatient basis.
- With serial hCG levels, TVU examinations and sometimes uterine curettage, tubal pregnancies can be diagnosed at early stages, often before symptoms become evident.

- Both conservative surgery and medical therapy may be viewed as appropriate first-line therapy and have comparable success rates.
- MTX as a single dose or multiple doses is the most widely used drug for medical management of tubal pregnancy.
- There have been no prospective randomized trials comparing salpingectomy versus salpingostomy for surgical treatment of tubal pregnancy.
- 60% of women with a history of a tubal pregnancy will subsequently achieve a normal intrauterine pregnancy.
- MTX-induced embryopathy is a serious and avoidable complication that may arise when a viable pregnancy is misdiagnosed as an ectopic pregnancy and exposed to MTX treatment.

References

1. Center for Disease Control and Prevention (CDC). Ectopic pregnancy—United States, 1990–1992. Maternal Mortality Weekly Report. 1995;44:46–8.
2. Hoover KW, Tao G, Kent CK. Trends in the diagnosis and treatment of ectopic pregnancy in the United States. Obstet Gynecol. 2010;115:495–502.
3. Van Den Eeden SK, Shan J, Bruce C, Glasser M. Ectopic pregnancy rate and treatment utilization in a large managed care organization. Obstet Gynecol. 2005;105:1052–7.
4. Ankum WM, Houtzager HL, Bleker OP. Reinier De Graaf (1641 – 1673) and the Fallopian tube. Hum Reprod Update. 1996;2:365–9.
5. Fritz MA, Speroff L. Ectopic pregnancy. In Clinical Gynecologic Endocrinology and Infertility. Fritz MA, Speroff L (Eds). 8th edition, Lippincott Williams and Wilkins, USA. 2011.pp.1383–1412.
6. Shaw JLV, Dey SK, Critchley HOD, Horne AW. Current knowledge of the aetiology of human tubal ectopic pregnancy. Hum Reprod Update. 2010;16:432–44.
7. Waylen AL, Metwally M, Jones GL, Wilkinson AJ, Ledger WL. Effects of cigarette smoking upon clinical outcomes of assisted reproduction: a meta-analysis. Hum Reprod Update. 2009;15:31–44.
8. Weigert M, Gruber D, Pernicka E, Bauer P, Feichtinger W. Previous tubal ectopic pregnancy raises the incidence of repeated ectopic pregnancies in in vitro fertilization-embryo transfer patients. J Assist Reprod Genet. 2009;26:13–7.
9. Dubuisson JB, Aubriot FX, Mathieu L, Foulot H, Mandlebrot L, de Joliere JB. Risk factors for ectopic pregnancy in 556 pregnancies after in vitro fertilization: implications for preventive management. Fertil Steril. 1991;56:686–90.
10. Verhulst G, Camus M, Bollen N, van Steirteghem A, Devroey P. Analysis of the risk factors with regard to the occurrence of ectopic pregnancy after medically assisted procreation. Hum Reprod. 1993;8:1284–7.
11. Butts S, Sammel M, Hummel A, Chittams J, Barnhart K. Risk factors and clinical features of recurrent ectopic pregnancy: a case control study. Fertil Steril. 2003;80:1340–4.
12. Job-Spira N, Coste J, Tharaux-Deneux C, Fernandez H. Chromosomal abnormalities and ectopic pregnancy? New directions for aetiological research. Hum Reprod. 1996;11:239–42.
13. Stovall TG, Ling FW, Carson SA, Buster JE. Nonsurgical diagnosis and treatment of tubal pregnancy. Fertil Steril. 1990;54:537–8.
14. Fritz MA, Guo SM. Doubling time of human chorionic gonadotropin (hCG) in early normal pregnancy: relationship to hCG concentration and gestational age. Fertil Steril. 1987;47:584–9.

15. Timor-Tritsch IE, Yeh MN, Peisner DB, Lesser KB, Slavik TA. The use of transvaginal ultrasonography in the diagnosis of ectopic pregnancy. Am J Obstet Gynecol. 1989;161:157–61.

16. Kadar N, Romero R. Observations on the log human chorionic gonadotropin-time relationship in early pregnancy and its practical implications. Am J Obstet Gynecol. 1987;157:73–8.

17. Barnhart KT, Sammel MD, Rinaudo PF, Zhou L, Hummel AC, Guo W. Symptomatic patients with an early viable intrauterine pregnancy: hCG curves redefined. Obstet Gynecol. 2004;104:50–5.

18. The Practice Committee of the American Society for Reproductive Medicine. Medical treatment of ectopic pregnancy. Technical Bulletin. Fertil Steril. 2008;90:S206–12.

19. Barnhart KT, Sammel MD, Rinaudo PF, Zhou L, Hummel AC, Guo W. Symptomatic patients with an early viable intrauterine pregnancy: hCG curves redefined. Obstet Gynecol. 2004;104:50–5.

20. Chung K, Sammel MD, Chalian R, Coutifaris C, Feedman M, Barnhart KT. Defining the rise of serum HCG in viable pregnancies achieved through use of IVF. Hum Reprod. 2006;213:823–8.

21. Kadar N, Freedman M, Zacher M. Further observations on the doubling time of human chorionic gonadotropin in early asymptomatic pregnancies. Fertil Steril. 1990;54:783–7.

22. Morse CB, Sammel MD, Shaunik A, Allen-Taylor L, Oberfoell NL, Takacs P, Chung K, Barnhart KT. Performance of human chorionic gonadotropin curves in women at risk for ectopic pregnancy: exceptions to the rules. Fertil Steril. 2012;97:101–6.

23. Barnhart K, Sammel MD, Chung K, Zhou L, Hummel AC, Guo W. Decline of serum human chorionic gonadotropin and spontaneous complete abortion: defining the normal curve. Obstet Gynecol. 2004;104:975–81.

24. Hönigl W, Lang PFJ, Weiß PAM, Winter R. Intrauterine pregnancy after the treatment of tubal pregnancy with local and systemic prostaglandins in a patient with a single oviduct. Hum Reprod. 1992;7:573–4.

25. Giuliani A, Hoenigl W, Schoell W, Tamussino K, Arikan G, Lang P. Reproductive outcome after laparoscopic instillation of hyperosmolar glucose into unruptured tubal pregnancies. Fertil Steril. 2001;76:366–9.

26. Maymon R, Shulman A, Maymon BB, Bar-Levy F, Lotan M, Bahary C. Ectopic pregnancy, the new gynecological epidemic disease: review of modern work-up and non-surgical treatment options. Int J Fertil. 1992;37:146–64.

27. Adam MP, Manning MA, Beck AE, Kwan A, Enns GM, Clericuzio C, et al. Methotrexate/misoprostol embryopathy: report of four cases resulting from failed medical abortion. Am J Med Genet A. 2003;123:72–8.

28. Rodi IA, Sauer MV, Gorrill MJ, Bustillo M, Gunning JE, Marshall JR, et al. The medical treatment of unruptured ectopic pregnancy with methotrexate and citrovorum rescue: preliminary experience. Fertil Steril. 1986;46:811–3.

29. Ory SJ, Villanueva AL, Sand PK, Tamura RK. Conservative treatment of ectopic pregnancy with methotrexate. Am J Obstet Gynecol. 1986;1546:1299–1306.

30. Stovall TG, Ling FW, Buster JE. Outpatient chemotherapy of unruptured ectopic pregnancy. Fertil Steril. 1989;51:435–8.

31. Pisarska MD, Carson SA, Buster JE. Ectopic pregnancy. Lancet. 1998;351:1115–20.

32. Lipscomb GH, Stovall TG, Ling FW. Nonsurgical treatment of ectopic pregnancy. N Engl J Med. 2000;343:1325–9.

33. Barnhart K, Coutifaris C, Esposito M. The pharmacology of methotrexate. Expert Opin Pharmacother. 2001;2:409–417.

34. Stovall TG, Ling FW, Gray LA. Single-dose methotrexate for treatment of ectopic pregnancy. Obstet Gynecol. 1991;77:754–7.

35. Lipscomb GH, Bran D, McCord ML, Portera JC, Ling FW. Analysis of three hundred fifteen ectopic pregnancies treated with single-dose methotrexate. Am J Obstet Gynecol. 1998;178:1354–8.

36. Barnhart KT, Sammel MD, Hummel A, Jain J, Chakhtoura N, Strauss J. A novel "two dose" regimen of methotrexate to treat ectopic pregnancy. [abstract] Fertil Steril. 2005;84(Suppl):S130.

37. Dudley PS, Heard MJ, Sangi-Haghpeykar H, Carson SA, Buster JE. Characterizing ectopic pregnancies that rupture despite treatment with methotrexate. Fertil Steril. 2004;82:1374–8.

38. Lipscomb GH, McCord ML, Stovall TG, Huff G, Portera SG, Ling FW. Predictors of success of methotrexate treatment in women with tubal ectopic pregnancies. N Engl J Med. 1999;341:1974–8.

39. Dudley P, Heard MJ, Sangi-Haghpeykar H, Carson SA, Buster JE. Characterizing ectopic pregnancies that rupture despite treatment with methotrexate. Fertil Steril. 2004;82:1374-8.

40. Fuh KC, Krieg S, Lathi RB. Misdiagnosis of ectopic pregnancies: the impact of heterophilic antibodies in infertile patients. Fertil Steril. 2008;90:S73.

41. Yao M, Tulandi T. Current status of surgical and nonsurgical management of ectopic pregnancy. Fertile Steril. 1997;67:421–33.

42. Clausen I. Conservative versus radical surgery for tubal pregnancy. Acta Obstet Gynecol Scand. 1996;75:8–12.

43. Pandis G, Cutner A. Laparoscopic management of ectopic pregnancies. In: The Fallopian Tube. Allahbadia GN, Saridogan E, Djahanbakhch O (Eds). Anshan Ltd. Kent, UK. 2009.pp.506–20.

44. Thornton K, Diamond M, DeCherney A. Linear salpingostomy for ectopic pregnancy. Obstet Gynecol Clin North Am. 1991;18:95–109.

45. Ng S, Hamontri S, Chua I, Chern B, Siow A. Laparoscopic management of 53 cases of cornual ectopic pregnancy. Fertil Steril. 2009;92:448–52.

46. Graczykowski JW, Mishell DR. Methotrexate prophylaxis for persistent ectopic pregnancy after conservative treatment by salpingostomy. Obstet Gynecol. 1997;89:118–22.

47. Gracia CR, Brown HA, Barnhart KT. Prophylactic methotrexate after linear salpingostomy: a decision analysis. Fertil Steril. 2001;76:1191–5.

Optimizing Ovulation Induction

Madhuri Patil

Introduction

One must understand the ovarian cycle well before knowing the ovulation induction protocols, as this will help in selecting the best protocol. The application of new forms of research in recent decades, as in the case of molecular biology, has contributed to a more in-depth and accurate understanding of the interaction of each of the inter and intracellular structures in the mechanics of human physiology. We know that folliculogenesis continues throughout life, right from before birth until menopause. Number of primordial follicles is recruited from the pool of resting follicles for further growth. The proportion of the pool of primordial follicles that is recruited for the development increases with age and is related inversely to the density of follicles in the ovary. During folliculogenesis oocyte and surrounding somatic cells undergo a series of changes that eventually result in development of a large antral follicle capable of ovulating a mature oocyte. There exists a 'folliculogenesis clock' that is set by the oocyte and a plethora of growth factors and cytokines are involved in the primordial follicle activation. Once activated to grow, oocytes orchestrate and coordinate the development of ovarian follicles and the rate of follicle development is controlled by oocyte. The primordial follicle activation appears to require close communication with somatic cells, i.e. granulosa cells which have a definite role to play in releasing oocytes into the growing pool. During folliculogenesis oocytes acquire molecular and cellular properties in a sequential manner that confers meiotic and developmental competence. Following the LH surge, a competent oocyte can complete meiosis, sustain fertilization and oocyte activation, and organize the transition from maternal transcripts to gene products of embryonic origin. At any time response to ovulation induction is determined by the ovarian reserve. We know that ovarian reserve is the total number of oocytes within the ovaries—growing follicles, small antral follicles, follicles that can be stimulated by FSH. There are certain putative predictors either biochemical or imaging variables, or dynamic tests of ovarian function that could predict the ovarian reserve and indirectly response to ovulation induction. One must remember that none of these putative markers of ovarian aging currently available are sufficiently accurate to provide a sound basis for clinical policies on eligibility for ART (Assisted Reproductive Techniques), as they reflect quantity and poorly reflect quality and fertility. Probably ovarian reserve markers can have a better focus on reproductive life span prediction.

Ovarian Cycle and its Physiology

A constant decline in the number of oocytes begins at 20 weeks gestation when the female fetus has approximately 6–7 million oogonia (largest lifetime endowment). The number of oocytes decreases to approximately 2–3 million at birth and decreases again to 300,000 – 400,000 at the time of puberty. Ironically, the human female has lost most of her eggs before she is able to reproduce. Of these only 300 – 400 oocytes will ovulate, and the remaining will undergo atresia or apoptosis. At menopause there are only 1000 primordial follicles remaining.

Hypothalamic GnRH plays a critical role in the neurohormonal control of reproduction by stimulating the secretion of the pituitary gonadotropins LH and FSH, which support the development of gonads, gametogenesis and the production and release of gonadal steroids.

After the onset of puberty and menses, the female human ovary recruits a cohort of follicles during each menstrual cycle. The initial follicular development occurs independently of hormone influence and is dependent on paracrine factors. This selection occurs 90 days before the cycle in which they are destined to ovulate. Once the growing follicle reaches the pre-antral stage, however, appropriate levels of gonadotropins, particularly follicle stimulating hormone (FSH) are required for development to the preovulatory stage (Table 5.1). The presence of FSH induces an increase in estrogen production from the follicle and synergistically, the estrogen and FSH increase the FSH receptor content of the growing follicle.

In a spontaneous cycle the levels of FSH rise immediately prior to and during menstrual cycle. The growth and maturation of the follicle depends on levels of follicle stimulating hormone (FSH) and luteinizing hormone (LH). With the onset of menstruation the FSH levels begin to rise and only those follicles that have a low threshold for FSH begin to grow. Usually selection of the dominant follicle happens in the mid-follicular phase that is 5–7 days. FSH increases the number of FSH receptors on granulosa cells, the number of LH receptors on theca cells, and granulosa cell aromatase activity. LH will increase the androgen production in theca cells. Androstenedione produced by the theca cells will diffuse into the granulosa cells, where it will be converted to estradiol by aromatase (Fig. 5.1).

The follicle that is at the appropriate pre-antral stage of development when the FSH begins to rise is selected to become an antral follicle. The antral follicles

TABLE 5.1 Function of follicle stimulating hormone

Recruitment of antral follicles
Selection and maturation of dominant follicle
Granulosa cell differentiation and growth
Activation of aromatase enzyme system resulting in E2 secretion
Exogenous FSH rescues follicles that would have undergone atresia

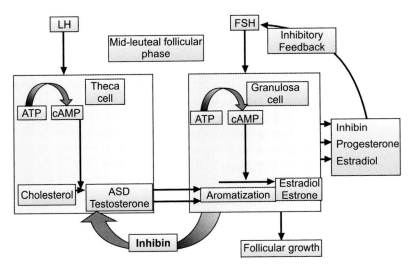

FIG. 5.1 Two cell two gonadotropin theory
Abbreviations: ASD, Atrial septal defect; ATP, Adenosine triphosphotase; CAMP, Cyclic
adenosine monophosphotase; FSH, Follicle stimulating hormone; LH, Luteinizing
hormone

compete with one another to become the dominant follicle. As this soon-to-be
dominant follicle begins to grow and produce increasing amounts of estrogen,
FSH production decreases through negative feedback, thus heralding the death (or
atresia) of the less developed follicles. This mid-follicular rise in estradiol exerts a
positivefeedbackinfluence on LH secretions resulting in an mid cyclic LH surge. The
estradiol rise also has a positive action on the bioactivity of both FSH and LH and
is responsible for a mid-cyclic small FSH surge. In the late follicular phase the FSH
induces receptors for LH on the granulosa cells. LH surge is primarily responsible
for inducing final follicular maturation by reinitiating the meiotic division. It also
results in synthesis of progesterone and prostaglandins (PG). Progesterone enhances
the proteolytic activity and PG results in digestion and rupture of follicular wall
that culminates in the release (ovulation) of a mature oocyte from the follicle
(Fig. 5.2). LH acting through its receptors also initiates luteinization and
progesterone production in the granulosa cells. Once ovulation occurs, progesterone,
estradiol and Inhibin A are secreted by the corpus luteum that acts centrally to
suppress gonadotropin production and inturn new follicular growth.

If pregnancy occurs human chorionic gonadotropin (hCG) rescues the corpus
luteum maintaining luteal function until placental steroidogenesis is established.
If there is no pregnancy there is demise of corpus luteum resulting in decrease
in circulating levels of estradiol, progesterone and inhibin A. This results in the
release of suppressive influence on FSH secretion in the pituitary and increase in
GnRH pulsatile secretion which in turn will result in greater secretion of FSH. This
increase in FSH will result in beginning of folliculogenesis by rescuing a cohort
of follicles that started growing 70–90 days prior.

This follicular response to the gonadotropins is also modulated by growth factors
and autocrine-paracrine peptides. Activin and Inhibin also play an important role.

Rise of FSH beyond certain threshold during luteal follicular transition

⬇

Follicular recruitment

⬇

Selection of dominant follicle – Follicle with GC
most responsive to FSH (lowest FSH thresh
hold), secrete Estrogens

⬇

Negative feedback to hypothalamo pituitary axis

⬇

Suppress FSH secretion

⬇

FSH insufficient to sustain development of other
follicles with higher FSH threshold

⬇

Non-ovulatory

⬇

Undergo atresia while dominant follicle continues to grow, secrete E2

⬇

Dominant follicle - > 10 mm

⬇

Increased synthesis of E2 with increased expression of LH receptor
on GC which are adequately stimulated by FSH

⬇

LH sustain pre-ovulatory follicular endocrine activity induced by FSH

⬇

LH plays primary role in complete maturation of follicle and
development of oocyte competence

⬇

Mid cycle LH surgery

⬇

LH follicle interaction disrupts GC contacts in cumulus
oophorus and induces oocyte maturation

⬇

Follicle rupture followed by GC luteinization

FIG. 5.2 Folliculogenesis
Abbreviations: FSH, Follicle stimulating hormone; GC, Ganglion cell;
LH, Lutienizing hormone

Activin originating in both pituitary and granulosa cells, augments FSH secretion and action in the ovary. Inhibin B secreted by the granulosa cells in response to FSH, directly suppresses pituitary secretion. Later in the follicular phase Inhibin enhances LH stimulation of androgen secretion in the theca cells.

Apart from activin and Inhibin B, Insulin like growth factor (IGF) both I and II also play an important role in folliculogenesis. Of the two IGF II is more important as it stimulates granulosa cell proliferation, aromatase activity and progesterone synthesis.

It is important to remember that follicular development at the beginning of each cycle occurs only if serum FSH concentration exceeds certain threshold and the

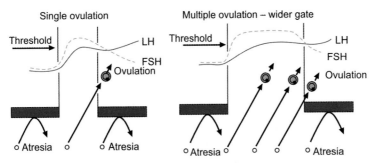

FIG. 5.3 Follicle stimulating hormone threshold and ovulation

number of follicles to ovulate is determined by length of time that the level of FSH remains above the threshold value (Fig. 5.3).

In view of the leading role that FSH plays in folliculogenesis, it is clear that the vast majority of women undergoing stimulation for single or multiple follicular developments only require a pharmaceutical preparation containing FSH or which indirectly increases the FSH secretion. The only possible exceptions are those women with hypothalamic hypogonadism, i.e. WHO group I infertile women and those who have an LH level < 1 IU/mL and also require external LH for optimal folliculogenesis.

How Much LH Is Required for Optimal Follicle Maturation? (Fig. 5.4)
Humaidan and colleagues (Rigshospitalet, Copenhagen, Denmark) 1 studied the IVF cycle outcomes with different stimulation by assessing day 8 LH levels. A total of 207 women were managed with luteal phase GnRH agonist (GnRHa) down regulation (0.8 mg sc) and recombinant FSH (rFSH) stimulation. The investigators found that estradiol production was positively correlated with LH levels, whereas the amount of rFSH used was negatively correlated with LH levels. Fertilization and pregnancy rates were lower when day 8 LH levels were below 0.5 IU/L or above 1.51 IU/L. Martin (Center for Assisted Reproduction, Bedford, Texas)[2] and colleagues evaluated the donor cycle outcome following oral contraceptive (OC) suppression by measuring day 1 LH levels. Stimulation was carried out with only rFSH in 52 cycles, but recombinant human chorionic gonadotropin (Rec hCG 250 mcg daily) was added to rFSH in 30 cycles. Rec hCG has LH-like activity; it has a longer half-life and therefore may provide a more stable gonadotropin environment for the follicles. Peak estradiol levels were higher when rec hCG was administered, both when day 1 LH levels were < 0.5 IU/L and when they were above this level. The number of eggs retrieved was also higher with rec hCG use and again this finding was not influenced by day 1 LH levels. Fertilization and blastulation rates were not affected by rec hCG. In cycles during which the LH level was < 0.5 IU/L, more embryos were available for freezing.

Low or high LH levels Vega-Cardenas (IECH, Monterrey, Mexico)[3] and associates discussed IVF cycle outcomes with different day 1 LH levels. They found that when GnRHa were used and LH levels were suppressed to a level < 1 IU/L, the pregnancy rates were significantly lower (10.7% vs 51.5%). When LH levels

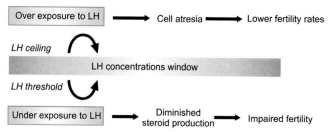

FIG. 5.4 The amount of lutienizing hormone (LH) required

were high (> 3 IU/L), similarly low pregnancy rates (12.5%) were seen, although there were fewer patients in this group. On the other hand, Cabrera (The Jones Institute for Reproductive Medicine, Norfolk, Virginia) and colleagues4, showed that with luteal phase GnRHa down regulation and rFSH stimulation, there were no differences in any IVF outcome parameters with various early- and mid-stimulation LH levels (< 1.0 IU/ L, 1.0-1.5 IU/L, and 1.5-2.0 IU/ L).

Lee (MizMedi Hospital, Seoul, South Korea) and co-workers[5] assessed the granulosa cell LH receptor mRNA content among poor and normal responders. They found significantly lower LH receptor mRNA expression among poor responders. Pregnancy rates were also lower with lower LH receptor mRNA expression.

On the basis of these and other previously reported studies, it seems that lower LH levels during IVF are associated with worse outcome. Similarly, high LH levels appear to be associated with poor outcome. The exact cut-off values have not been determined, but most likely LH has to be suppressed to a level < 0.5 IU/L to see an adverse effect. It is unclear whether there are subgroups of patients with different LH needs. There probably are patients whose cycle is not affected by lower LH levels. It is also unclear from these reports whether LH affects oocyte quality or embryo quality or has effects on the endometrium. Any of these effects could alter the clinical outcome.

Ovulation Induction

Aim of ovulation induction is to overcome natural follicular selection process to increase the number of oocytes available for fertilization. Ovulation induction aims to restore normal fertility to anovulatory women by generating normo-ovulatory cycles (i.e. to mimic physiology and induce single dominant follicle selection and ovulation). Representing one of the most common interventions for the treatment of infertility (Collins and Hughes, 1995),[6] ovulation induction can achieve excellent cumulative pregnancy rates if normal menstrual cyclicity is restored. This is enhanced if more than one oocyte is released.

The role of ovulation-inducing agents for in vitro fertilization is to disturb this normal relationship by increasing the amounts of FSH available to follicles other than the dominant follicles and thus to increase the total number of follicles that reach the pre-ovulatory stage (Fig. 5.5).

It is important to determine when one should commence ovulation induction. We know that the selection of dominant follicle occurs in the early follicular phase and

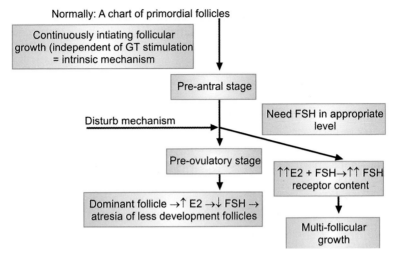

FIG. 5.5 Physiological key point

so OI (Ovulation Induction) drugs should be initiated within 3 days of menstrual cycle. The dose of all the drugs used—CC/Letrozole/GT should be tailored to each individual.

The success of ovulation induction and in vitro fertilization embryo transfer (IVF-ET) is dependent on an adequate response of the ovaries to exogenous gonadotropin stimulation. Treatment cancellation owing to poor ovarian response or ovarian hyper stimulation syndrome (OHSS) is a significant problem during ovulation induction that makes it mandatory to individualize the dose and protocol used.

The Choice of Treatment will Depend on

- Body weight
- Body mass index (BMI)
- Female age
- Cause of infertility
- Duration of infertility
- Results of the test done to predict ovarian response
- Previous treatment modalities used
- Available resources
- Risk tolerance
- Type of anovulation (WHO I – hypogonadotropic hypogonadal anovulation; WHO II – normogonadotropic normoestrogenic anovulation; WHO III – hypergonadotropic hypoestrogenic anovulation and hyperprolactinemic anovulation).

The WHO I anovulation require treatment with both FSH and LH for optimal folliculogenesis and steroidogenesis. Women with WHO II anovulation who fail to ovulate or conceive following ovulation induction with anti-estrogens can be successfully treated with exogenous gonadotropins. However, the challenge presented by the small therapeutic window for achieving monofollicular development is further complicated by variability in response to gonadotropin treatment.[7] WHO III is very difficult to treat and usually ovulation induction is unsuccessful.

There are clear advantages of identifying women at risk of a poor response or excessive response to ovulation induction before commencement of an *in vitro* fertilization (IVF) treatment cycle. We know that IVF is expensive and invasive, and should not be performed if there is not a realistic chance of pregnancy. Determining the ovarian reserve helps in predicting the response to ovarian stimulation and thus modulating the drug and the dose used. Putative predictors may be biochemical or imaging variables, or dynamic tests of ovarian function.

The availability of an accurate screening test of ovarian reserve would also allow those predicted to under-respond to be given higher dose of gonadotropin without risk of ovarian hyperstimulation syndrome (OHSS), possibly improving oocyte yield.[8]

Whether declining fecundity might be advanced or retarded in some women can be addressed by prediction studies on the association between assumed markers of ovarian aging and conception or a related outcome. By estimating ovarian reserve, prediction of number of remaining years of reproductive life could be made along with likely hood of success with ART.

Prediction of Ovarian Response/Reserve is based on following Tests

- Age
- Day 2/3 FSH - Indirect measure of the size of follicle cohort[9]
- Day 2/3 E2
- Basal FSH:LH ratio
- Intercycle variability in basal FSH
- P4 – Day 10 of COH
- Day 3 Inhibin-B
- Anti-Müllerian hormone (AMH)
- Transvaginal USG – AFC
- Abnormal dynamic testing – Clomiphene citrate challenge test (CCCT), GnRH agonist stimulation test (GAST), Exogenous FSH ovarian reserve test (EFORT)
- Response to ovarian stimulation in previous cycles.

These tests help us to predict response to tailor correct stimulation regimen for adequate response. But it is important to remember that most ovarian reserve tests are adequate in predicting ovarian response, but fail to predict the occurrence of pregnancy.

Female fertility declines with age and can affect both quantity and quality of oocytes. However, age *per se* can be a poor determinant of female fertility, since there is wide range in the relationship between ovarian reserve and age. We need to identify women of relatively young age with diminished reserve and those around the mean age at which natural fertility on average is lost (41 years) but still have adequate ovarian reserve.

Markers of High Response

- AFC – Optimum Cut-off value for AFC = >14 with sensitivity of 82% and specificity 89%[10]
- AMH – At an optimal cut-off 3.36 ng/mL AMH has sensitivity of 90.5% (95% CI 69.6–98.5) and specificity of 81.3% (95% CI 75.8–86.0)[11]
- Dynamic tests – CCCT, EFORT - E2 increment in EFORT, CCCT, and bFSH at different cut-off levels were of less clinical relevance compared with inhibin B increment in the EFORT at the cut off level of 130 ng/L.[12]

Markers of Low Response

- Age – > 36 years - PRs significantly higher (P < 0.05) in women with normal FSH those aged < 36 years compared to those aged ≥ 36 years[13]
- Day 2/3 – FSH > 10 mIU/mL Elevated day 3 FSH – heterogeneous group
  - true reduced ovarian reserve
  - due to the presence of heterophylic antibodies
- FSH receptor polymorphism in patients with otherwise normal ovaries[14]
- Elevated day 2 E2 (> 75 – 80 pg/mL) indicates an inappropriately advanced stage of follicular development, consistent with ovarian aging or simply reflect the presence of functional ovarian cysts
- Basal FSH:LH ratio > 1.5 (Basal FSH < 10 mIU/mL)—associated with inferior outcome in IVF treatment cycles and may be used as an additional predictor for decreased ovarian response
- Large intercycle variability inbasal FSH
- P4 – Day 10 of COH > 1.1 ng/mL
- Day 3 Inhibin – B< 45 pg/mL, has a sensitivity of 87% and specificity of 49%
- AMH – < 0.35 ng/mL – Optimum cut off value for poor response for AMH is 0.99 ng/mL. Post-test probability was highest at cut off levels of 0.59ng/mL.[15]
- Low antral follicle count – Optimum cut off value for poor response for AFC is < /= 10 but the post-test probability was highest at cut off levels of < 8[15]
- Low ovarian volume – Ovarian volume correlates with number of growing follicles, but not with number of oocytes retrieved.[16] Women with small ovaries- < 3 cm[3] – High cancellation rate of IVF.[17]
- Dynamic tests—CCCT, EFORT: CCCT appeared to have the best discriminative potential for poor response, as expressed by the largest ROC-AUC (0.88) followed by Inhibin increment in EFORT. CCCT at the cut off level of 18 IU/L has a positive predictive Value.[12]
- AFC and AMH are significant single predictors of poor response. Evaluation of AFC and AMH as a combined test did not significantly improve the level of prediction (AUC < 0.946).[15]

Pre-requisite to ovulation induction therapy is complete infertility evaluation of the couple with evaluation of male factor, tubal factor or any other pathology, which could prevent fertility. Ovulation induction could be optimized by utilizing individualized protocols and medication based on ovarian reserve testing, previous response to COS and type of anovulation.

Drugs Used for Ovulation Induction

- Clomiphene citrate (CC)
- Tamoxifen (TMX)
- Aromatase inhibitors – Letrozole, Anastrazole
- Gonadotropins (GT) – human menopausal gonadotropin (hMG), follicle stimulating hormone (FSH), luteinizing hormone (LH). These preparations could be either urinary (purified or ultra-purified) or recombinant.

With Ovulation inducing agents the stimulation may occur either at the pituitary levelviz GnRh, GnRha, CC, Tamoxifen and Letrozole or ovarian level viz hMG, FSH, Recombinant FSH and Letrozole. Combination therapies have action at both pituitary and ovarian level.

Clomiphene Citrate

Blocks (down regulates) estrogen receptors on hypothalamus,increasing the FSH secretion from pituitary resulting in follicular growth. Estradiol levels increase with follicular growth resulting in LH surge and ovulation. The dose of CC is 50-200 mg/day, starting from day 2, 3, 4 or 5 for 5 days. Monitoring with ultrasound, basal body temperature (BBT), LH kits, day 21 progesterone will indicate the response of the patient.

The least effective dose to induce ovulation is used for at least 4–6 cycles to consider the clomiphene trial "effective".

Hypothalamic Amenorhea (Hypogonadotrophic Hypogonadism) will not respond to Clomiphene citrate and therefore should not be used in such cases.

Ovulation is seen in 70 – 85% with a pregnancy rate of 30 – 40% and multiple pregnancy rate of 5%.About 10–30% of the patients will be 'clomiphene resistant' i.e. will remain anovulatory after 6 months of treatment.[18] Obese women with hyperandrogenemia are less likely to respond to clomiphene.[19]

When pregnancy is not achieved despite ovulation, the term 'clomiphene failure' is used. Important parameters for prediction of conception include patient age and cycle history.[20]

In clomiphene resistance, some advocate a treatment period of more than 5 days to induce ovulation.[21,22]

Combinations with other drugs have been also used and proved to be beneficial. Beneficial effects have been reported during coadministration of clomiphene with dexamethasone[23] or when clomiphene was preceded by the oral contraceptive pills.[24]

Sequential CC and GT therapy is useful in CC resistant and failure and in those women where minimal or mild stimulation protocol is indicated. Clomiphene citrate is given in the dose of 100 mg from days 2 to 6. GT (37.5 – 75 IUis started on day 5 or 7 of menstrual cycle. In certain patients ovarian drilling is the option to improve ovulation in women with CC resistance or failure. In obese patients aggressive weight loss regimens may be recommended to improve response to CC. In CC resistance, one could try other oral ovulation induction agents like Tamoxifen in the dose of 20 or 40 mg for five days starting on day 2 or 3 of the menstrual cycle. Aromatase inhibitor letrozole in the dose of 2.5 – 5 mg may be given for 5 days starting from day 3 of menstrual cycle. Metformin may be started in the presence of abnormal glucose tolerance test in women with polycystic ovarian syndrome.

Its side effects include thick, dry cervical mucus, abnormal endometrial thickness, hot flashes, nausea, breast tenderness, headache, blurring of vision, depression, mood swings, ovarian cysts formation and pelvic discomfort.

The goal of therapy is to achieve 3 ovulatory cycles; 40–50% of women should become pregnant in this time frame in the absence of any other abnormality that can prevent conception. If conception has not occurred after 3 clomiphene citrate cycles, one should investigate for other causes of infertility. No more than six consecutive cycles are recommended because of the theoretical risk of borderline ovarian tumors and extremely low pregnancy success rates after this point.

Evidence suggests that starting clomiphene citrate earlier (day 2 or 3) is more beneficial because this conforms to a more typical cycle length of 28 days. Beginning clomiphene citrate cycle on day 2 or 3 also promotes ovulation around days 12–16, which is more physiologic and may avoid delayed ovulation and excessive maturity of the oocyte. Evidence also demonstrates that a day 2 or 3 clomiphene citrate start allows the endometrium to thicken to a more normal and physiologic range. We know that endometrial thinning is a well-known adverse effect of clomiphene citrate and an endometrial thickness less than 7–8 mm has been associated with a lower pregnancy rates.

Studies have also showed that delayed ovulation (after cycle day 16) had a higher relative miscarriage rate. This was believed to be caused by meiotic dysfunction within the oocyte.

Tamoxifen Citrate

May be used alone orin combination with CC or gonadotropins to act in synergy for better response or in cases resistant to CC alone. It is a nonsteroidal compound structurally related to DES. It is a triphenyl-ethylene derivative and acts primarily on hypothalamic pituitary axis. Its 20 mg from Day 2 or 3 of spontaneous or progesterone induced bleeding for 5 days. At times combination treatment of CC 50 mg and Tamoxifen 20 mg from Day 2 or 3 of menstrual cycle for 5 days may be used. If no response is seen to 20 mg the dose can be increased to maximum of 40 mg. It is discontinued if patients anovulatory despite 40 mg in 2 consecutive cycle.

Aromatase Inhibitors

Today in India aromatase inhibitor – letrozoleis banned to be used for ovulation induction still one needs to have some knowledge on it as it is still being used in the other parts of the world. Oral administration of the aromatase inhibitor letrozole is effective for ovulation induction in anovulatory infertility.

Mechanism of Action

- Suppresses estrogen biosynthesis and releases hypothalamopituitary axis from estrogen negative feedback resulting in GnRh and GT secretion that leads to follicular development and ovulation

- Increases follicular sensitivity to FSH
- Increases blood flow in the uterus and endometrial thickness.

Advantages

- Requires minimal monitoring
- Minimal risk OHSS
- Nil/minimal peripheral anti-estrogenic effect
- Improve implantation and pregnancy rate by amelioration of deleterious effects of supra physiological levels of estrogen during ovarian stimulation.

Letrozole

With a short half-life of 45 hours is a good ovulation induction drug with minimal antiestrogenic properties. It has a ovulation rate of 75% and pregnancy rate of 17–20%. When used with GT, it reduces the dose of FSH and or hMG. It increases the follicle recruitment in ovulatory infertility and avoids the unfavorable effects on the endometrium frequently seen with anti-estrogen use for ovulation induction. It is indicated for induction of ovulation in women in whom clomiphene citrate (CC) treatment was unsuccessful. It is given orally in the dose of 2.5 to 5 mg from day 3 to 7 of menstrual cycle or as a single dose of 20 mg on day 3 of menstrual cycle.

Side effects of letrozole include vasomotor symptoms, visual symptoms, headache, nausea/vomiting, abdominal distention, ovarian enlargement with or without cyst formation and multiple gestations.

Anastrozole

A third generation aromatase inhibitor used in the dose of 1 mg from day 3 to day 7 of the menstrual cycle. Ovulation was seen in 67% of the patients with a pregnancy rate of 12%. There was no difference in the miscarriage rate though it was associated with fewer mature and growing follicles, lower serum estradiol levels as compared to clomiphene citrate. Anastrozole may be helpful in situations in which multiple pregnancies are not desirable or when risk of ovarian hyperstimulation syndrome is high.[25]

Gonadotropins

Human gonadotropins are used as first line of treatment in WHO group I anovulation and as a second line of treatment for ovulation induction in WHO group II anovulation in cases of clomiphene resistance or failure. The dose of gonadotropins needs to be modulated depending on whether the woman is polycystic ovary syndrome (PCOS) or not and whether she is for timed intercourse, intra uterine insemination or *in vitro* fertilization. In the earlier days, the starting dose of 150 IU/day HMG was used in patients belonging to WHO group II. With this dose the success rate was significantly lower and the rate of the OHSS significantly higher than in patients belonging to WHO group I.[26,27] For these reasons, protocols involving chronic low doses of HMG were introduced in the early 1980s.[28]

Follicle stimulating hormone (FSH) and hMG can be used alone or in combination with CC/Letrozole. When used in combination CC/Letrozole stimulates recruitment of number of small follicles and GTs sustains the growth of recruited follicles. GTs should be initiated only if follicule size on day 2 is less than 10 mm and estradiol levels are less than 35 pg/mL.

Initial dose of GTs depends on

- Weight/BMI
- Age
- Basal FSH levels
- AMH
- Response to previous stimulation.

Indications for use of gonadotropin therapy are clomiphene or letrozole resistance and failure, persistent hypersecretion of LH, assisted conception and negative post coital test or poor cervical mucus. It is more difficult to induce ovulation in patients with more severe PCOS, characterized by obesity, insulin resistance and PCO appearance.

Regimens of Gonadotropin Therapy

Conventional Step-up protocol (Fig. 5.6)

Supra-physiological doses of FSH in this protocol provoke initial development of a large cohort, stimulate additional follicles and even rescue those follicles destined for atresia resulting in large number of dominant follicles on the day of hCG.

This protocol has an ovulation rate of 70% and a cumulative pregnancy rate of 21–75%. But it is associated with a high incidence of ovarian hyperstimulation syndrome (OHSS) and multiple pregnancies. The incidence of severe OHSS is as high as 7–14% and that of multiple pregnancies is 36%.

Chronic Low Dose Protocol (Fig. 5.7)[29]

- Low FSH dose of 37.5–75 IU used daily initially and increased by 50% or 37.5 IU after 14 days if no ovarian response
- Any further FSH increment thereafter is made by 37.5 IU at weekly intervals to a maximum of 225 IU/day
- Once dominant follicle emerges, dose of FSH is maintained same until the follicle reaches 18–20 mm

With this protocol 69% cycles were mono ovulatory with a very low incidence of OHSS (1.4%) and a multiple pregnancy rate of only 5.7%.[30,31]

Low Dose Protocol (Figs 5.8 and 5.9)

In this protocol the increment in the gonadotropin dose either by 100 or 50% is made every 7 days in case of no response with GT dose of 37.5–75 IU.

Step-down Protocol (Fig. 5.10)

Loading FSH dose is anywhere between 112.5 to 187.5 0 IU per day. The dose is decreased by 37.5 IU every 3–5 days till criteria for hCG administration is reached.

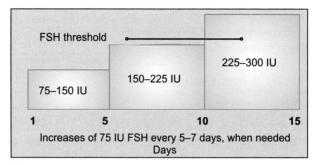

FIG. 5.6 Conventional step-up protocol

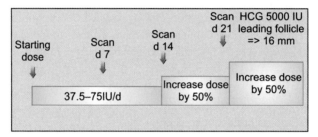

FIG. 5.7 Chronic Low dose protocol

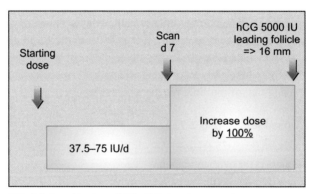

FIG. 5.8 Low (37.5–75 IU/d) FSH dose increased by 100% every 7 days

Sequential Protocol (Fig. 5.11)

The initial dose of gonadotropin is 37.5 to 75 IU daily for first 14 days, thereafter the dose is increased by 50% every 7 days till the dominant follicle is 14 mm. FSH threshold dose decreased by 50% once the leading follicle is 14 mm.

Principle

- FSH dependence of leading follicle decreases as follicle grows
- Decrease in FSH threshold contributes to the escape of the leading follicle from atresia when FSH concentrations start to decrease because of negative feedback of rising E2.

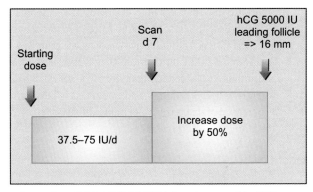

FIG. 5.9 Low (37.5–75 IU/d) FSH dose increased by 50% every 7 days

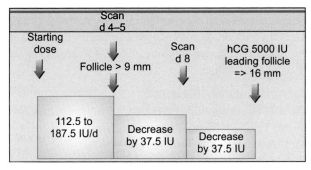

FIG. 5.10 Step down protocol

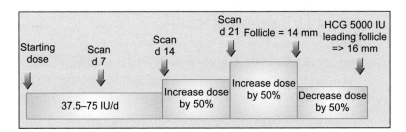

FIG. 5.11 Sequential Protocol

Adjustment of GT dose depends on:
- Serial E2 levels
- Serial USG findings.

Initial dose is changed after 4–5 days of GT therapy. On day 4 of ovulation, induction if the number of follicles are less than 4 or rise in E2 is less than 50%, one needs to increase the dose by 37.5 to 75 IU. On the contrary, if the number of follicles is more than 8 or rise in E2 is more than 100% we need to decrease the dose by 37.5 to 75 IU. On day 7 of ovulation induction one needs to repeat a scan and only if required does an E2 level. The normal rate of growth of follicles is 2–3 mm per day. If follicles are less than 4 with a diameter of less than 12 mm or rise in E2 of less than 50% increase the dose by 37.5–75 IU. On the contrary, if on day 7 of ovulation induction if rate of follicular growth is more than 2–3 mm/day and the number of follicles with a diameter of more than 12 mm are more than 10 or rise in E2 level is more than 100% reduce dose by 37.5–75 IU. The same dose is continued if follicular growth 2–3 mm/day and rise in E2 is between 50–100%. Thereafter, the dose increased or decreased depending on rate of growth and number of dominant follicles along with E2 levels.

Newer Gonadotropins

1. *Corifollitropin Alfa*

It is a recombinant fusion molecule of FSH and the carboxy terminal peptide (CTP) of human chorionic gonadotropin beta (βhCG) subunit with sustained follicle stimulating activity. Development of corifollitropin alfa is the first step towards a new generation of recombinant gonadotropins with longer terminal half-life (t1/2) and slower absorption to peak serum levels. Such a molecule will increase the efficiency, decrease the side effects, will be easy to administer and increases patient convenience.

i. Method of Administration (Fig. 5.12)

Corifollitropin alfa is developed in two therapeutic strengths after the Engage (150 µg) and Ensure (100 µg) dose finding trial
- 100 µg for patients with body weight ≤ 60 kg
- 150 µg for patients with body weight > 60 kg.

Initial follicular response, reflects response to corifollitropin alfa and number of oocytes reflects response to regimen. With the use of corifollitropin alpha there is a 3 days of injection free period.

ii. Mechanism of Action

Single injection induces and sustains multi-follicular development during the first week of stimulation and if criteria for hCG administration is not reached one's need to add recombinant FSH in the dose of 150 IU. Corifollitropin alfa is effective in stimulation of multi-follicular growth for IVF but less suitable for induction of monofollicular growth and therefore cannot be used for women undergoing intra- uterine inseminations (IUI).

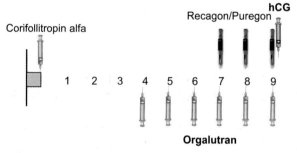

FIG. 5.12 Method of administration of corifollitropin alfa

2. *Combination of Follitropin Alfa and Lutropin Alfa* in ratio of 2:1 available as Pergoveris (r-hFSH 150IU and r-hLH 75IU). Two multicentric studies done in Spain and Germany showed its beneficial effect in suboptimal patients thats included young poor responders and older women (>35 years). The German study also included women with low LH levels. Multicentric prospective observation study was done in 487 patients from 19 Spanish centers in suboptimal patients, that included young poor responders and older women (>35 years). This study reported a pregnancy rate of 25.9% per initiated cycle and 33.2% per transfer.[32]

Another multicentric study from 19 German centers was done in young poor responders and older women (>35 years) with low basal LH. This study reported a pregnancy rate of 27.5% per transfer.[33]

3. *Recombinant LH*

Recombinant LH has a definite role in women with LH deficiency, that include gonadotropin deficient (WHO group I) anovulation and patients treated with GnRH agonists or antagonist.

No significant difference was observed in the probability of live birth rate with or without recombinant LH addition to FSH in a study published by Kolibianakis et al.[34] There was also no significant difference observed in the gonadotropin consumption, duration of stimulation, estrogen and progesterone levels on the day of hCG, number of COCs retrieved, fertilization rate and number of 2PN embryos. So the available evidence does not support the hypothesis that the addition of recombinant LH increases the live birth rate in patients treated with FSH and GnRH analogs (agonist and antagonist) for IVF.

Studies of gonadotropin therapy have shown that the duration of treatment, the amount of gonadotropins administered, the associated risks of cycle-to-cycle variability, multifollicular development, OHSS and multiple pregnancies might all be reduced if the starting dose were individualized depending on the ovarian reserve tests. More than the ovarian reserve tests response to previous controlled ovarian stimulation (COS) can predict the correct dose of FSH as it is only at COS the individual FSH threshold for stimulation is determined. In a recent meta-analysis, obesity and insulin resistance was shown to beassociated with higher gonadotropin dose requirements.[35,36]

A prediction model has recently been developed that may be used to determine the individual FSH response dose.[37] In multivariate analysis, body mass index (BMI), ovarian response to preceding clomiphene citrate medication [clomiphene citrate resistant anovulation (CRA), or failure to conceive despite ovulatory cycles], initial free insulin-like growth factor-I (free IGF-I) and serum FSH concentrations were included in the final model.

The GT therapy is contraindicated in presence of tumors of ovary, breast, pituitary or hypothalamus, pregnancy or lactation, undiagnosed vaginal bleeding, primary ovarian failure, ovarian cyst and malformation of sexual organs / fibroid uterus incompatible to pregnancy.

Disadvantages of Controlled Ovarian Hyperstimulation

- Time consuming and stressful to the couple
- Imposes heavy financial burden
- Result in OHSS that may be life-threatening at times
- Detrimental effect on embryo implantation may be seen because of altered estrogen progesterone balance
- Higher incidence of multiple pregnancy
- Excess embryos require cryopreservation that could induce ethical and moral problems.

Luteal Phase Support

Luteal phase support (LPS) is required to optimize the results of ovulation induction. LPS is required in all controlled ovarian stimulation (COS) cycles that use either GnRH agonist or antagonist, but is given empirically in other ovulation induction cycles because of lack of clearly defined treatment goals either morphologic or hormonal that relate to appropriate endometrial preparation for implantation during luteal phase of COH cycles. We know that both estrogens and progesterone play crucial role in process of implantation. Estradiol is essential for modulating effect on secretory endometrial progesterone receptors as it serves to replenish and maintain a requisite level of progesterone receptors to mediate and complete progesterone response. Endometrium is sensitive to decreased steroid levels as altered estradiol and progesterone ratio results in subnormal mid-luteal estradiol and progesterone concentrations which in turn is associated with delayed endometrial maturation and reduced endometrial receptivity.

Thus optimal balance of estradiol and progesterone is necessary for implantation and normal progression of early pregnancy.

Luteal Phase Support can be Given with the Following

Human chorionic gonadotropin: 1000–2000 IU every 3 days from 4th day of ovulation or oocyte retrieval (OR) (Day 4, 7, 10,13)

Progesterone 200–400 micrograms vaginal pessaries or pure progesterone injections in the dose of 50–100 mg IM daily or oral dydrogesterone 10 mg twice daily from day of ovulation or oocyte retrieval for 16–17 days till the serum beta hCG levels are done to confirm pregnancy.

Combination of hCG and progesterone: Progesterone IM, vaginally or orally for 15 days with hCG in the dose of 1000 – 2000 IU day 4 onwards every 3 days for a total of 4 doses

Progynova 2 mg 8 or 12 hourly 7 days after OR/ovulation if estradiol levels are more than 2500 pg/mL on day of hCG or in an hormone replacement cycle (HRT) to be started on day 2 of the cycle.

Adjuncts to Ovulation Induction Drugs: At times one needs to use adjuvant drugs along with ovulation induction medication to optimize ovulation.

1. GnRH analogs –Agonist or antagonists
   GnRH agonists are used both for stimulation and down regulation whereas GnRH antagonists are used to prevent LH surge
2. Estrogen/Progesterone pretreatment
3. Growth hormone in poor responders
4. Pulsatile GnRH in hypothalamic deficiency
5. Dexamethasone for elevated androgen levels—DHEAs
6. hCG/GnRH agonist—initiation of oocyte maturation and induction of ovulation
7. Dopamine agonist
8. Metformin—in polycystic ovarian syndrome (PCOS) with abnormal glucose tolerance test (GTT)
   GnRH analogs—Both GnRH agonist and antagonist prevent premature LH surge thus improving the outcome of infertility treatment.

GnRH Agonist

Mechanism of Action

Occupy GT receptors to cause initial stimulation, then results in internalization of receptors and down regulation with continuous use over a few days. It can be administered either as a nasal spray, subcutaneous injection or intramuscular injection (avoided for OI because of erratic action). Of these the subcutaneous route is the most reliable.

Advantages of GnRH agonist

- Better synchronization of follicular recruitment
- Higher yield of oocytes
- Problems associated with raised tonic LH levels and occurrence of premature LH surge adequately controlled
- Better scheduling of the ART program
- Fewer cycles cancelled
- Widens the window of uterine implantation thus increasing pregnancy rates.

Disadvantages of GnRH agonist

- Requirement of GT increases by 50%
- Results in luteal phase defects and has a higher incidence of ovarian cyst formation and OHSS
- May result in atypical response or poor response.

Protocols of GnRH Agonist

Ultrashort or flare protocol utilizes the initial boost of endogenous FSH.

Dose:
500 mg/day from D1 or 2 for 3 days.

Short protocol:
The initial flare response provides initial folliculogenesis boost whilst subsequently preventing the endogenous LH surge (Fig. 5.13). The dose used is 250–300 µg/day from day 2 till hCG injection.

Long protocol or Flare down: Initial stimulation is followed by pituitary desensitization with reversible inhibition of GT secretion (Fig. 5.14). It is started in the dose of 500 – 600 µg/day from day 21 of previous cycle till menses. Dose is then reduced to 100 to 300 µg/day after initiation of GT till hCG injection.

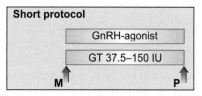

FIG. 5.13 GnRH agonist short protocol

Micro-dose GnRH-a flare-up regimen (Fig. 5.15)

Oral contraceptive pills are initiated from day 1 to 21 of previous cycle. On day 24, GnRH agonist is started in dose of 40 µg twice a day for 3 days. The dose is then made once a day and GT is started with a dose of 225 IU per day. One could use either hMG or FSH. Increase or decrease the dose by 75–150 IU after day 7 depending on estradiol level and follicular growth at USG till the dominant follicle is 16 to18 mm.

Successful down-regulation after administration of GnRH agonist is confirmed by day two LH and estradiol levels. Successful down regulation is confirmed by serum LH level of less than 2 mIU/mL, serum estradiol level of less than 50 pg/mL, absence of ovarian cyst and on transvaginal sonography endometrial thickness is less than or equal to 6 mm and no follicles greater than 8 mm exist.

Usually the side effects are similar to menopausal symptoms and include hot flashes, headache, vaginal dryness, dyspareunia, decreased breast size, bone loss, insomnia and mood swings.

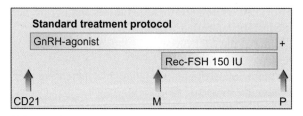

FIG. 5.14 GnRH agonist long protocol

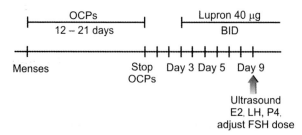

FIG. 5.15 Microdose protocol of GnRH agonist

GnRH Antagonists

The aim of using GnRH antagonists in IVF is to inhibit the occurrence of premature LH surge that could lead to premature luteinization and follicular rupture, follicle maturation arrest and asynchrony of oocyte maturation. The use of GnRH antagonists in IVF has both advantages and disadvantages. It immediately suppresses GT secretion by blocking GnRH receptor restricting treatment only to those days when LH surge is likely to occur. Mechanism of action is dependent on equilibrium between endogenous GnRH and dose of applied antagonist. Addition of LH or increase in the dose of GT used from initiation of stimulation or from antagonist administration does not appear to be necessary.

The GnRH agonist can be used instead of hCG to trigger final oocyte maturation in GnRH antagonist cycles.[38] Replacing hCG with GnRH agonist has been claimed to lead to a decreased risk of developing OHSS in high-risk patients.[39]

The existing literature suggests that there is a lower probability of pregnancy when a single dose of GnRH agonist is used instead of hCG for triggering final oocyte maturation.[40-42]

Advantages

i. Prevention of premature LH surge is easier and takes less time. GnRH antagonists act within a few hours after their administration[43] in contrast to GnRH agonists where pituitary down-regulation occurs only after 7–10 days.

ii. GnRH antagonists are not associated with an acute stimulation of gonadotropins and steroid hormones, that occurs with GnRH agonist administration.

iii. The initial stimulation by GnRH agonists can induce cyst formation, that is avoided with GnRH antagonists.

iv. No hot flushes are observed with GnRH antagonists as their use does not result in profound hypo-estrogenemia observed with GnRH agonists.[44]

v. Inadvertent administration of the GnRH analog in early pregnancy can be avoided as GnRH antagonist is administered in the mid-follicular phase.

vi. Requirement for exogenous gonadotropins is reduced, making ovarian stimulation less costly.

vii. Duration of ovarian stimulation protocols is shortened, improving patient discomfort. Total cycle treatment duration of 9–13 days against 26 days for agonist.

viii. Lower risk of OHSS with ability to use bolus GnRH agonist to trigger mid-cycle LH surge which in turn will decrease the severity of OHSS.

ix. Recent studies have reported similar implantation rate and pregnancy rates with antagonist and agonist.

Disadvantages

i. Knowledge accumulation is necessary for GnRH antagonist co-treatment in ovarian stimulation for IVF for its optimization.

ii. GnRH antagonists offer less flexibility regarding cycle programming as compared with the long, but not with the short, GnRH agonist protocol.

   iii. Most comparative studies earlier report a minor reduction in pregnancy rates per cycle with GnRH antagonists as compared with GnRH agonists.
   iv. Number of oocytes retrieved was 7.9 versus 9.6 for antagonist and agonist respectively.
   v. Number of embryos obtained was 4 versus 4.7 for antagonist and agonist respectively.

Regimens

Two GnRH antagonist protocols were developed involving either multiple (Fig. 5.16)[45] or single (Fig. 5.17) administration.[46] The minimal dose shown to prevent the occurrence of a premature LH rise in the great majority of patients was shown to be 0.25 mg.[47, 48]

   One could use either a fixed or flexible protocol. In fixed protocol, the antagonist is started on day six of gonadotropin stimulation. In flexible protocol, antagonist is started daily once the dominant follicle reaches a diameter of 13–14 mm until hCG administration. The clinical pregnancy rates are superior in the fixed protocol as compared to flexible.

   In the single dose protocol, a 3 mg dose of GnRH antagonist given on cycle day 7 during ovarian stimulation was shown to prevent a premature LH surge.[48] In case of the need to delay HCG, low daily doses of GnRH antagonists could be added 4 days after the single antagonist dose.

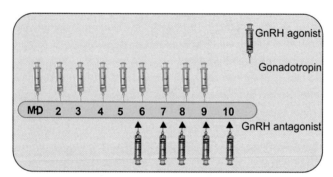

FIG. 5.16 Multiple dose GnRH antagonist protocol

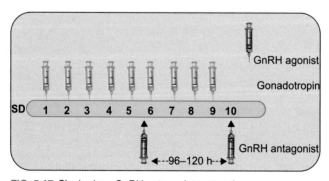

FIG. 5.17 Single dose GnRH antagonist protocol

Pros for the single dose GnRH antagonist protocol: Potential for fewer injections, although in 10% of cycles additional daily doses of GnRH antagonist are necessary.[49]

Cons for the single dose: Besides inhibiting premature LH surge, the single dose protocol results in an excessive and potentially harmful suppression of endogenous LH. However, no significant difference in pregnancy rates was shown in a randomized- controlled trial (RCT) that compared the two antagonist protocols.[50]

Oral Contraceptive Pill Pre-treatment in Ovarian Stimulation with GnRH Antagonists

The use of Oral contraceptive pills (OCP) has been advocated as a means for programming IVF cycles using GnRH antagonists.[51, 52] In addition, it has been speculated that the use of OCP pre-treatment may result in improved synchronization of the recruitable cohort of ovarian follicles. Its use in ovarian stimulation for IVF is associated with advantages and disadvantages.

Use of oral contraceptives results in easier scheduling of the cycle that is not based in this case on the occurrence of menstruation but on the discontinuation of the OCP. But pre treatment with OC pills has been associated with a longer duration of treatment.[53]

ii. An increased gonadotropin requirement has been observed with the use of OCP.[54]

iii. Administration of OCP might be emotionally disturbing, since OCP is mainly used to prevent conception. No significant effect of OCP pre-treatment on the probability of pregnancy in GnRH antagonist cycles was shown in a large RCT55, suggesting that programming of IVF cycles with the use of OCP is feasible. The effect of the time interval from OCP discontinuation to initiation of stimulation on IVF outcome[56] still needs to be assessed.

Estrogen/Progesterone Pre-treatment

Down regulation with ovarian steroids can reduce the cost and result in synchronized follicular growth.

- Oral contraceptives are started from Day 1 of menstrual cycle and continued for 21 to 28 days. Ovulation induction medication is started 5 days after discontinuation of pill either with CC/Letrozole/GT (Fig. 5.18).
- Norethisterone 10–40 mg from day 2 or day 15 of spontaneous menstrual cycle for 10 to 25 days after which ovulation induction done with CC/GT.

Growth Hormone (GH) Augmentation

This is useful in GT resistant and poor responders though costly. Improved stimulation is because of increased granulosa cell response to growth hormone (GH) and insulin like growth factor.

It is given in the dose of 0.2–0.4 μg or 8 IU at night from day 2 to 12 of menstrual cycle after GnRH agonist down regulation or with GnRH antagonist.

In non poor responder women undergoing IVF, there is no evidence from RCTs to support the use of GH, but in poor responders the use of GH has shown to significantly improve the live birth and pregnancy rate. Although the exact sub-

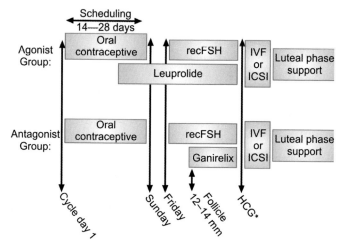

FIG. 5.18 Use of oral contraceptive pills
* ≥ follicles ≥ 16–18 mm

group of poor responders who would benefit from GH augmentation needs to be identified.

GnRH for Anovulation Because of Hypothalamic Factor

Pulsatile GnRH

This treatment is suitable for women with intact pituitary gland and especially for those with idiopathic hypogonadotropic hypogonadism and weight loss-related amenorrhea.[57]

The infusion of GnRH is performed by a computerized minipump at pulse intervals between 60 and 180 minutes, although a successful outcome is more likely with pulse frequencies of 90 and 120 minutes.[58]

Although there has been a debate as to whether the intravenous (IV) route (15 ug/pulse) is more successful than the subcutaneous (SC) one (20–25 µg/pulse),[59] no prospective randomized comparisons exist. For monitoring of treatment, Serum progesterone measurements could verify normal luteal phase, while ultrasound scans of the ovaries can monitor folliculogenesis and predict the risk of multiple pregnancies and OHSS. The treatment is discontinued if pregnancy occurs, although adverse effects in early pregnancy have not been reported. Overall, treatment results in ovulation in more than 90%, with a cumulative pregnancy rate up to 96% after six cycles.[57, 60] The miscarriage rate appears similar to that in the normal population[61,62] but higher rates have been shown in smaller series.[60]

An advantage of GnRH treatment over the use of gonadotropins is the low rate of multiple pregnancy.[59, 60]

Disadvantages of this mode of treatment include the need for the pump to be connected to the body all day for a considerable number of days, the necessity to refill the pump at frequent intervals and the possible reactions of the skin at the site of injection, particularly during the s.c. administration. Finally, the formation of antibodies against the synthetic GnRH seems to be a rare possibility.[59]

Adjuncts to Ovulation inducing Drugs

Glucocorticoids

Glucocorticoids have been proposed as a useful adjuvant to both CC and gonadotropin ovulation induction in women with PCOS. The therapeutic rationale is based on reducing ovarian androgen concentrations, improving ovulatory function and reducing resistance to ovulation induction agents.[63] In order to normalize (without suppressing) adrenal steroid production, daily oral doses of dexamethasone 0.25–0.5 mg or 5–10 mg prednisone have been employed from day 2 to 11 of the menstrual cycle in a continuous regime. In a study of women with PCOS, the chance of ovulation after glucocorticoid suppression of adrenal androgens was not predicted by either basal dehydroepiandrosterone sulfate (DHEAS) concentrations or suppressed concentrations and limited effects on ovulation were observed.[64] Major problem from the adjuvant use of lowdose glucocorticoids are rare, but weight gain may be seen. Use of dexamethasone in the dose of 0.5 mg at night for 4 months leads to a weight gain of more than 5 kg in 70–80% of the patients.[65] Other reported side effects include glucose intolerance[66] and osteoporosis. Given possible side effects and in particular the negative influence of weight gain on ovulation induction, their use should remain as a second line therapy subject to further research.

Prolactin Reducing Medications

The two most common dopamine agonist used are bromocriptine and cabergoline. The former needs to be given once in twelve hours while the latter has an action which lasts for seven days.It is indicated for ovulatory dysfunction associated with hyperprolactinemia. Bromocriptine is given in the dose of 2.5 mg once or twice a day depending on the prolactin levels. Cabergoline is given in the dose of 0.25 to 0.5 mg either once or twice a week, again depending on the prolactin levels. With the above dose it usually normalizes the prolactin level in 60–85% of hyperprolactinemic women. Cyclic menstrual cycle is established in 70 to 90% within 6 to 8 weeks once treatment is initiated. Ovulatory cycles are seen in 50 to 75% of these treated women. Side effects with dopamine agonist include dizziness, nausea, vomiting, nasal stuffiness and orthostatic hypotension. These side effects are much less with cabergoline as compared to bromocriptine.

Insulin Sensitizers

Metformin

Metformin hydrochloride a dimethylbiguanide is an oral anti-hyperglycemic agent used in the management of patients with Type-2 diabetes mellitus, either alone or in combination with sulfonylureas or other agents. It is used as an adjuvant in women with PCOS. Its action is by inhibiting gluconeogenesis in the liver with enhanced peripheral uptake of glucose and increased intestinal use of glucose. It also decreases fatty acid oxidation. In the ovaries, it restores normal ovarian activity. Metformin positively modulates the reproductive axis (namely GnRH-LH episodic release) but there is no evidence that adding metformin is beneficial in achieving pregnancy either in the obese or non obese.[70-75]

The Cochrane[70] review published that there is no evidence that metformin improves live birth rates whether it is used alone (pooled OR = 1.00, 95% CI 0.16–6.39) or in combination with clomiphene (pooled OR = 1.05, 95% CI 0.75–1.47).

Since women with WHO type II anovulatory infertility frequently demonstrate a hyper-response to FSH, it has been proposed that metformin may also have an adjuvant role to gonadotropin in ovulation induction by correcting hyperinsulinemia, and hence normalizing the response of the patient to gonadotropin stimulation. Few prospective studies are available to support this, however a randomized trial compared metformin co-administration versus placebo during r-FSH treatment in CC-resistant women with PCOS.[76] No differences were observed in indices of insulin sensitivity or ovarian response during r-FSH treatment. More adequately powered studies are now required to further elucidate the role of metformin as an adjunctive therapy to ovulation induction with gonadotropins.

The use of metformin in improving reproductive outcome appears to be limited. It is indicated in patients with glucose intolerance and for those patients who have metabolic syndrome for cardiovascular protection.

Bromocriptine, Lisuride, Cabergoline

Some women ovulate irregularly because their pituitary glands secrete too much prolactin. Prolactin by altering FSH and LH secretion can stop the normal ovulatory cycle. High prolactin levels and thyroid dysfunction go hand-in-hand and in the presence of galactorrhea, it is mandatory to assess the thyroid function. With addition of prolactin lowering agents in 90% women, prolactin levels revert to normal with ovulation occurring in 85% and many achieve pregnancy. One may add ovulation induction medication along with prolactin lowering drugs to get better results.

Ovulation Induction in Special Situations

Hypergonadotropic Hypogonadism

In this group, the induction of a multi-follicular response is a challenge and a frustrating problem. Success rate with different modalities have been tried but the success rate has been poor. High dose of gonadotropins, natural cycle IVF (Fig. 5.19) and, mild stimulation protocols (Fig. 5.20) either with GnRH agonist or antagonist have been used but with limited success. Ovum donation and hormone replacement therapy to prevent osteoporosis and cardiovascular disease remains a mainstay in this group.

Natural Cycle IVF

Results comparable with those obtained with stimulated cycles in true poor responders[77-81] reported higher pregnancy rate in natural cycle IVF. It is a simple treatment with nomultiple pregnancies and OHSS. It reduced financial, social and emotional costs and consecutive cycles were possible. A premature LH surge with spontaneous ovulation can occur in 30–60% of the patients. The other disadvantages are that in 5 to 15% no oocytes are obtained at oocyte pick up (OPU) and despite getting one oocyte in 50% there could be no embryo transfer. Natural cycles are difficult to schedule and with only one embryo to transfer it would have low pregnancy rates.

Natural Cycle IVF with Minimal Stimulation (Fig. 5.20)

One could add 75–150 IU of FSH once the follicle reaches 14 mm along with GnRH antagonist till criteria for hCG administration is reached that is the follicular diameter is 17- 18 mm. This protocol with hormonal add back had better pregnancy rates than a natural cycle and also had lesser cancellation rates. The pregnancy rates were better in poor responders who were less than 38 years as compared to those women who were more than 38 years of age (Ubaldi et al, RBM Online 2007).

Mild Stimulation

In mild stimulation (Fig. 5.21) we can use oral compounds (Clomiphene citrate, letrozole or tamoxifen) with or without gonadotropins but with GnRH antagonist to prevent LH surge, hCG for follicular maturation and luteal phase support.

Mild stimulation aims at 1-7 oocytes at OR with comparable PRs as conventional stimulation where > 8 oocytes are obtained. Figure 5.22 shows the difference in spontaneous, conventionally stimulated and minimally stimulated cycle.

The FSH window is widest in conventional stimulated cycle resulting in more number of dominant follicles being formed with more than eight oocytes retrieved. It is shortest in the natural cycle and intermediate in the mild stimulation cycles.

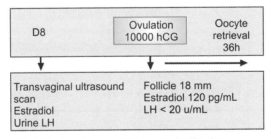

FIG. 5.19 Natural cycle IVF in vitro fertilization

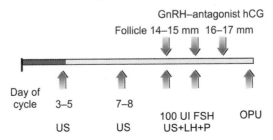

FIG. 5.20 Natural cycle IVF with minimal stimulation

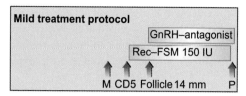

FIG. 5.21 Mild stimulation protocol

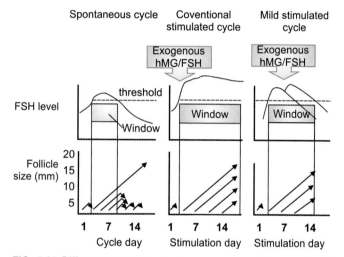

FIG. 5.22 Difference between spontaneous, conventional and mild stimulated cycles

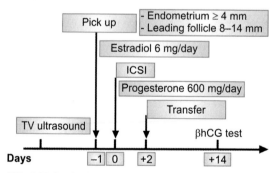

FIG. 5.23 In vitro maturation cycle

Stimulation for In Vitro Maturation (IVM)

The IVM is done in healthy regular cycling women and mostly in PCOS with anovulation. Collection of oocyte done in the follicular phase at the leading follicular diameter of 10–14 mm. Luteal phase is supported by both estradiol and progesterone (Fig. 5.23). One could use a natural cycle without priming (Fig. 5.24) or use hCG 10,000 IU (Fig. 5.25) or FSH 150 IU (Fig. 5.26) or combination of FSH 150 IU and hCG 10,000 IU (Fig. 5.27). Priming with FSH may improve the implantation rate.

Protocols for In Vitro Maturation

1. IVM without priming (Fig. 5.24)
2. IVM with hCG priming (Fig. 5.25)
3. IVM with FSH priming (Fig. 5.26)
4. IVM with FSH and hCG priming (Fig. 5.27)

The IVM/IVF is an established clinical technique that reduces the incidence of OHSS and can now be the treatment of choice for PCOS.

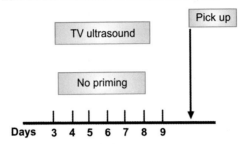

FIG. 5.24 No priming

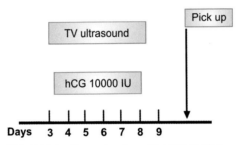

FIG. 5.25 In vitro maturation with hCG priming

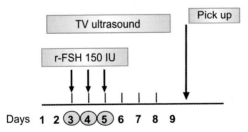

FIG. 5.26 In vitro maturation with FSH priming

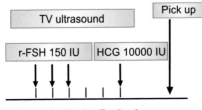

FIG. 5.27 In vitro maturation with FSH and hCG priming

Concerns of IVM

- Disrupted synchronization between nuclear and cytoplasmic maturation
- Higher frequency of abnormal spindle organization[82-87]
- Possible imprinting defects
- Difference in protein synthesis
- DNA fragmentation
- Cumulus cells might be more resistant to removal in immature oocytes matured *in vitro* and thus require more handling than *in vivo* matured oocytes
- Significantly lower rates of fertilization and blastocyst formation compared with *in vivo* matured oocytes.[88]

The first birth after IVM specifically in patients with polycystic ovaries was published by Trounson in 1994.[89] Initial IVM success rates were relatively low and only sporadic pregnancies were reported,[90,91] though more recent studies have demonstrated success rates of 21.5%,[92] 22.5%,[93] and 38.5%.[94]

The continued lower success rate of IVM could be explained by suboptimal oocyte maturation and/or impaired endometrial receptivity as at IVM the follicles are aspirated at 14 mm diameter, the endometrium is exposed to lower levels of endogenous E2 than with conventional IVF.[95] Suboptimal and asynchronized nuclear and cytoplasmic maturation has been postulated as a cause of IVM implantation failure.[96]

To improve IVM results, FSH priming, hCG priming, prolonged hCG interval, or freezing all the oocytes of embryos after IVM to proceed in a delayed transfer in a subsequent and prepared cycle.[97,98] No neurodevelopmental concerns during infancy and early childhood were found.[99] Most studies have reported gestational age at birth and birth weight that is comparable with the general population.[100]

The IVM is not ready as a routine treatment because of unsolved problems such as epigenetic modifications. When oocytes were matured in culture, meiotic spindle and cytoplasmic phenotypic properties of M-II oocytes were affected relative to in vivo conditions and between strains. Specifically, measures of meiotic spindle size, shape, polar pericentric distribution and cytoplasmic MTOC number all revealed characteristic variations.

COH in Cancer Patients

Fertility preservation should be considered for all young people undergoing potentially gonadotoxic treatment. The age and relationship status of the patient, the type of cancer and stage at diagnosis, the type and dose of chemotherapy and radiotherapy required and the time available before initiation of cancer treatment will influence individual patient management. Therefore, a variety of safe and effective options for fertility preservation are required.

Sperm, oocyte and embryo cryopreservation are considered standard practice and is method of choice as compared to other available fertility preservation methods that are considered investigational and be performed in centers with the necessary expertise. For oocyte and embryo cryopreservation, we require protocols that will

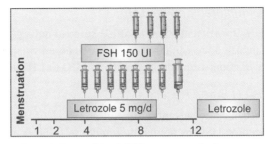

FIG. 5.28 Protocol for COH in cancer patients

result in follicular growth with as low as possible estradiol levels. For this, we could use the combination of letrozole or tamoxifen with FSH (Fig. 5.28). The Letrozole or tamoxifen is continued after oocyte retrieval.

GnRH Antagonists are given when the dominant follicle is ≥14 mm.

GnRH agonist is given for trigger when at least 3 follicles are more than 17 mm and estradiol levels are more than 250 pg/mL. Letrozole 5 mg or tamoxifen 20 to 40 mg has to be continued till estradiol level reach less than 50 pg/mL or in patients with breast cancer for longer time if ER/PR is positive.

Monitoring Ovulation Induction Cycles

It helps the physician to choose the most suitable protocol, to obtain best possible outcome, determine response to ovulation induction drugs and the dose and length of gonadotropin therapy. It also helps to confirm the down-regulation after GnRH agonist therapy, determine optimal time of hCG administration, detect ovulation, time oocyte retrieval, identify poor and hyper responders and avoid complications.

What to Monitor?

- Patient's initial parameters—determine ovarian morphology and reserve, uterine and adnexal pathology and decide the stimulation protocol for adequate response.
- Ovarian response to ovulation induction.
- Endometrial thickness that is a reliable bioassay of the patient's estrogenic status and endometrial pathology if any.
- Completion of the treatment course.
- Complications of ovulation stimulation drugs.
  In the form of premature luteinization, endogenous surge, poor response and hyperstimulation should be prevented.

Complications of Ovulation Induction

Premature Luteinization

It is because of premature and suboptimal LH surge where there is progesterone production but no ovulation. Oocyte maturation without follicular rupture occurs and if oocyte retrieval is done, the oocytes and embryos are of poor quality. Endometrium is also out of phase that reduces the implantation rate.

Luteinized Unruptured Follicle (LUF)

It is because of insufficient strength of LH surge to induce follicular rupture but sufficient to induce oocyte maturation. It is diagnosed when dominant follicle is still apparent 48 hours after administration of hCG or LH surge.

Endogenous LH Surge Results

In compromised oocytes and embryo quality as a result of exposure to inappropriate LH levels. Seen on USG as premature rupture of follicles at diameter < 16 – 17 mm. Requires extensive endocrine monitoring to prevent endogenous LH surge. It can be prevented with use of GnRH agonist or antagonist.

Poor Response

Could be idiopathic or because of ovarian failure or antibodies to exogenous gonadotropins. It could be treated either by modified stimulation protocols addition of growth hormone, though success is limited.

Ovarian Hyperstimulation Syndrome (OHSS)

The pathogenesis of which is dependent on ovarian renin-angiotensin system. It is excessive response to ovulation induction. Small and thin patient, polycystic ovarian syndrome and high dose of GT early in follicular phase are predisposing factors for OHSS. Experience with OI therapy and recognition of risk factors for OHSS is an important factor for prevention. Highly individualized OI regimens with use of minimum dose and duration of GT therapy necessary to achieve the therapeutic goal are essential along with careful monitoring of folliculogenesis with USG and E2. In patients with high estradiol level, high number of small and intermediate follicles along with dominant follicles one could cost the patient and use GnRH agonist instead of hCG in an antagonist cycle. Despite maintaining the input and output if the OHSS increase, it is best to cryopreserve the embryos to be transferred in the subsequent cycle. One could continue GnRH antagonist post-cryofreezing to reduce the severity or use dopamine agonist. Apart from cancellation; none of the approaches were totally efficient, although they decrease the severity. hCG is primary stimulus for the syndrome and withholding hCG is the main preventive measure.

Functional Cyst

It is presence of cyst at pre-stimulation base line scan following GnRH agonist stimulation for down regulation. Characterized by sharp edges and an echogenic contents and is because of initial FSH surge when GnRH agonist is commenced in the luteal phase.

Persistent Corpus Luteum (CL) or Retention Cyst

It is presence of cyst at baseline scan that could be follicle from previous cycle or persistent CL. Normally requires no treatment and should be followed by ultrasound. No ovulation induction drug should be given in that cycle and if required may be given oral contraceptives.

Conclusion

Ovarian superovulation is of paramount importance to obtain a good reproductive outcome. Selection of the correct stimulation protocol to produce adequate number of mature follicles (generally > 3 follicles >17 mm), so as to obtain optimal number of oocytes for fertilization in a spontaneous or IUI cycle or at oocyte retrieval for in vitro fertilization and embryo transfer. Before treatment with gonadotropins, evaluation generally should exclude abnormalities of thyroid function and hyperprolactinemia, and should include hysterosalpingography, transvaginal ultrasonography and evaluation of the male partner by semen analysis.

The balance between success and complications resulting from ovulation induction is dependent on many factors. These include patient characteristics, gonadotropin preparations and dose regimens used, the intensity of monitoring ovarian response to stimulation and willingness to cancel the cycle in case of hyper-response.

Refining ovulation induction therapy by individualizing the drug and dose used offers the prospect of improving safety, reducing the risk of multiple pregnancies and improving the efficiency of ovulation induction. Thus success with ovulation induction with minimal complications can be obtained with the use of simple predictive factors such as increased age, duration of infertility, etiology of infertility with associated factors and conventional markers of ovarian reserve like antral follicle count, AMH, FSH, Inhibin B, estradiol, ovarian volume and Doppler. Though these conventional markers to predict exact response and egg quantity are not perfect, but they allow us to counsel women regarding complications and poor prognosis. A normal test has little predictive value, but an abnormal test requires critical evaluation before recommending that a patient abandon fertility treatment. At any stage if any doubt exists one should always give treatment a try.

The AFC and AMH are equally accurate predictors of high ovarian response to COH and allow us to identify the patients who are at increased risk of OHSS. AMH best single marker and Day 3 FSH, E2, AFC and Inhibin B are best combined markers to predict poor response to GT stimulation.

Available tests reflect, directly or indirectly, the size of the antral (2–5 mm) follicle pool and response to ovulation induction drugs, but cannot predict the occurrence of pregnancy. Relationship between AFC and AMH concentrations is more reliable than that observed with FSH, inhibin B and estradiol on cycle day 3. Basal FSH should not be used as a screening tool but instead used to counsel patients appropriately regarding the realistic chance of conception and aiding determination of appropriate GT dose. In ART population, first cycle IVF still remains the most informative test in terms of how a woman will respond to ovarian stimulation.

Among women not previously treated with exogenous gonadotropins, treatment generally should begin at a relatively low dose (e.g. 37.5–75 IU/day). In subsequent cycles, treatment generally begins at the threshold of response previously determined.

The last century has seen tremendous advances in the treatment of infertility with progress made in ovulation induction, laboratory techniques and oocyte retrieval and embryo transfer. Technology has come a long way since the era of animal, human pituitary- and urinary-derived hormones, and new pharmaceutical products will offer safest option for ovarian stimulation during assisted reproductive techniques.

The application of new preparations such as recombinant LH, long-acting FSH, fixed combinations of recombinant LH and recombinant human FSH, recombinant hCG and an increasing emphasis on individualized treatment regimens should lead to further improvements in outcome from gonadotropin ovulation induction. Today technologies that are developed for monitoring ovulation induction cycles have decreased the incidence of ovarian hyperstimulation and high-order multiple pregnancies and improved the outcome of infertility treatment.

Great progress in ovulation induction has been achieved during the last 20 years. Although conventional regimens are still in use, new modalities have been developed that may open up new methods in the treatment of anovulation. Improvement for prediction models to tailor and optimize the treatment outcomes will improve safety and efficacy compared with classical ovulation induction strategies.

Case Studies

Case 1

A 30-year-old female, married since 10 years with irregular cycles and primary infertility 5 years. Had menarche at 13 years with irregular cycles every 3 – 4 months with bleeding for 4 – 5 days. HSG was normal with one intrauterine polyp. A hysterolaparoscopy with polypectomy and laparoscopic ovarian drilling (LOD) was done. Semen analysis and hormonal evaluation was normal. She was obese with BMI of 33.8, had moderate hirsutism and acne. On ultrasound, the uterus was normal with both ovaries being enlarged with a volume of 21 and 19 cu mm with multiple small follicles. Ovulation induction with clomiphene citrate using maximum dose of 200 mg and letrozole 5 mg was tried without any success. Ovulation induction with GnRH agonist Short protocol and FSH 75 IU was planned. No follicular growth was seen till the 10th day and E2 level was only 100 pg/mL, so the dose was increased to 150 IU. 3 days later multiple folliculogenesis with an E2 of 3500 pg/mL was seen. The dose of FSH was reduced to 75 IU and was counseled for IVF. hCG given on day 16 when there were 20 follicles with 18 mm, 8 follicles with 16 mm and several small follicles. On the day of hCG, E2 level was 9850 pg/mL and progesterone 4.3 ng/mL. 23 oocyte cumulus complexes (OCC) were obtained, 17 fertilized and 14 cleaved with 5 blastocyst frozen. Embryo transfer was not done in view of OHSS. She conceived in the second frozen embryo transfer cycle. It was a twin pregnancy and she had a preterm twin delivery at 32 weeks. From this case we know that women with PCOS are difficult to treat and the response is unpredictable. Initially the ovaries may be resistant to stimulation but with increase in the dose there is over response. Though the AMH, LH and androgen levels were normal there was over response on increasing the dose. So in PCOS one cannot predict response using the conventional markers.

Case 2

A 25-year-old female, married since 4 years with irregular cycles every 2–3 months. She had not conceived with five cycles of ovulation induction (3 with CC and 2 with Letrozole). Her natural cycles were anovulatory. She had mild hirsutism and was not obese. On ultrasound, uterus was normal with enlarged ovaries with increased stroma and multiple small follicles. Semen analysis was normal with all hormonal levels being normal except for LH, free testosterone and DHEAS, that were elevated. At hysterolaparoscopy, the endometrium had polypoidal hyperplasia with unhealthy tubes and mild endometriosis. Laparascopic ovarian drilling (LOD) was done.

In view of severe PCOS, IVF with long protocol COS with Rec FSH 150 IU was planned. On day 4 of stimulation, E2 was168.26 pg/mL but on day 6 it increased to 671.74 pg/mL with multiple folliculogenesis (> 20 per ovary). Dose of FSH reduced to 75 IU but surprisingly on day 8 E2 dropped to 96.86 pg/mL and on day 10 dropped further to 72 pg/mL. So hMG 75 IU was added that was further increased to 150 IU from day 12. On day 13, with 6 follicles more than 12 mm, E2 was 710 pg/mL. On day 16, there was only 1 dominant follicle of 21 mm and 8 follicles between 11–16 mm.

Thereby, a decision was taken to convert the cycle to IUI, which was done on day17. Patient conceived but had a missed abortion at gestational age of 10 weeks. As she conceived with IUI, the patient wanted to try few more cycles of IUI. No conception was seen with CC or Letrozole. In view of CC and Letrozole failure, a gonadotropin cycle was done. There was no response to Rec FSH 37.5 IU that was increased to 50 IU and then 75 IU. The E2 level was also low so Rec FSH was replaced by hMG 75 IU. One dominant follicle ovulated, IUI done but failed to conceive. Second cycle of IVF with GnRH agonist long protocol and COS with Rec FSH 100 IU planned. On day 5, E2 was 115 pg/mL and on day 7 there were more than 25 small follicles with E2 of 497 pg/mL, so the dose reduced to 75 IU. On day 9, E2 reduced to 419 pg/mL, on day 12 it was 171 pg/mL and on Day 15 E2 102 pg/mL with about 20 – 25 follicles of 10 – 13 mm in size. The stimulation was changed from FSH to hMG 150 IU for 3 days but E2 dropped further to 117 pg/mL, so the cycle was cancelled.

Third cycle of IVF was done in GnRH agonist long protocol with COS using uFSH 150 IU and hMG 75 IU. On day 5 E2 was 306 pg/mL. In view of drop in E2 level once the dose was reduced, the gonadotropin was continued in the same dose. On day 8 E2 was 1130 pg/mL but dropped onday 10 to 895 pg/mL and progesterone was 1.49 ng/mL. hCG 250 µg was given subcutaneously when 5 follicles >17 mm, 6 follicles between 15–16 mm and 8 follicles <14 mm. 10 oocytes were obtained, 8 fertilized, Two 8 cell with Grade 1 embryos were transferred with failed conception.

The patient was given Diane 35 for 2 months prior to next IVF. This time we decided a GnRH antagonist in a fixed protocol. COS with uFSH 150 IU. On day 5, E2 188 pg/mL with multiple small follicles, which dropped to 138 pg/mL once the antagonist were started, so hMG 75 IU added. On day 11, E2 was 199 pg/mL, so hMG increased to 150 IU. The patient had breakthrough bleeding for 3 days so estrogel was given for skin application. On day 15 of COS hCG was administered when 2 follicles were 18 mm and E2 was 542 pg/mL. Two oocytes were obtained, ICSI was done and both fertilized. Day 3 embryo transfers was done, two 8 cell Grade 1 embryos, which were laser hatched and transferred. Patient conceived and delivered female child 2.4 kg. During pregnancy she was admitted for anemia as she had thalassemia trait and had also developed gestational diabetes mellitus.

Here in this case, we can see that PCOS patients behave very differently to COS. Despite using hMG instead of recombinant FSH estradiol levels remained low and on the contrary decreased as follicles gained dominance. The low estradiol levels could probably be because of granulosa cell dysfunction as they were seen in both GnRH agonist and antagonist cycle.

Case 3

A 25-year-old female, married since 4 years presented with primary infertility and irregular cycles every 2 – 3 months. Her HSG was normal, semen analysis had a normal count but motility was only 28% and hypo osmotic swelling test (HOS) was only 15. Her LH, androstenedione, total and free testosterone, 17 hydroxyprogesterone and AMH were elevated. The AMH level was 11.6 ng/mL. On transvaginal ultrasound, both ovaries were enlarged with a volume of 27.4 and 33.6 cu mm with increased stroma and multiple small follicles. She was on metformin for three years and had undergone ovulation induction with CC and letrozole for three years. In view of PCOS with asthenospermia, ovulation induction with IUI was planned. She failed to ovulate with 200 mg of CC so a gonadotropin cycle was planned. Recombinant FSH was started on day two of the cycle in the dose of 37.5 IU with 250 µg of GnRH agonist as baseline LH was high. After 14 days of COS all follicles were small and the E2 level was only 65 pg/mL, so the dose was increased to 50 IU. Seven days later the follicles were still less than 10 mm with the E2 level of 49 pg/mL decision was taken to give hMG instead of Rec FSH in the dose of 75 IU. On day 28 of COS despite 75 IU of hMG the E2 level was only 60 pg/mL, so the dose was increased to 150 IU. After seven days of 150 IU of hMG, on the right there were three follicles 11 – 12 mm in diameter with an E2 of 140 pg/mL, so the dose was increased to 225 IU. On day 42 of COS the follicles in both ovaries were still small with five follicles between 12 – 14 mm in diameter and E2 level of 162 pg/mL, so the dose was increased to 300 IU. Once the dose was increased to 300 IU several follicles started growing and a decision was taken to convert the IUI cycle into an IVF cycle. hCG was given on day 50 of COS when there were 21 follicles 17 – 18 mm, 6 follicles between 15 – 16 mm and the rest were between 12 – 15 mm. The estradiol level on day of hCG was 3164 pg/mL and progesterone level was 1.6 ng/mL. At oocyte retrieval we obtained 18 follicles out of which 13 were MII. IVF was done and ten out of thirteen fertilized. Six blastocysts formed on day five, two 4AA were transferred and four were frozen. She was monitored strictly for input and output, weight gain and abdominal distension in view of multiple small and intermediate follicles on day of hCG, so as to diagnose OHSS early. Patient conceived and delivered at 38 weeks. Thus, in PCOS it is not necessary that low dose could result in mono folliculogenesis. We have to administer a gonadotropin dose that is more than the follicular threshold for FSH for folliculogenesis to occur.

All the above three cases were PCOS and we saw that each patient responded differently. Only when we stimulate the patient do we know the FSH threshold, so that in the next cycle we start the threshold dose right from the beginning so that the duration of treatment is shorter. Again in PCOS one should not stop the gonadotropins if there is no response after 14 days, but gradually increase the dose to the threshold level that will result in folliculogenesis.

Case 4

A 33-year-old woman, married since 9 years presented in 2007 with primary infertility and trying to conceive for 8 years. She had regular cycles with normal flow. She had undergone ovulation induction with timed intercourse for seven years and 3 cycles of IUI. She had a variable FSH level from 7.2 mIU to 15 mIU/mL and at ultrasound both ovaries were small with a volume of 1.8 and 2.1 cu mm and AFC of five. In view of treatment taken for 8 years and low ovarian reserve, IVF was planned. First cycle was a short agonist cycle to take advantage of the initial flare effect. The COS was with FSH 150 IU and hMG 150 IU. After seven days the follicles were small with an E2 of 150 pg/mL, the hMG dose was increased to 300 IU. Five days after increasing the dose criteria for hCG administration was reached with two follicles being 17 – 18 m in diameter. Two oocytes obtained but only one was MII, and a day three transfer of an 8 cell Grade B embryo was done, but no pregnancy was achieved. She came regularly on day two of each cycle for FSH levels for eleven months, but the levels were between 15 – 22 mIU/mL. In the 12th month the FSH level was 6.8 mIU/mL, ICSI cycle was done with Letrozole (day 3 – 7) with FSH 150 IU and hMG 300 IU in an antagonist cycle. Total days of COS were 9 with two MII oocytes at retrieval, both fertilized and cleaved. Day three ET, two 11 cell grade 1 embryos transferred, but no pregnancy. We know that odd cell embryos may have aneuploidy. Five months later when FSH was 7.1, one more antagonist cycle done, but despite the use of antagonist the follicle ruptured prematurely and so an IUI was done. Next cycle of ICSI was done three months later when the FSH was 9.1. COS done with Letrozole (day 3 – 7) with FSH 150 IU and hMG 300 IU in an antagonist cycle. The number of days of COS was 8 and E2 on the day of hCG was 390 pg/mL. Four oocytes obtained, three MII, and 1 GV. All three MII fertilized and cleaved. Three embryos 10 cell grade 1, 8 cell grade 2 and 11 cell grade 1 transferred on day three. Singleton pregnancy with live birth at 37 weeks. This patient was an ideal case for oocyte donation but the patient insisted on using her own oocytes, so we targeted a cycle where the FSH values were low and were able to achieve pregnancy.

So using proper drugs after proper evaluation and investigations at its proper timing and dose is the key to the success of infertility management.

References

1. Humaidan P, Bungum L, Bungum M, Andersen CY. Ovarian response and pregnancy outcome related to mid-follicular LH levels in women undergoing assisted reproduction with GnRH agonist down-regulation and recombinant FSH stimulation. Hum Reprod. 2002;17:2016–21.

2. Martin L, Marek D, Doody K, et al. Daily low dose recombinant HCG and recombinant FSH: a novel stimulation protocol for IVF. Fertil Steril. 2002;76(suppl 1):1.

3. Vega-Cardenas J, Hernandez-Ayup S, Galache-Vega P, et al. Biologic effect of leuprolide acetate on luteinizing hormone (LH) in human reproduction. Fertil Steril. 2002;76(suppl 1):S124.

4. Cabrera RA, Stadtmauer L, Mayer JF, Gibbons WE, Oehninger S. Follicular phase serum levels of luteinizing hormone do not influence delivery rates in in vitro fertilization cycles down-regulated with a gonadotropin-releasing hormone agonist and stimulated with recombinant follicle-stimulated hormone. Fertil Steril. 2005;83:42–8.

5. Lee JB, Do BR, Lee KH, et al. The role of LH receptor in human IVF-ET program. Fertil Steril. 2002;76(suppl 1):S216.

6. Collins JA, Hughes EG. Pharmacological interventions for the induction of ovulation. Drugs. 1995;50(3):480–95.

7. Fauser BC, Macklon NS. Medical approaches to ovarian stimulation for infertility. In:Strauss JF, Barbieri RL, editors. Yen and Jaffe's Reproductive Endocrinology. Philadelphia: Elsevier Saunders, 2004.pp.965–1012.

8. Arslan M, Bocca S, Mirkin S, Barroso G, Stadtmauer L, Oehninger S. Controlled ovarian hyperstimulation protocols for in vitro fertilization: two decades of experience after the birth of Elizabeth Carr. Fertil Steril. 2005;84:555–69.

9. Te Velde and Pearson PL. The variability of female reproductive ageing. Hum Reprod Update. 2002;8(2):141–54.

10. Kwee J, Elting ME, Schats R, McDonnell J, Lambalk CB. Ovarian volume and antral follicle count for the prediction of low and hyper responders with in vitro fertilization. Reprod Biol Endocrinol. 2007;5:9.

11. Lee TH, Liu CH, Huang CC, Wu YL, Shih YT, Ho HN, et al. Serum anti-Müllerian hormone and estradiol levels as predictors of ovarian hyperstimulation syndrome in assisted reproduction technology cycles. Hum Reprod. 2008;23:160–7.

12. Kwee J, Schats R, McDonnell J, Schoemaker J, Lambalk CB. The clomiphene citrate challenge test versus the exogenous follicle-stimulating hormone ovarian reserve test as a single test for identification of low responders and hyperresponders to in vitro fertilization. Fertil Steril. 2006;85:1714–22.

13. Julie Galey-Fontaine, Isabelle Cédrin-Durnerin, Rachid Chaïbi, Nathalie Massin, Jean-Noël Hugues. Age and ovarian reserve are distinct predictive factors of cycle outcome in low responders. Reproductive BioMedicine Online. 2005.

14. Lambalk CB. Value of elevated basal follicle-stimulating hormone levels and the differential diagnosis during the diagnostic subfertility work-up. Fertil Steril. 79:489–90.

15. Jayaprakashan K, Campbell D, Hopkisson K, Johnson I, Raine F. A prospective comparative analysis of anti mullerian hormone, inhibin B and 3 dimensional ultrasound determinants of ovarian reserve in the prediction of poor response to contrilled ovarian stimulation. Fertil Steril. 2008.

16. Tomas C, Nupjua-Huttunen S, Martikainen H. Pretreatment transvaginal ultrasound examination predicts ovarian responsiveness to gonadotropins in in vitro fertilization. Hum. Reprod. 1997;12:220–3.

17. Sharara FI, McClamrock HD. The effect of ageing on ovarian volume measurements in infertile women. Obstet. Gynecol. 1999;94:57–60.

18. Hughes E, Collins J, Vandekerckhove P. Clomiphene citrate for ovulation induction in women with oligo-amenorrhoea. Cochrane Database Syst Rev 2: CD000056, 2000.
19. Imani B, Eijkemans MJ, te Velde ER, Habbema JD, Fauser BC. Predictors of patients remaining anovulatory during clomiphene citrate induction of ovulation in normogonadotropic oligoamenorrheic infertility. J Clin Endocrinol Metab, 1998;83:2361–5.
20. Imani B, Eijkemans MJ, te Velde ER, Habbema JD, Fauser BC. Predictors of changes to conceive in ovulatory patients during clomiphene citrate induction of ovulation in normogonadotropic oligoamenorrheic infertility. J Clin Endocrinol Metab. 1999;84:1617–22.
21. O'Herlihy C, Pepperell RJ, Brown JB, Smith MA, Sandri L, McBain JC. Incremental clomiphene therapy: A new method for treating persistent anovulation. Obstet Gynecol. 1981;58:535–42.
22. Fluker MR, Wang IY, Rowe TC. An extended 10-day course of clomiphene citrate (CC) in women with CC-resistant ovulatory disorders. Fertil Steril. 1996;66:761–4.
23. Trott EA, Plouffe L Jr, Hansen K, Hines R, Brann DW, Mahesh VB. Ovulation induction in clomiphene-resistant anovulatory women with normal dehydroepiandrosterone sulfate levels: beneficial effects of the addition of dexamethasone during the follicular phase. Fertil Steril. 1996;66:484–6.
24. Branigan EF, Estes MA. Treatment of chronic anovulation resistant to clomiphene citrate (CC) by using oral contraceptive ovarian suppression followed by repeat CC treatment. Fertil Steril. 1999;71:544–6.
25. Badawy A, Abdel Aal I, Abulatta M. Clomiphene citrate or anastrozole for ovulation induction in women with polycystic ovary syndrome? A prospective controlled trial. Fertil Steril. 2009;92:860–3.
26. Wang CF, Gemzell C. The use of human gonadotropins for the induction of ovulation in women with polycystic ovarian disease. Fertil Steril. 1980;33:479–86.
27. Messinis IE, Bergh T, Wide L. The importance of human chorionic gonadotropin support of the corpus luteum during human gonadotropin therapy in women with anovulatory infertility. Fertil Steril. 1988;50:31–5.
28. Kamrava MM, Seibel MM, Berger MJ, Thompson I, Taymor ML. Reversal of persistent anovulation in polycystic ovarian disease by adminis- tration of chronic low-dose follicle-stimulating hormone. Fertil Steril. 1982;37:520–3.
29. Polson DW, Mason HD, Saldahna MB, Franks S. Ovulation of a single dominant follicle during treatment with low-dose pulsatile follicle stimulating hormone in women with polycystic ovary syndrome. Clin Endocrinol (Oxf). 1987;26:205–12.
30. Homburg R, Howles CM. Low-dose FSH therapy for anovulatory infertility associated with polycystic ovary syndrome: rationale, results, reflections and refinements. Hum Reprod Update. 1999;5:493–9.
31. Franks S, White D. Low-dose gonadotropin treatment in polycystic ovary syndrome: the step-up protocol. In: Tarlatzis B (ed) Ovulation Induction. Elsevier, Paris, 2002. pp.98–107.
32. Ruiz Balda JA, Caballero JL, Roque A, Ezcurra D. Clinical experience with pergoveris™, a new formulation of rFSH and rLH in a 2:1 ratio, for the treatment of suboptimal patient populations: Spanish preliminary results. Fertility and Sterility 2009;92(3):Supplement S163–4.
33. Buhler K, Naether OGJ. Large multicentre, observational study of a new 2:1 formulation of follitophin alfa and lutropin alfa in assisted reproductive technology (ART) in routine practice. Fertility and Sterility 2009;92(3) Supplement S54.
34. Kolibianakis EM, Collins J, Tarlatzis BC, Devroey P, Diedrich K, Griesinger G. Among patients treated for IVF with gonadotropins and GnRH analogues, is the probability

of live birth dependent on the type of analogue used? A systematic review and meta-analysis. Hum Reprod Update 2006;12:651–71.

35. Mulders AG, Eijkemans MJ, Imani B, Fauser BC. Prediction of chances for success or complications in gonadotropin ovulation induction in normogonadotrophic anovulatory infertility. Reproductive Biomedicine Online 2003;7:170–8.

36. Mulders AG, Laven JS, Eijkemans MJC, Hughes EG, Fauser BC. Patient predictors for outcome with gonadotropin ovulation induction in women with normogonadotrophic anovulatory infertility: a meta-analysis. Human Reproduction Update 2003;9:429–49.

37. Imani B, Eijkemans MJ, Faessen GH, et al. Prediction of the individual follicle-stimulating hormone threshold for gonadotropin induction of ovulation in normogonadotropic anovulatory infertility: An approach to increase safety and efficiency. Fertility and Sterility 2002;77:83–90.

38. Felberbaum RE, Reissmann T, Kupker W, Bauer O, al Hasani S, Diedrich C, et al. Preserved pituitary response under ovarian stimu- lation with HMG and GnRH antagonists (Cetrorelix) in women with tubal infertility. Eur J Obstet Gynecol Reprod Biol. 1995;61:151–5.

39. Kol S. Luteolysis induced by a gonadotropin-releasing hormone agonist is the key to prevention of ovarian hyperstimulation syndrome. Fertil Steril. 2004;81:1–5.

40. Humaidan P, Ejdrup Bredkjaer H, Bungum L, Bungum M, Grondahl ML, Westergaard L, et al. GnRH agonist (buserelin) or hCG for ovulation induction in GnRH antagonist IVF/ICSI cycles: a prospective randomized study. Hum Reprod. 2005;20:1213–20.

41. Griesinger G, Diedrich K, Devroey P, Kolibianakis EM. GnRH agonist for triggering final oocyte maturation in the GnRH antagonist ovarian hyperstimulation protocol: A systematic review and meta-analysis. Hum Reprod Update. 2005b;12:159–68.

42. Kolibianakis EM, Schultze-Mosgau A, Schroer A, van Steirteghem A, Devroey P, Diedrich K. A lower ongoing pregnancy rate can be expected when GnRH agonist is used for triggering final oocyte maturation instead of HCG in patients undergoing IVF with GnRH antagonists. Hum Reprod. 2005b;20:2887–92.

43. Klingmuller D, Schepke M, Enzweiler C, Bidlingmaier F. Hormonal responses to the new potent GnRH antagonist Cetrorelix. Acta Endocrinol (Copenh). 1993;128:15–8.

44. Varney NR, Syrop C, Kubu CS, Struchen M, Hahn S, Franzen K. Neuropsychologic dysfunction in women following leuprolide acetate induction of hypoestrogenism. J Assist Reprod Genet. 1993;10:53–7.

45. Diedrich K, Diedrich C, Santos E, Zoll C, al-Hasani S, Reissmann T, et al. Suppression of the endogenous luteinizing hormone surge by the gonadotropin-releasing hormone antagonist Cetrorelix during ovarian stimulation. Hum Reprod. 1994;9:788–91.

46. Olivennes F, Fanchin R, Bouchard P, de Ziegler D, Taieb J, Selva J, et al. The single or dual administration of the gonadotropin-releasing hormone antagonist Cetrorelix in an in vitro fertilization-embryo transfer program. Fertil Steril. 1994;62:468–76.

47. Albano C, Smitz J, Camus M, Riethmuller-Winzen H, Van Steirteghem A and Devroey P. Comparison of different doses of gonadotropin-releasing hormone antagonist Cetrorelix during controlled ovarian hyperstimulation. Fertil Steril, 1997;67:917-22.

48. Olivennes F, Alvarez S, Bouchard P, Fanchin R, Salat-Baroux J, Frydman R. The use of a GnRH antagonist (Cetrorelix) in a single dose proto- col in IVF-embryo transfer: a dose finding study of 3 versus 2 mg. Hum Reprod. 1998;13:2411–4.

49. Olivennes F, Belaisch-Allart J, Emperaire JC, Dechaud H, Alvarez S, Moreau L, et al. Prospective, randomized, controlled study of in vitro fertilization-embryo transfer with a single dose of a luteinizing hormone-releasing hormone (LH-RH) antagonist (cetrorelix) or a depot formula of an LH-RH agonist (triptorelin). Fertil Steril. 2000;73:314–20.

50. Wilcox J, Potter D, Moore M, Ferrande L, Kelly E. Prospective, randomized trial comparing cetrorelix acetate and ganirelix acetate in a programmed, flexible protocol for premature luteinizing hormone surge prevention in assisted reproductive technologies. Fertil Steril. 2005;84:108–17.
51. Fischl F, Huber JC, Obruca A. Zeitliche optimierung der kontrolli- erten hyperstimulation (koh) in kombination mit gnrh-antagonisten und ovulationshemmer in einem ivf-programm. J Fertilität Reproduktion. 2001;11:50–1.
52. Cedrin-Durnerin I, Grange-Dujardin D, Laffy A, Parneix I, Massin N, Galey J, et al. Recombinant human LH supplementation during GnRH antagonist administration in IVF/ICSI cycles: A prospective randomized study. Hum Reprod. 2004;19:1979–84.
53. van Loenen ACD, Huirne JAF, Schats R, Donnez J, Lambalk CB. An open-label multicentre, randomized, parallel, controlled phase II study to assess the feasibility of a new programming regimen using an oral contraceptive prior to the administration of recombinant FSH and a GnRH-antagonist in patients undergoing ART (IVF-ICSI) treatment. Hum Reprod. 2001;16:144.
54. Bendikson K, Milki A, Speck-Zulak A, Westphal L. Comparison of GnRH antagonist cycles with and without oral contraceptive pill pretreatment in poor responders. Fertil Steril. 2003;80(Suppl. 3):S188.
55. Kolibianakis EM, Papanikolaou EG, Camus M, Tournaye H, Van Steirteghem AC, Devroey P. Effect of oral contraceptive pill pretreatment on ongoing pregnancy rates in patients stimulated with GnRH antagonists and recombinant FSH for IVF. A randomized controlled trial. Hum Reprod. 2006;21:352–7.
56. van Heusden AM, Fauser BC. Residual ovarian activity during oral steroid contraception. Hum Reprod Update. 2002;8:345–58.
57. Homburg R, Eshel A, Armar NA, Tucker M, Mason PW, Adams J. One hundred pregnancies after treatment with pulsatile luteinising hormone releasing hormone to induce ovula- tion. Br Med J. 1989;298:809–12.
58. Letterie GS, Coddington CC, Collins RL, Merriam GR. Ovulation induction using SC. pulsatile gonadotropin-releasing hormone: effectiveness of different pulse frequencies. Hum Reprod. 1996;11:19–22.
59. Shoham Z, Homburg R, Jacobs HS. Induction of ovulation with pulsatile GnRH. Baillières Clin Obstet Gynaecol. 1990;4:589–608.
60. Martin KA, Hall JE, Adams JM, Crowley WF Jr. Comparison of exogenous gonadotropins and pulsatile gonadotropin-releasing hormone for induction of ovulation in hypogonadotropic amenorrhea. J Clin Endocrinol Metab. 1993;77:125–9.
61. Filicori M, Flamigni C, Meriggiola MC, Ferrari P, Michelacci L, Campaniello E, et al. Endocrine response determines the clinical outcome of pulsatile gonadotropin-releasing hormone ovulation induction in different ovulatory disorders. J Clin Endocrinol Metab. 1991;72:965-72.
62. Homburg R, Insler V. Ovulation induction in perspective. Hum Reprod Update. 2002;8:449–62.
63. Hoffman D, Lobo RA. Serum dehydroepiandrosterone sulfate and the use of clomiphene citrate in anovulatory women. Fertility Sterility. 1985;43:196–9.
64. Azziz R, Black VY, Knochenhauer ES, et al. Ovulation after glucocorticoid suppression of adrenal androgens in the polycystic ovary syndrome is not predicted by the basal dehydroepiandrosterone sulfate level. Journal of Clinical Endocrinology and Metabolism. 1999;84:946–50.
65. Azziz R. Glucocorticoid suppression in the treatment of androgen excess. In: Azziz R, Nestler JE, Dewailly D (eds) Androgen Excess Disorders in Women. Lippencott Williams and Wilkins, Philadelphia, USA, 1997.pp.737–47.

66. Buyalos RP, Geffner ME, Azziz R, Judd HL. Impact of overnight dexamethasone suppression on the adrenal androgen response to an oral glucose tolerance test in women with and without polycystic ovary syndrome. Human Reproduction. 1997;12:1138–41.

67. Al Inany H, Aboulghar M, Mansour R, Proctor M. Recombinant versus urinary human chorionic gonadotropin for ovulation induction in assisted conception. Cochrane Database Syst RevCD003719, 2009.

68. Kolibianakis EM, et al. Human Reproduction, 2005;20(10):2887–92.

69. Humaidan P, et al. Human Reproduction Update, 2011;17(4):510–24.

70. Tang T, Lord JM, Norman RJ, et al. Insulin-sensitising drugs (metformin, rosiglitazone, pioglitazone, D-chiro-inositol) for women with polycystic ovary syndrome, oligo amenorrhoea and subfertility. Cochrane Database of Systematic Reviews, Issue 1. Art. No.: CD003053, 2010.

71. Stefano Palomba, Francesco Orio Jr, Angela Falbo, Tiziana Russo, Achille Tolino, Fulvio Zullo. Clomiphene Citrate Versus Metformin as First-Line Approach for the Treatment of Anovulation in Infertile Patients with Polycystic Ovary Syndrome JCEM, 2007;92:3498-3503; doi: 10.1210/jc.2007–1009.

72. Moll E, Bossuyt PM, Korevaar JC, Lambalk CB, van der Veen F. Effect of clomifene citrate plus metformin and clomifene citrate plus placebo on induction of ovulation in women with newly diagnosed polycystic ovary syndrome: randomised double blind clinical trial. BMJ 2006;332:1485.

73. Legro RS, Barnhart HX, Schlaff WD, Carr BR, Diamond MP, Carson SA, et al. Clomiphene, metformin, or both for infertility in the polycystic ovary syndrome. N Engl J Med. 2007;356:551–66.

74. The Thessaloniki ESHRE/ASRM-Sponsored PCOS Consensus Workshop Group Consensus on infertility treatment related to polycystic ovary syndromeHum. Reprod, 2008;23(6):1474/Fertil Steril. 89(3):505–22.

75. Johnson NP, Stewart AW, Falkiner J, Farquhar CM, Milsom S, Singh VP, Okonkwo QL, Buckingham KL and on behalf of REACT-NZ (Reproduction And Collaborative Trials in New Zealand), a multi-centre fertility trials group PCOSMIC: A multi-centre randomized trial in women with PolyCystic Ovary Syndrome evaluating Metformin for Infertility with Clomiphene. Hum. Reprod. 2010;25(7):1675–83.

76. Yarali H, Yildiz BO, Demirol A, et al. Co-administration of metformin during rFSH treatment in patients with clomiphene citrate-resistant polycystic ovarian syndrome: a prospective randomized trial. Hum. Reprod. 2002;17:289–94.

77. Bassil S, Godin PA, Donnez J. Outcome on in-vitro fertilization through natural cycles in poor responders. Human Reprod. 1999;14:1262–5.

78. Feldman B, Seidman DS, Levron J, Bider D, Shulman A, Shine S, et al. In vitro fertilization following natural cycles in poor responders. Gynecol Endocrinol. 2001;15:328–34.

79. Kolibianakis E, Zikopoulos K, Camus M, Tounaye H, Van Steirteghem A, Devroey P. Modified natural cycle for IVF does not offer a realistic chance of parenthood in poor responders with high day 3 FSH levels, as a last resort prior to oocyte donation. Hum Reprod. 2004;19:2545–9.

80. Morgia F, Sbracia M, Schimberni M, Giallonardo A, Piscitelli C, Giannini P, et al. A controlled trial of natural cycle versus microdose gonadotropin-releasing hormone analog flare cycles in poor responders undergoing in vitro fertilization. Fertil Steril. 2004;81:1542–7.

81. Ubaldi FM, Rienzi L, Ferrero S, et al. Management of poor responders in IVF. Reproductive BioMedicine Online. 2005;10:23.

82. Li Y, Feng H-L, CaoY-J, Zheng G-J, Yang Y, Mullen S, et al. Confocal microscopic analysis of the spindle and chromosome configurations of human oocytes matured in vitro. Fertil Steril. 2006;85:827–32.

83. Mullen SF, Agca Y, Broermann DC, Jenkins CL, Johnson CA, Critser JK. The effect of osmotic stress on the metaphase II spindle of human oocytes, and the relevance to cryopreservation. Hum Reprod. 2004;19:1148–54.

84. Zenzes MT, Bielecki R, Casper RF, Leibo SP. Effects of chilling to 0 degrees C on the morphology of meiotic spindles in human metaphase II oocytes. Fertil Steril. 2001;75:769–77.

85. Pickering SJ, Braude PR, Johnson MH, Cant A, Currie J. Transient cooling to room temperature can cause irreversible disruption of the meiotic spindle in the human oocyte. Fertil Steril. 1990;54:102–8.

86. Wang WH, Meng L, Hackett RJ, Oldenbourg R, Keefe DL. Rigorous thermal control during intracytoplasmic sperm injection stabilizes the meiotic spindle and improves fertilization and pregnancy rates. Fertil Steril. 2002;77:1274–7.

87. Wang WH, Keefe DL. Predictions of chromosome alignment among in vitro matured human oocytes by spindle imaging with the Polscope. Fertil Steril. 2002;78:1077–81.

88. Moon JH, Jee BC, Ku SY, Suh CS, Kim SH, Choi YM, et al. Spindle positions and their distributions in in vivo and in vitro matured mouse oocytes. Hum Reprod. 2005;20:2207–10.

89. Trounson A, Wood C, Kausche A. In vitro maturation and the fertilization and developmental competence of oocytes recovered from untreated polycystic ovarian patients. Fertil Steril. 1994;62:353–62.

90. Cha KY, Chian RC. Maturation in vitro of immature human oocytes for clinical use. Hum Reprod Update. 1998;4:103–20.

91. Barnes FL, Kausche A, Tiglias J, Wood C, Wilton L, Trounson A. Production of embryos from in vitro matured primary human oocytes. Fertil Steril. 1996;65:1151–6.

92. Child TJ, Phillips SJ, Abdul-Jalil AK, Gulekli B, Tan SL. A comparison of in vitro maturation and in vitro fertilization for women with polycystic ovaries. Obstet Gynecol. 2002;100:665–70.

93. Le Du A, Kadoch IJ, Bourcigaux N, Doumerc S, Bourrier MC, Chevalier N, et al. In vitro oocyte maturation for the treatment of infertility associated with polycystic ovarian syndrome: the French experience. Hum Reprod. 2005;20:420–4.

94. Chian RC, Buckett WM, Tulandi T, Tan SL. Prospective randomized study of human chorionic gonadotropin priming before immature oocyte retrieval from unstimulated women with polycystic ovarian syndrome. Hum Reprod. 2000;15:165–70.

95. Russell JB, Knezevich KM, Fabian KF, Dickson JA. Unstimulated immature oocyte retrieval: early versus midfollicular endometrial priming. Fertil Steril. 1997;67:616–20.

96. Moor RM, Dai Y, Lee C, Fulka J Jr. Oocyte maturation and embryonic failure. Hum Reprod Update. 1998;4:223–36.

97. Son WY, Chung JT, Chian RC, Herrero B, Demirtas E, Elizur S, et al. A 38- hour interval between hCG priming and oocyte retrieval increases in vivo and in vitro oocyte maturation rate in programmed IVM cycles. Hum Reprod. 2008;23:2010–6.

98. Mikkelsen AL, Smith SD, Lindenberg S. In-vitro maturation of human oocytes from regularly menstruating women may be successful without follicle stimulating hormone priming. Hum Reprod. 1999;14:1847–51.

99. Shu-Chi M, Jiann-Loung H, Yu-Hung L, Tseng-Chen S, Ming-I L, Tsu-Fuh Y. Growth and development of children conceived by in-vitro maturation of human oocytes. Early Hum Dev. 2006;82:677–82.

100. Buckett WM, Chian RC, Holzer H, Dean N, Usher R, Tan SL. Obstetric outcomes and congenital abnormalities after in vitro maturation, in vitro fertilization, and intracytoplasmic sperm injection. Obstet Gynecol. 2007;110:885–91.

Third Party Reproduction

6

Chapter

Duru Shah, Anita Soni, Seeru Garg

Introduction

> *The Parents construct the Child biologically,*
> *While the Child constructs the Parents socially.*
>
> *But*
>
> *"Just because we can do this doesn't mean we should."[1]*

What modern science has wrought is an increasingly complex and intentionally non-traditional definition of family. As Liza Mundy comments in her investigative report *Everything Conceivable*, "science has given us something new: families that are designed, from the start, to have only a single parent; to have quite a few parents; to have two parents, only one of whom is biologically related to the child, the other of whom is biologically unrelated, with a third party out there who is biologically related but, often, unknown. Families with these qualities have spontaneously arisen in the past, and still do, of course [by war, adultery, epidemics, childbed fever, remarriage, slavery, stepparents, social upheaval, and shifts in gender roles], but now they are being consciously formed."[2]

Third party reproduction refers to the use of eggs, sperm, or embryos that have been donated by a third person (donor) to enable an infertile individual or couple (intended recipient) to become parents. Donors may be known or anonymous to the intended recipient. "Third party reproduction" also includes traditional surrogacy and gestational carrier arrangements.[3]

Third party reproduction is a complex process requiring consideration of social, ethical, and legal issues. The increased utilization of egg donation has required a reconsideration of the social and ethical impact this technology has had on prospective parents, their offspring, and the egg donors themselves. Surrogacy has been acknowledged within the reproductive medicine community in India as well as by the American Society for Reproductive Medicine (ASRM).

There are no detailed figures of the extent of infertility prevalent in India but a multinational study carried out by WHO that included India, places the incidence of infertility between 10 and 15%. Out of a population of 1000 million Indians, an estimated 25% (250 million individuals) may be conservatively estimated to be attempting parenthood at any given time; by extrapolating the WHO estimate, approximately 13 to 19 million couples are likely to be infertile in the country at any given time.

Important Definitions

Surrogacy: It is a method of assisted reproduction in which a woman carries a pregnancy and gives birth to a baby for another woman. It is gaining popularity as it may be the only method for a couple to have their own child.

Surrogate or Surrogate mother: The word surrogate is derived from the Latin *subrŏg are* and simply means 'to substitute'. Surrogate pregnancy (the practice of which is generally referred to as is a form of assisted conception, and is defined as the practice whereby one woman (the surrogate mother) carries a child for another person(s) (the commissioning couple) as the result of an agreement prior to conception that the child should be handed over to that person after birth.[4]

Traditional or partial surrogacy: Here surrogate is the genetic mother (straight surrogacy) i.e. surrogacy using her own egg and she is inseminated with sperm from the male partner of intended parent couple. The implanted embryo could also result from anonymous donor insemination. The child that results is genetically related to the surrogate and the male partner but not the female partner.

Gestational surrogacy: Surrogate has a fertilized embryo (created by egg and sperm of intended parents) by using in vitro fertilization (IVF)techniques implanted in her womb by embryo transfer ('host' or 'full' surrogacy).[4] the child is not genetically linked to the surrogate.

Gestational carrier (GC) or Gestational surrogate: The surrogate who has no genetic relationship with the fetus.

Commercial Surrogacy: Commercial surrogacy is a form of surrogacy in which a gestational carrier is paid to carry a child to maturity in her womb and is usually resorted to by higher income infertile couples who can afford the cost involved or people who save or borrow in order to complete their dream of being parents. Commercial surrogacy is also known as 'wombs for rent', outsourced pregnancies or baby farms.

Altruistic Surrogacy: Altruistic surrogacy is a situation where the surrogate receives no financial reward for her pregnancy or the relinquishment of the child (although usually all expenses related to the pregnancy and birth are paid by the intended parents such as medical expenses, maternity clothing, accommodation, diet and other related expenses).

The Intended Parents (IPs) or The Commissioning couple: The commissioning couple are the people (or in some cases, person) who wish to bring up the child after his or her birth. They may both be the genetic parents (gestational surrogacy), or one of them may be, or neither of them may be genetically related to the child. The woman for whom the child is to be carried (the commissioning mother) may be the genetic mother in that she provides the egg. The genetic father may be the husband or partner of the commissioning mother or he may be an anonymous donor.[4] Any reproduction involving three or more parties is termed "collaborative reproduction." To complicate this "collaboration" further, there may be more than three parties involved in "parenting" a desired child. The IP(s) may provide all or none of the gametes that make up the embryo. In an extreme case, the IP(s) may choose a male donor to provide sperm, a female donor to provide eggs, and a GC to carry and deliver the child. This type of reproductive "collaboration" thus includes five potential "parents."

It is likely that surrogacy has been used through the ages to help women who are unable to have children themselves to have families, but no specific incidences are recorded in the medical history texts. Until the introduction of modern assisted reproductive techniques, traditional or partial surrogacy was the only means of helping women who had no uterus or major abnormalities of the uterus to have children. Then, artificial insemination, either intracervical or intrauterine, was used to inseminate surrogate hosts with the semen of the male partner of the couple wishing to have the child; this being more socially acceptable than by the 'natural way'.

Historical Context

Despite the instinct to classify surrogacy as a modern issue, the practice of surrogacy is alluded to in the Bible. The following quote is taken from the book of Genesis: 'Abram's wife Sarah said "the Lord has restrained me from bearing children. Please go to my maid; perhaps I shall obtain children by her." Hagar bore Abrahm a son'. In chapter 30 of book of Genesis Isaac and his infertile wife Rachel, ask the same of their maid Bilbah.

The first ever report of a baby being born following treatment by gestational surrogacy was from the US.[5] The largest experience of both partial and gestational surrogacy is in the US, where commercial surrogacy arrangements are allowed.

In the UK, one of the few countries in Europe that allows surrogacy,[6] there was a great deal of controversy following the birth of a child in 1985 in a partial surrogacy arrangement and legislation was rapidly passed to limit but not ban the practice (Surrogacy Arrangements Act, 1985).[7] Under this law, commercial surrogacy arrangements were made illegal. The Human Fertilization and Embryology Act[8] was passed in the UK Parliament in 1990 and surrogacy was not banned. The most recent report from the British Medical Association (1996)[9] states: 'Surrogacy is an acceptable option of last resort in cases where it is impossible or highly undesirable for medical reasons for the intended mother to carry a child herself' Mr Patrick Steptoe and Professor Robert Edwards treated the first couple to request treatment by gestational surrogacy in Europe at Bourn Hall Clinic after extensive discussion. The treatment was initiated, their host became pregnant and a child was born to them in 1989.[10]

The roots of surrogacy can be traced long back in Indian history. The field of assisted reproductive technology (ART) has developed rapidly in India. There are an estimated 250 IVF clinics in India today.

There are still relatively few publications in the literature of experience with gestational surrogacy; the majority of them come from the US.[5, 11] There have also been very few long-term follow-up studies of the babies or the couples involved in surrogacy arrangements.[12]A few follow-up studies on the children, hosts and commissioning couples have been published, all of which show reassuring data and positive outcomes.[11, 13]

Reproductive Tourism in India

Increasingly common is a type of "reproductive tourism" in which relatively wealthy infertile couples send their embryos to be gestated by foreign women for a fraction of the cost of this practice in the United States.[14] India is currently the favored location for this practice, as surrogacy is legal with acceptable guidelines (surrogacy is not legal in many countries). There is easy availability of gestational carriers and very well equipped ART (Artificial reproductive technology) clinics, some have arisen specifically to cater to this "reproductive tourism".

India's surrogacy journey began in 2002 with the Supreme Court of India recognizing surrogacy as legal. India has a robust fertility tourism industry which started in 2005. For the childless gay couples, India provides a legally hassle-free means of achieving parenthood through surrogacy. At present the agreement between the parties based on the ICMR Guidelines are the guiding force. With the recent growth in the intended parents opting for surrogacy here, India has become the much sought after surrogacy destination. With the acceptance of same sex marriages/union and the recognition of the basic human right to have family and children has given rise to surrogacy manifold. However, at the same time nations all across the globe are condemning commercial surrogacy as it results in commercialization of human reproductive system and co-modification of children. For its various socio-ethical reasons, surrogacy has become a topic of deep interest amongst the government of different nations, medico-legal luminaries as well as public at large.

The intended parents (commissioning couple) generally seek a surrogacy arrangement because of:

- Infertility: Female infertility, absent uterus or other medical issues, which may make the pregnancy or delivery risky.
- The intended mother could also be fertile and healthy, and prefer the convenience of someone else undergoing pregnancy and labor for her.
- Same sex couple: Surrogacy can help the same sex couples realize their dream of having their own child which is otherwise not possible for them to have a child of their own by natural way.
- Single parent (man or woman): For those who want to fulfill their desire of having a child without a partner, surrogacy is a ray of hope.

Advantages of Surrogacy in India

- As mentioned earlier, the cost of surrogacy in India is merely a fraction of the cost of surrogacy in the developed countries, such as the US.
- The surrogate mothers in India are healthy females with their own families.
- Indian hospitals that offer surrogacy employ good medical practices for the surrogacy process.
- Reputable surrogacy clinics in India are equipped with the latest technology.
- The surrogate mothers in India are chosen after a rigid screening that also includes a thorough medical screening.
- Under the guidelines issued by the Indian Council of Medical Research, surrogate mothers sign away their rights to any children.
- The guidelines in India give utmost importance to the privacy of the couple that wishes to have a surrogate baby in India.

Surrogacy and Law

In the US, the majority of problems arising out of surrogacy have been associated with natural surrogacy. The earliest major case was known as the `Baby M case' in New Jersey in 1988 in which the judge decided that the genetic couple would have precedence for custody of the child over the birth mother.[6] Because of such risks, most collaborative reproductive arrangements now preclude such traditional surrogacy, and most clinics and agencies do not provide these services. Like the US, Australia has different regulations in different states. The only countries in Europe which allow surrogacy are the UK, Belgium, Holland and Finland.[6]

In the UK, treatment by gestational surrogacy is already fully regulated. Because the creation of embryos is involved, it can only be practised in centers licensed by the HFEA. Treatment cannot take place outside of the legal cover provided by the Human Fertilisation and Embryology Act (1990).

In India, there are no surrogacy laws but India follows the ICMR guidelines for surrogacy. Assisted reproductive technology has enabled both partners in a relationship to use their own gametes to create their own unique embryos and for these embryos to be transferred to a surrogate host. This has meant that, although the female partner of the couple wanting the child may have no uterus, she is able to have her own genetic child or children. Since most couples want their own genetic children, 'IVF surrogacy' has become an accepted treatment option for women in certain countries with these unique circumstances. The penalty paid, however, is that the sophistication of the treatment is very much greater than it is for 'partial surrogacy' and therefore the degree of commitment and the costs are very much higher.

In India, ICMR (Indian Council of Medical research) guidelines for ART clinics are followed for third party reproduction.[15]

Clinics which should be Registered

Clinics involved in any one of the following activities should be regulated, registered and supervised by the State Accreditation Authority/State Appropriate Authorities

1. Any treatment involving the use of gametes which have been donated or collected or processed *in vitro, except for* AIH (artificial insemination by husband's semen), and for IUI by Level 1A clinics that will not process the gametes themselves.
2. Any infertility treatment that involves the use and creation of embryos outside the body.
3. The processing or /and storage of gametes or embryos.
4. Research on human embryos.

The term ART clinic used in this document refers to a clinic involved in any one of the first three of the above activities.

Responsibilities of the Clinic

- To give adequate information to the patients.
- To explain to the patient the rationale of choosing a particular treatment and indicate the choices the patient has (including the cheapest possible course of treatment), with advantages and disadvantages of each choice. To help the patient exercise a choice, which may be best for him/her, taking into account the individual's circumstances.
- To maintain records in an appropriate Performa (to be prescribed by the authority) to enable collation by a national body.
- When commercial DNA fingerprinting becomes available, to keep on its record, if the ART clinic desires and couple agrees, DNA fingerprints of the donor, the child, the couple and the surrogate mother should be done.
- To keep all information about donors, recipients and couples confidential and secure. The information about the donor (including a copy of the donor's DNA fingerprint if available, but excluding information on the name and address—that is, the individual's personal identity) should be released by the ART clinic after appropriate identification, only to the offspring and only if asked by him/her after he/she reaches the age of 18 years, or as and when specified and required for legal purposes, and never to the parents (excepting when directed by a court of law).
- To maintain appropriate, detailed record of all donor oocytes, sperm or embryos used; the manner of their use (e.g. the technique in which they are used, and the individual/couple/surrogate mother on whom they are used). These records must be maintained for at least ten years after which the records must be transferred to a central depository to be maintained by the ICMR. If the ART clinic/center is wound up during this period, the records must be transferred to the central repository in the ICMR.
- To have the schedule of all its charges suitably displayed in the clinic and made known to the patient at the beginning of the treatment. There must be no extra charges beyond what was intimated to the patient at the beginning of the treatment.
- To ensure that no technique is used on a patient for which demonstrated expertise does not exist with the staff of the clinic.

- To be totally transparent in all its operations. The ART clinics must, therefore, let the patient know what the success rates of the clinic are in regard to the procedures intended to be used on the patient.
- To have all consent forms available in English and local language(s).

Information and Counseling to be given to Patients

- Information must be given to couples seeking treatment, on the following points:
- The basis, limitations and possible outcome of the treatment proposed, variations in its effectiveness over time, including the success rates with the recommended treatments obtained in the clinic as well as around the world (this data should be available as a document with references, and updated every 6 – 12 months).
- The possible side-effects (e.g. of the drug used) and the risks of treatment to the women and the resulting child, including (where relevant) the risks associated with multiple pregnancy.
- The need to reduce the number of viable fetuses, in order to ensure the survival of at least two fetuses. Possible disruption of the patient's domestic life which the treatment may cause.
- The techniques involved, including (where relevant) the possible deterioration of gametes or embryos associated with storage, and possible pain and discomfort.
- The cost (with suitable break-up) to the patient of the treatment proposed and of an alternative treatment, if any (there must be no other "hidden costs").
- The importance of informing the clinic of the result of the pregnancy in a pre-paid envelope.
- To make the couple aware, if relevant, that a child born through ART has a right to seek information (including a copy of the DNA fingerprint, if available) about his genetic parent/surrogate mother on reaching 18 years, excepting information on the name and address—that is, the individual's personal identity—of the gamete donor or the surrogate mother. The couple is not obliged to provide the information to which the child has a right, on their own to the child when he/ she reaches the age of 18, but no attempt must be made by the couple to hide this information from the child if occasion arises when this issue becomes important for the child.
- The advantages and disadvantages of continuing treatment after a certain number of attempts.
- Pamphlets (one-page on each technique in all local languages and English) which give clear, precise and honest information about the procedure recommended to be used will help the couple make an informed choice.

Desirable Practices/Prohibited Scenarios

- A third party donor of sperm or oocytes must be informed that the offspring will not know his/her identity. There would be no bar to the use of ART by single woman who wishes to have a child, and no ART clinic may refuse to offer its services to the above, provided other criteria mentioned in this document are satisfied.

- The child thus born will have all the legal rights on the woman or the man.
- The ART clinic must not be a party to any commercial element in donor programs or in gestational surrogacy.
- A surrogate mother carrying a child biologically unrelated to her must register as a patient in her own name. While registering, she must mention that she is a surrogate mother and provide all the necessary information about the genetic parents such as names, addresses, etc. She must not use /register in the name of the person for whom she is carrying the child, as this would pose legal issues, particularly in the untoward event of maternal death (in whose names will the hospital certify this death?).
- The birth certificate shall be in the name of the genetic parents. The clinic, however, must also provide a certificate to the genetic parents giving the name and address of the surrogate mother. All the expenses of the surrogate mother during the period of pregnancy and post-natal care relating to pregnancy should be borne by the couple seeking surrogacy. The surrogate mother would also be entitled to a monetary compensation from the couple for agreeing to act as a surrogate; the exact value of this compensation should be decided by discussion between the couple and the proposed surrogate mother. An oocyte donor cannot act as a surrogate mother for the couple to whom the ecotype is being donated.
- A third-party donor and a surrogate mother must relinquish in writing all parental rights concerning the offspring and vice versa.
- No ART procedure shall be done without the spouse's consent. The provision or otherwise of AIH or ART to an HIV-positive woman would be governed by the implications of the decision of the Supreme Court in the case of X – vs. – Hospital 2 (1998) Sec. 269 or any other relevant judgement of the Supreme Court, or law of the country, whichever is the latest. Gametes produced by a person under the age of 21 shall not be used.
- The accepted age for a sperm donor shall be between 21 and 45 years and for the donor woman between 18 and 35 years.
- Sex selection at any stage after fertilization, or abortion of fetus of any particular sex should not be permitted, except to avoid the risk of transmission of a genetic abnormality assessed through genetic testing of biological parents or through preimplantation genetic diagnosis (PGD).
- No ART clinic shall offer to provide a couple with a child of the desired sex.
- Collection of gametes from a dying person will only be permitted if the widow wishes to have a child.
- No more than three eggs or embryos should be placed in a woman during any one treatment cycle, regardless of the procedure used, excepting under exceptional circumstances {such as elderly women (above 37 years), poor implantation (more than three previous failures), advanced endometriosis, or poor embryo quality} which should be recorded.
- Use of sperm donated by a relative or a known friend of either the wife or the husband shall not be permitted. It will be the responsibility of the ART clinic to obtain sperm from appropriate banks; neither the clinic nor the couple shall

have the right to know the donor identity and address, but both the clinic and the couple, however, shall have the right to have the fullest possible information from the semen bank on the donor such as height, weight, skin color, educational qualification, profession, family background, freedom from any known diseases or carrier status (such as hepatitis B or AIDS), ethnic origin, and the DNA fingerprint (if possible), before accepting the donor semen. It will be the responsibility of the semen bank and the clinic to ensure that the couple does not come to know the identity of the donor. The ART clinic will be authorized to appropriately charge the couple for the semen provided and the tests done on the donor semen.

- What has been said above also would be true of oocyte donation.
- When DNA fingerprinting technology becomes commercially available, the ART clinic may offer to the couple, a DNA fingerprint of the donor without revealing his/her identity, against appropriate payment towards the cost of the DNA fingerprint. An ART clinic will then have DNA fingerprinting done of the couple and keep the DNA fingerprints on its records.
- Trans-species fertilization involving gametes of two species is prohibited.
- Ova derived from fetuses cannot be used for IVF but may be used for research.
- Semen from two individuals must never be mixed before use, under any circumstance.
- Transfer of human embryo into a human male or into any animal belonging to any other species, must never be done and is prohibited.
- The data of every accredited ART clinic must be accessible to an appropriate authority of the ICMR for collation at the national level.
- Any publication or report resulting out of analysis of such data by the ICMR will have the concerned members of the staff of the ART clinic as co-authors.
- The consent on the consent form must be a true informed consent witnessed by a person who is in no way associated with the clinic.

Requirements for a Sperm Donor

1. The individual must be free of HIV and hepatitis B and C infections, hypertension, diabetes, sexually transmitted diseases, and identifiable and common genetic disorders such as thalassemia.
2. The age of the donor must not be below 21 or above 45 years.
3. An analysis must be carried out on the semen of the individual, preferably using a semen analyzer, and the semen must be found to be normal according to WHO method manual for semen analysis, if intended to be used for ART.
4. The blood group and the Rh status of the individual must be determined and placed on record.

Other relevant information in respect of the donor, such as height, weight, age, educational qualifications, profession, color of the skin and the eyes, record of major diseases including any psychiatric disorder, and the family background in respect of history of any familial disorder, must be recorded in an appropriate Performa.

Requirements for an Oocyte Donor

1. The individual must be free of HIV and hepatitis B and C infections, hypertension, diabetes, sexually transmitted diseases, and identifiable and common genetic disorders such as thalassemia.
2. The blood group and the Rh status of the individual must be determined and placed on record.
3. Other relevant information in respect of the donor, such as height, weight, age, educational qualifications, profession, color of the skin and the eyes, and the family background in respect of history of any familial disorder, must be recorded in an appropriatePerforma.
4. Age of donor must not be less than 21 or more than 35 years.

How may Sperm and Oocyte Donors and Surrogate Mothers be Sourced?

1. Semen banks
- Either an ART clinic or a law firm or any other suitable independent organization may set up a semen bank. If set up by an ART clinic, it must operate as a separate identity.
- The bank will ensure that all criteria mentioned (requirements for a sperm donor) are met and a suitable record of all donors is kept for 10 years after which, or if the bank is wound up during this period, the records shall be transferred to an ICMR repository.
- A bank may advertise suitably for semen donors who may be appropriately compensated financially.
- On request for semen by an ART clinic, the bank will provide the clinic with a list of donors (without the name or the address but with a code number) giving all relevant details. The semen bank shall not supply semen of one donor for more than ten successful pregnancies. It will be the responsibility of the ART clinic or the patient, as appropriate, to inform the bank about a successful pregnancy. The bank shall keep a record of all semen received, stored and supplied, and details of the use of the semen of each donor. This record will be liable to be reviewed by the accreditation authority.
- The bank must be run professionally and must have facilities for cryopreservation of semen, following internationally accepted protocols. Each bank will prepare its own Standard Operating Procedures (SOP) for cryopreservation.
- Semen samples must be cryopreserved for at least six months before first use, at which time the semen donor must be tested for HIV and hepatitis B and C.
- The bank must ensure confidentiality in regard to the identity of the semen donor.
- A semen bank may store a semen preparation for exclusive use on the donor's wife or on any other woman designated by the donor. An appropriate charge may be levied by the bank for the storage. In the case of non-payment of the charges when the donor is alive, the bank would have the right to destroy the

semen sample or give it to a bonafide organisation to be used only for research purposes. In the case of the death of the donor, the semen would become the property of the legal heir or the nominee of the donor at the time the donor gives the sample for storage to the bank. All other conditions that apply to the donor would now apply to the legal heir, excepting that he cannot use it for having a woman of his choice inseminated by it. If after the death of the donor, there are no claimants, the bank would have the right to destroy the semen or give it to a bonafide research organisation to be used only for research purposes.

- All semen banks will require accreditation.

2. **Sourcing of oocytes and surrogate mothers**

Law firms and semen banks will be encouraged to obtain (for example, through appropriate advertisement) and maintain information on possible oocyte donors and surrogate mothers as per details mentioned elsewhere in this document.

The above organizations may appropriately charge the couple for providing an oocyte or a surrogate mother. The oocyte donor may be compensated suitably (e.g. financially) by the law firm or semen bank when the oocyte is donated.

However, negotiations between a couple and the surrogate mother must be conducted independently between them.

3. **Oocyte sharing**

The system of oocyte sharing in which an indigent infertile couple that needs to raise resources for ART agrees to donate oocytes to an affluent infertile couple wherein the wife can carry a pregnancy through but cannot produce her own oocyte, for in-vitro fertilization with the sperm of the male partner of the affluent couple, for a monitory compensation that would take care of the expenses of an ART procedure on the indigent couple, must be encouraged.

Surrogacy: General Considerations

1. A child born through surrogacy must be adopted by the genetic (biological) parents unless they can establish through genetic (DNA) fingerprinting (of which the records will be maintained in the clinic) that the child is theirs.
2. Surrogacy by assisted conception should normally be considered only for patients for whom it would be physically or medically impossible/ undesirable to carry a baby to term.
3. Payments to surrogate mothers should cover all genuine expenses associated with the pregnancy. Documentary evidence of the financial arrangement for surrogacy must be available. The ART center should not be involved in this monetary aspect.
4. Advertisements regarding surrogacy should not be made by the ART clinic. The responsibility of finding a surrogate mother, through advertisement or otherwise, should rest with the couple, or a semen bank.
5. A surrogate mother should not be over 45 years of age. Before accepting a woman as a possible surrogate for a particular couple's child, the ART clinic must ensure (and put on record) that the woman satisfies all the testable criteria to go through a successful full-term pregnancy.

6. A relative, a known person, as well as a person unknown to the couple may act as a surrogate mother for the couple. In the case of a relative acting as a surrogate, the relative should belong to the same generation as the women desiring the surrogate.
7. A prospective surrogate mother must be tested for HIV and shown to be sero negative for this virus just before embryo transfer. She must also provide a written certificate that (a) she has not had a drug intravenously administered into her through a shared syringe, (b) she has not undergone blood transfusion; and (c) she and her husband (to the best of her/his knowledge) has had no extramarital relationship in the last six months.
   (This is to ensure that the person would not come up with symptoms of HIV infection during the period of surrogacy.) The prospective surrogate mother must also declare that she will not use drugs intravenously, and not undergo blood transfusion excepting of blood obtained through a certified blood bank.
8. No woman may act as a surrogate more than thrice in her lifetime.

Preservation, Utilization and Destruction of Embryos

1. Couples must give specific consent to storage and use of their embryos.
   The Human Fertilisation & Embryology Act, UK (1990), allows a 5- year storage period which India would also follow.
2. Consent shall need to be taken from the couple for the use of their stored embryos by other couples or for research, in the event of their embryos not being used by themselves. This consent will not be required if the couple defaults in payment of maintenance charges after two reminders sent by registered post.
3. Research on embryos shall be restricted to the first fourteen days only and will be conducted only with the permission of the owner of the embryos.
4. No commercial transaction will be allowed for the use of embryos for research.

Rights of a Child Born through Various ART Technologies

1. A child born through ART shall be presumed to be the legitimate child of the couple, having been born in wedlock and with the consent of both the spouses. Therefore, the child shall have a legal right to parental support, inheritance, and all other privileges of a child born to a couple through sexual intercourse.
2. Children born through the use of donor gametes and their "adopted" parents shall have a right to available medical or genetic information about the genetic parents that may be relevant to the child's health.
3. Children born through the use of donor gametes shall not have any right whatsoever to know the identity (such as name, address, parentage, etc.) of their genetic parent(s). A child thus born will, however, be provided all other information about the donor as and when desired by the child, when the child becomes an adult. While the couple will not be obliged to provide the above "other" information to the child on their own, no deliberate attempt will be made by the couple or others concerned to hide this information from the child as and when asked for by the child.

4. In the case of a divorce during the gestation period, if the offspring is of a donor program – be it sperm or ova – the law of the land as pertaining to a normal conception would apply.

Responsibilities of the Drug Industry

1. Drug companies must not make exaggerated claims for infertility drugs and market them only to qualified specialists. All available information on the drug must be provided to the specialist.
2. Infertility drugs must be sold only on prescription by a qualified doctor/ ART specialist.
3. There has been a spurt of new media introduced for in vitro culture of gametes and embryos. Companies dealing with culture media do not give full details of the composition because they wish to retain this as a trade secret. This poses problems for those dealing with human embryos.

The future life of the products created in the laboratory is dependant, to a certain extent, on the culture media used. ART centers should not encourage companies that do not give details of the full composition of the culture media. This will also make it possible to take legal action against a company supplying something different from what it is stated to be.

General Considerations

1. **Minimum age for ART:** For a woman between 20 and 30 years, two years of cohabitation/ marriage without the use of a contraceptive, excepting in cases where the man is infertile or the woman cannot physiologically conceive. For a woman over 30 years, one year of cohabitation/marriage without use of contraceptives. Normally, no ART procedure shall be used on a woman below 20 years.
2. **Advertisements of an infertility center:** False claims via hoardings and paper advertisements are a cheap way of attracting a clientele that is vulnerable and, therefore, easily swayed. Such advertisements shall be banned. An honest display at appropriate places or publicity of statistics, fee structure, quality of service and of service provided, will be encouraged, provided the guidelines lay down by the Medical Council of India in this regard, are not violated.
3. As already mentioned, sperm banks where a complete assessment of the donor has been done, medical and other vital information stored, quality of preservation ensured, confidentiality assured, and strict control exercised by a regulatory body, must be set up. Donor sperm would be made available only through such specialized banks/centers.
4. In the light of a recent technological breakthrough where a fertilized ovum containing ooplasm (including mitochondria) from a donor ovum has been successfully cultured, the embryo or the future child may now have three genetic parents. In such cases, the ooplasm donor must sign a waiver relinquishing all rights on the child, and must be screened for and declared free of known mitochondrial genetic abnormalities.

5. No new ART clinic may start operating unless it has obtained a temporary registration to do so. This registration would be confirmed only if the clinic obtains accreditation (permanent registration) from the Center or State's appropriate accreditation authority within two years of obtaining the temporary registration. The registration must be renewed every seven years.
6. Existing ART clinics must obtain a temporary registration within six months of the notification of the accreditation authority, and appropriate accreditation (permanent registration) within two years of the notification.
7. The Center/State Government would close down any unregistered clinic not satisfying the above criteria.
8. If the ART clinic that has applied for a temporary registration to the appropriate accreditation authority, does not receive the registration (or a reply) within two months of the receipt of the application from the concerned office of the authority, the ART clinic would be deemed to have received the registration. The same would apply for the permanent registration after the above-prescribed period.
9. The technique of ICSI has never undergone critical testing in animal models, but was introduced into the human situation directly. Defects in spermatogenesis and sperm production can be often traced to genetic defects. Such individuals are normally prevented from transmitting these defects to their offspring because of their natural infertility. ICSI by-passes this barrier and may help in transmitting such defects to the offspring, which sometimes may be exaggerated in the offspring. In view of this, the ART clinic must point out to the prospective parents that their child born through ICSI may have a slightly higher risk over and above the normal risk, of suffering from a genetic disorder.
10. Human cloning for delivering replicas must be banned.
11. Stem cell cloning and research on embryos (less than 15 days old) needs to be encouraged.
12. All the equipments/machines should be calibrated regularly.

Responsibilities of the Accreditation Authority

A State Accreditation Authority will be set up by the State Government through its Department of Health and/or Family Welfare to oversee all policy matters relating to Accreditation, Supervision and Regulation of ART Clinics in the States in accordance with the National Guidelines. The State Government may also set up appropriate authorities for implementation of the Guidelines for the whole or a part of State having regard to the number of the ART Clinics. The appropriate authority would have right to visit individually or collectively, any ART Clinic/Center(s) accredited or not accredited, once a year with or without prior information to the clinic/center, to determine if the ethical guidelines and operative procedures mentioned here are being followed. If not, the appropriate authority will point out the lapses to the clinic/center in writing. If these lapses continued for a maximum period of six months (during which period the clinic shall not engage in any activity related to the lapses), the appropriate authority would recommend to the State Accreditation Authority that the clinic/center may be ordered to be closed.

The State Accreditation Authority will have the powers to order the closing of such a clinic or a center. The appropriate authority may be delegated powers to impose a fine or a penalty on the center/clinic. The above-mentioned appropriate authority would consist of appropriately qualified scientists, technologists and sociologists. The appropriate authority will also be authorized to visit and regulate semen banks in the manner mentioned above. In addition to the above, the Ministry of Health and Family Welfare, Govt. of India, will set up a National Advisory Committee. The National Advisory Committee may be headed by the Secretary, Health and Family Welfare as chairman and the Director General of ICMR as cochairman.

The National Advisory Committee will advise the Central Government on policy matters relating to regulation of ART clinics. The State Accreditation Authority will have the rights and the responsibility of fixing the upper limit of charges for gamete donation and surrogacy and of revising these charges from time to time.

Legal Issues

1. A child born through ART shall be presumed to be the legitimate child of the couple, born within wedlock, with consent of both the spouses, and with all the attendant rights of parentage, support and inheritance. Sperm/oocyte donors shall have no parental right or duties in relation to the child and their anonymity shall be protected.

2. **Adultery in the case of ART:** ART used for married woman with the consent of the husband does not amount to adultery on part of the wife or the donor. Aid without the husband's consent can, however, be a ground for divorce or judicial separation.

3. **Consummation of marriage in case of AIH:** Conception of the wife through AIH does not necessarily amount to consummation of marriage and a decree of nullity may still be granted in favor of the wife on the ground of impotency of the husband or his willful refusal to consummate the marriage. However, such a decree could be excluded on the grounds of approbation.

4. **Rights of an unmarried woman to AID:** There is no legal bar on an unmarried woman going for AID (artificial insemination with donor semen). A child born to a single woman through AID would be deemed to be legitimate. However, AID should normally be performed only on a married woman and that, too, with the written consent of her husband, as a two-parent family would be always better for the child than a single parent one, and the child's interests must outweigh all other interests.

5. **Posthumous AIH through a sperm bank:** Though the Indian Evidence Act, 1872, says that a child born within 280 days after dissolution of marriage (by death or divorce) is a legitimate child since that is considered to be the gestation period, it is pertinent to note that this Act was enacted as far back as 1872 when one could not even visualize ART. The law needs to take note of the scientific advancements since that time. Thus a child born to a woman artificially inseminated with the stored sperms of her deceased husband must be considered

to be a legitimate child notwithstanding the existing law of presumptions under our Evidence Act. The law needs to move along with medical advancements and suitably amended so that it does not give rise to dilemma or unwarranted harsh situations.

Institutional Ethics Committees

Each ART clinic of Levels 1B, 2 and Level 3 must have its own ethics committee constituted according to ICMR guidelines, comprising reputed ART practitioners, scientists who are knowledgeable in developmental biology or in clinical embryology, a social scientist, a member of the judiciary and a person who is well-versed in comparative theology. Should the local ART clinic have difficulty in establishing such a body, the state accreditation authority should constitute such a body, co-opting a representative of the ART clinic.

Egg (Ovum) Donation

The first pregnancy achieved with egg donation was reported in 1984. Since that time, there has been increasing utilization of egg donation to help infertile couples/individuals conceive. Egg donors are identified and through the process of IVF, eggs are obtained from the donor's ovaries and donated to the intended recipient. It requires ovarian stimulation with monitoring with oocyte retrieval and hence discomfort to the donor. Sperm obtained from the recipient's partner is used to fertilize these eggs, and embryos are transferred into the recipient's uterus. If pregnancy occurs, the recipient will have a biological but not genetic relationship to the child; her partner will be both biologically and genetically related.

Indications for use of Donor Oocytes[16]

- Women with hypo-gonadotropic hypogonadism
- Women with advanced reproductive age
- Women with diminished ovarian reserve
- Women who are known to be affected by or a carrier of a genetic condition or have a significant family history of a disease whose carrier state cannot be determined
- Women who have poor oocyte and/or embryo quality or multiple failed attempts to conceive by ART.

Types of Ovum Donors

Anonymous donors: Women who are not known to the recipient. Donors may be recruited through established egg donation programs, or may be identified through agencies.

Known or directed donors: Women who are known to the recipient. The donor is generally a close relative or friend. In some instances, recipients advertise directly for donors in newspapers or on the Internet. In these circumstances, the recipient couple and the donor are known to each in a limited way, having met without an intermediary program or agency. Recipients should exercise caution about recruiting donors directly without having an intermediary program or agency screen donors, or without seeking legal counselor agency screen donors, or without seeking legal counsel.

IVF programs: Women undergoing IVF may agree to donate their excess eggs to infertile patients. This source of donors is limited.

Evaluation of the recipient couple is similar to that of couples undergoing routine IVF.

Preparation of the Donor for Egg Retrieval

In order to retrieve multiple eggs from the donor's ovaries, the donor must be given ovulation induction. When the eggs are mature, the eggs are harvested from the ovary approximately 34–36 hours after injection. through a process called trans vaginal ultrasound aspiration. The eggs are obtained, evaluated for maturity, and then are inseminated with the male partner's sperm (donor sperm may also be used) which has been processed in the laboratory.

Preparation of the Recipient for Embryo Transfer

In order for embryos to implant into the recipient's uterus, the endometrium must be appropriately prepared and synchronized with the donor reproductive cycle. Embryos are transferred into the recipient's uterus usually within three to five days after the eggs are fertilized in the laboratory by process of embryo transfer. If the recipient couple has extra embryos, these embryos may be cryopreserved (frozen) for utilization at a later time for additional attempts to achieve a pregnancy.

Success Rates of Egg Donation

The success rates of egg donation depend on many factors but are generally independent of the age of the recipient. Success rates compiled by the Centers for Disease Control for the year 2000 show the average live birth rate per transfer of 43% for all egg donor programs. The major risk for donor egg programs is multiple gestations. In 2000, of the 3,436 pregnancies conceived with egg donation in the US 2,992 resulted in a live birth. Of these, the multiple pregnancy rate was 40% with 36.6% being twins and 3.7% being triplets or greater. Because many of the pregnancies miscarry before the actual number of fetuses can be determined, the percentage of multiple pregnancies may actually be higher. The current trend is to reduce the number of embryos transferred in an effort to reduce the risk of multiple gestations.

Sperm Donation

Artificial insemination using donor sperm has been practised for over a century, although the first published reports about the practice were in 1945. Over the past 10 years, the utilization of donor sperm has decreased as the utilization of intracytoplasmic sperm injection (ICSI) for the treatment of male infertility has become widespread. Since the late 1980s with the emergence of AIDS, artificial donor insemination has been performed exclusively with frozen and quarantined sperm. Current FDA and ASRM guidelines recommend that sperm be quarantined for at least six months before being released for use.

Indications for Use of Donor Sperm[16]

- The male partner has a zoospermia, severe oligospermia or other semen or seminal fluid abnormalities.
- The male partner has ejaculatory dysfunction
- The male partner demonstrates significant male factor infertility (i.e. significant oligoasthenospermia or prior failure to fertilize after insemination in vitro and ICSI is not elected or feasible.
- The male partner has a significant genetic defect or the couple has previously produced an offspring with defect for which carrier status cannot be determined.
- The male partner has a sexually transmissible infection which cannot be eradicated.
- The female partner is Rh negative and severely Rh isoimmunized and male partner is Rh positive.
- Females without male partners.

Procedure

Intra cervical insemination specimens (ICI) are prepared for intra cervical inseminations only and must be washed if used for intrauterine inseminations. Intrauterine insemination specimens (IUI) are pre-washed for intrauterine insemination. ICI or IUI semen samples are frozen and quarantined for a minimum of 180 days. They are not released until the donor is retested for communicable diseases and the results are negative.

Success Rates

The success rates with donor insemination depend on many factors. These include the female age and the presence of other female fertility factors such as endometriosis, tubal disease, or ovulatory dysfunction. In general, the monthly chance of pregnancy ranges from 8% to 15%. A number of studies have demonstrated that the success rates with IUI are greater than ICI when frozen donor semen is used. The risk of birth defects as a result of conceiving with donor insemination is no different than from conceiving naturally, and is in the range of 2% to 4%.

Embryo Donation

Embryo donation is a procedure that enables embryos either that were created by couples undergoing fertility treatment or that were created from donor sperm and donor eggs specifically for the purpose of donation to be transferred to infertile patients in order to achieve a pregnancy. Indications for embryo donation include untreatable infertility that involves both partners, untreatable infertility in a single woman, recurrent pregnancy loss thought to be related to embryonic factors, and genetic disorders affecting one or both partners. The process of embryo donation requires that the recipient couple undergo the appropriate medical and psychological screening recommended for all gamete donor cycles. In addition, the female partner undergoes an evaluation of her uterine cavity and then her endometrium is prepared with estrogen and progesterone in anticipation of an embryo transfer. In India, embryo donation must meet established ICMR guidelines for screening of the donors. For embryos that are created specifically for donation, the sperm donor and egg donor must be screened and tested as any other sperm and egg donors who are not intimate sexual partners of the recipients.

Embryo donation is a controversial process from both an ethical as well as legal standpoint. What differentiates embryo donation from either egg or sperm donation is that the child born to the couple will have no genetic link with them, yet all parties will benefit from the biologic relationship they share through the commitment the parents have made to gestate this embryo. Of paramount importance is that informed consent and counseling be provided to both the donors of the embryos and the recipient couple to address all of the potential issues embryo donation might raise. In addition, due to the absence of explicit laws regarding embryo donation, couples should consult with legal counsel regarding the necessity of a pre-donation agreement as well as to seek a judicial determination or recognition of parentage.

Success rates with embryo donation depend on the quality of the embryos that were frozen, the age of the woman who provided the eggs, and the number of embryos transferred.

Number of Embryos to be Transferred

It is shown in Table 6.1.
- In donor egg cycles the age of the donor should be used to calculate the appropriate number of eggs to be transferred.
- In frozen embryo transfer cycles the number of good quality thawed embryos transferred should not exceed the recommended number of embryos transferred.

TABLE 6.1 Recommended limit on the number of embryos to transfer (ASRM)[17]

	Age (years)			
Prognosis	< 35	35–37	38–40	41–42
Cleavage stage embryo				
Favorable	1–2	2	3	5
All others	2	3	4	5
Blastocysts				
Favorable	1	2	2	3
All others	2	2	3	3

*Favorable = first cycle of IVF, good embryo quality, excess embryos available for cryopreservation, or previous successful IVF cycle.

Types of Surrogacy

Surrogacy is both a medically and emotionally complex process that involves careful evaluation by medical professionals, mental health professionals, and legal professionals to ensure that the procedure is successful for both the surrogate as well as the intended parents. There are two types of surrogacy arrangements: traditional surrogacy in which the surrogate is inseminated with sperm from the male partner of the intended parent couple (donor sperm may be used as well) and gestational surrogacy in which the surrogate carries a pregnancy created by transferring an embryo created with the sperm and egg of the intended parent (donor sperm or donor eggs may be used as well).

Indications for Gestational Surrogacy[18]

Gestational carriers may be used when a true medical condition precludes a woman from carrying a pregnancy or if it poses a threat of death or harm to the intended parent or fetus. The indication for surrogacy should be clearly mentioned in the patient's documents. Examples of such conditions are:

- Absence of uterus (congenital or acquired)
- Significant uterine anomaly like irreparable Asherman's syndrome or unicornuate uterus with recurrent pregnancy loss.
- Absolute medical contraindication to pregnancy, e.g. pulmonary hypertension.
- Serious medical condition that could get exacerbated by pregnancy or cause significant risk to the fetus.
- Biologic inability to conceive and bear a child such as single male or homosexual male couple.

Gestational carriers may be considered when an unidentified endometrial factor exists such as for those women who had multiple IVF failures in spite of transfer of good quality embryos.

No owner, operator, laboratory director or employee of the practice may act as a gestational carrier or intended parent in that practice.

Selection of a Gestational Surrogate

Gestational surrogates may be known to the intended parents or may be anonymous. Known surrogates are typically relatives or friends who volunteer to carry the pregnancy. Anonymous surrogates are identified through agencies that specialize in recruiting women to become surrogates. It should be done according to ICMR guidelines.

Counseling of Gestational Surrogates and the Intended Parents

Counseling of surrogates is intended to provide the surrogate with a clear understanding of the psychological issues related to pregnancy. With the assistance of a mental health professional (MHP), the gestational surrogate, and her partner should explore issues such as managing a relationship with the intended parents, coping with attachment issues to the fetus, and the impact of a gestational surrogacy arrangement on her children and her relationships with her partner, friends and employers. The intended parents should be counseled regarding their ability to maintain a respectful relationship with the surrogate.

The surrogate, the intended parents, and the MHP should also meet to discuss the type of relationship they would like to have. In addition, expectations they have regarding a potential pregnancy should be discussed. This includes a discussion of the number of embryos for transfer, prenatal diagnostic interventions, fetal reduction and therapeutic abortion, as well as managing the relationship while respecting the carrier's right to privacy.

What is the Success Rate of Surrogacy in India?

The success rate (carry home baby) of surrogacy is around 45% in case of fresh embryos. In case of frozen embryos, it is about 25%. High success rates and low medical costs are the highlights of surrogate pregnancy in India. No wonder many couples from the US, Australia, UK, Israel and other European countries seek surrogacy in India.

The laws regarding third party reproduction are either non-existent or different from one state to another. Thus, all couples are advised to consult with an attorney knowledgeable in the area of reproductive law within their individual states.

Our Experience with Gestational Surrogacy

Dr LH Hiranandani Hospital in Mumbai is the tertiary care center where maximum number of gestational carriers are referred from various IVF centers for their antenatal follow-up, antenatal management and delivery.

What is the Nine Months Journey like with the Gestational Surrogate?

The surrogate is treated as a high-risk pregnancy and is cared for by consultant gynecologists. Appointments are scheduled with the consultants every two weeks for the first 6 months, then every week for the next 2 months and then weekly / biweekly in the last month. Blood tests and ultrasound are done as and when required. Routine blood tests like hemoglobin, blood group, blood sugars, thyroid function tests, VDRL, HCV, HBs AG & HIV and also urine routine examination are done. Special care is given, and tests are done to pick up any obstetric or medical complications like hypertension, diabetes, etc. at the earliest. Two doses of injection Tetanus are given during pregnancy. The baby's growth is monitored stringently. Ultrasound is done at 6 weeks to confirm pregnancy and the viability of the pregnancy, then at 12 weeks to assess growth and certain parameters like nuchal fold translucency. At 18–20 weeks, a detailed level III anomaly scan is done to detect any abnormalities in the fetus. At 16 weeks, after counseling and with the consultation of the genetic parents, amniocentesis is performed, if indicated. Complete blood count is done frequently and GTT and thyroid function tests are done at 28 weeks. At 28 weeks and 34 weeks, ultrasound with color Doppler is performed to assess the growth of the baby and rule out intrauterine growth retardation, every 4 weekly in case of multiple gestation. Fetal wellbeing tests, like nonstress test, are done as per the requirement. Detailed information is given to the surrogates about nutrition and diet during pregnancy. They are regularly provided with supplements from their center. Thus, adequate care and precaution is taken, to ensure that sufficient and optimum nutrition reaches the baby. The IVF center is regularly updated on the progress of the pregnancy.

Labor room for delivery is equipped to handle any obstetric emergency. NICU setup is also completely equipped to handle any neonatal complications, with a neonatologist who is available round the clock.

What are the Different Ways Children Born through Surrogacy may Receive Breast Milk?

Just because the baby is born through surrogacy does not mean he or she cannot receive breast milk and the many health benefits it provides. Breastfed babies have been found to have higher IQ, are better protected from leukemia and are less likely to have problems regarding obesity. Breast milk protects babies from getting diarrhea, ear infections and respiratory disorders such as asthma. Premature babies who receive breast milk are more protected from infections and high blood pressure later in life. Breast milk contains the protein CD14 which works to develop B cells, which are immunity cells that are essential for the production of antibodies in an infant, to build the babies' immune system.

The babies may drink breast milk acquired through a milk bank, breast milk donor may be located or the intended mother may induce lactation before the birth of the baby. Induced lactation has been embraced by the nursing community as a welcome method to enhance the bonding relationship between a new mother and baby born through surrogacy. Prolactin and oxytocin are the two pituitary hormones that cause lactation to occur. They may be stimulated despite the woman's inability to carry a child. Lactation may be induced in a number of ways, and the amount of milk a nonlactating woman can produce through inducement varies from woman to woman. The most common way women induce lactation is through manual or mechanical stimulation. With this method lactation is induced by massage, nipple manipulation and sucking either by the baby or breast pump. The second common method used is drug therapy whereby a woman uses herbal remedies such as fenugreek, lactare capsules and granules or is prescribed medications such as domperidone and metoclopromide to induce and increase her milk supply. Induced lactation milk skips the colostrum phase and resembles mature breast milk.

Manual stimulation of lactation usually takes between two and seven weeks and drug therapy usually takes between one to four months. For this reason intended mothers usually begin during the final trimester of their surrogate mother's pregnancy.

Surrogacy: A High-Risk Pregnancy

A retrospective analysis of 330 surrogate mothers who delivered at Dr L H Hiranandani Hospital over three years from January 2009 to December 2011 was done. This is the unpublished data of the co-authors. Out of these 330 cases there were 193 singleton pregnancies (58%) and 137 twins pregnancies (42%).

We found that in surrogate mothers, 276 underwent cesarean section (83%) and 54 had vaginal delivery (17%). Among mothers 45 had pre-eclampsia, 23 had anemia, and 17 had gestational diabetes, 12 had placentaprevia, 3 had placental abruption, 62 had preterm delivery, 30 had premature rupture of membranes. Postpartum hemorrhage was seen in 43 cases out of which 22 required blood transfusion. Cesarean hysterectomy was needed in 2 cases, intrauterine fetal death was seen in 4 cases, postoperative fever in 7 cases and wound infection in 6 cases. In the neonates, average gestational age at delivery was 35 weeks in twins and 37 weeks in singletons. Average weight was 2.14 kg in twins and 2.76 kg in singletons. Twins delivered after 36 weeks had average birth weight of 2.68 kg while singletons delivered after 37 weeks had average birth weight of 3.24 kg. Out of 463 neonates, 84 twins had birth weight < 2 kg and 50 singletons had birth weight < 2.5 kg.

Out of 463 neonates, 30 had jaundice, 52 had tachypnea, 23 had respiratory distress syndrome, 30 had retinopathy of prematurity, 12 had sepsis, 17 had necrotizing enterocolitis, 24 had apnea, 41 had hypoglycemia and 64 neonates required NICU care.

The incidence of various obstetrical complications was noted which is compared with WHO/HRP values. Four years ago HRP launched a systematic review aimed at determining the global burden of maternal mortality and morbidity. This project involved systematic review of 2443 studies providing information on frequency of 19 major maternal disorders.[19]In this review, biological mothers were taken for study whereas in the above mentioned analysis the surrogate mothers were studied. It is mentioned in Table 6.2.

Table 6.3 shows the various complications in neonates delivered by surrogate mothers at Dr LH Hiranandani hospital.

It was noted that 62 patients had a preterm delivery. Figure 6.1 shows the picture

TABLE 6.2 Incidence of various maternal complications in surrogate mothers delivered at our hospital

Maternal complication (% Incidence)	WHO/HRP	Our study
Pre-eclampsia	14.9	13.63
Anemia	4.5	6.9
Gestational diabetes mellitus	3.8	5.15
Preterm delivery	8.2	18.7
Hemorrhage (Antepartum, Postpartum)	6.2	17.5
Intrauterine fetal death	13.9	1.2
Premature rupture of membranes	2.4	9
Puerperal infection	1.5	3.9
Placenta previa, Placental abruption	4.1	4.5

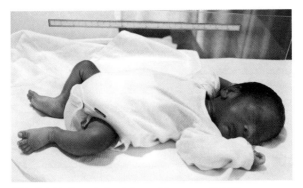

FIG. 6.1 Preterm baby delivered from a surrogate
(For color version see Plate 1)

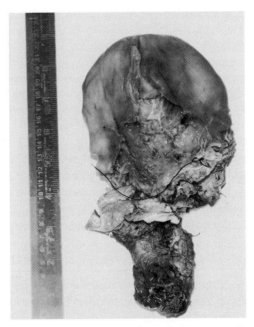

FIG. 6.2 Hysterectomy specimen of a term surrogate
for placenta accretra *(For color version see Plate 1)*

of preterm baby delivered by a surrogate at 29 weeks in view of preterm labor who required NICU care.

Obstetric complication rate is much high in GCs as evident by Table 6.2.

Figure 6.2 shows the obstetric hysterectomy specimen recently done in case of a term surrogate pregnancy with placenta accreta.

Surrogate mothers hail from a lower socio-economic class. Poor nutrition, pre-existing anemia, repeated pregnancies predispose to poor reserves. Thus complications like anemia, preterm delivery and hemorrhage take a significant toll on their obstetric outcome. These patients need more attention to catch such

TABLE 6.3 Incidence of various complication in neonates delivered by surrogate mothers at Dr LH Hiranandani hospital

Neonatal complications	% Incidence
Jaundice	6.4
Tachypnea	11.2
Respiratory distress syndrome	4.9
Retinopathy of prematurity	6.4
Sepsis	2.5
Necrotizing enterocolitis	3.6
Apnea	7.2
Hypoglycemia	8.8

complications in early stage and rectify them. Hence they should be managed with strict vigilance.

Conclusion

The options available through third party reproduction provide many couples the opportunity to make their dream of parenthood a reality. The comprehensive nature of the screening and counsel-ing of intended parents and their donors or surrogates ensures that the process meets the needs of all involved. Finally, as third party reproduction is more widely used, there continues to be a broader understanding of the ethical, moral and legal issues involved. The ultimate goal of physicians, mental health professionals, and attorneys specializing in reproductive law is to enable this process to move forward as smoothly as possible and bring joy and satisfaction to all parties involved in ensuring the conception and delivery of a healthy child.

Glossary

Cryopreserved: Freezing at a very low temperature, such as in liquid nitrogen (-196°C), to keep embryos viable so as to store them for future transfer into a uterus or to keep sperm viable for future insemination or assisted reproductive technology procedures. At present, cryopreservation of eggs is experimental.

Donor eggs: The eggs taken from the ovaries of a fertile woman and donated to an infertile woman to be used in an assisted reproductive technology procedure.

Eggs: The female sex cells (ova) produced by the female's ovaries, which, when fertilized by a male's sperm, produce embryos, the early form of human life.

Embryo: The earliest stage of human development arising after the union of the sperm and egg (fertilization).

Embryo transfer: Placement of an embryo into the uterus through the vagina and cervix or, in the case of zygote intrafallopian transfer (ZIFT) or tubal embryo transfer (TET), into the fallopian tube.

Endometriosis: A condition where endometrial-like tissue (the tissue that lines the uterus) implants outside of the uterine cavity in abnormal locations, such as the ovaries, fallopian tubes, and abdominal cavity. Endometriosis can grow with hormonal stimulation and cause pain, inflammation, and scar tissue. It may also be associated with infertility.

Endometrium: The lining of the uterus that is shed each month with the menstrual period. The endometrium thickens and thus provides a nourishing site for the implantation of a fertilized egg.

Fertilization: The fusion of sperm and egg.

Gestational carrier: A woman who carries an embryo to delivery. The embryo is derived from the egg and sperm of persons not related to the carrier; therefore the carrier has no genetic relationship with the resulting child.

Hepatitis B and C: Viruses that may be sexually transmitted, or transmitted by contact with blood and other bodily fluids, that can cause infection of the liver leading to jaundice and liver failure.

Human chorionic gonadotropin (hCG): A hormone that increases early in pregnancy. This hormone is produced by the placenta; its detection is the basis of most pregnancy tests. It can also be used as an LH substitute to trigger ovulation in conjunction with clomiphene or gonadotropin therapy.

Human immunodeficiency virus (HIV): A retrovirus that causes acquired immune deficiency syndrome (AIDS), a disease that destroys the body's ability to protect itself from infection and disease. It is transmitted by the exchange of bodily fluids or blood transfusions.

In vitro fertilization (IVF): A method of assisted reproduction that involves combining an egg with sperm in a laboratory dish. If the egg fertilizes and begins cell division, the resulting embryo is transferred into the woman's uterus where it will hopefully implant in the uterine lining and further develop. IVF may be performed in conjunction with medications that stimulate the ovaries to produce multiple eggs in order to increase the chances of successful fertilization and implantation. IVF bypasses the fallopian tubes and is often the treatment choice for women who have badly damaged or absent tubes.

Ovulation: The release of a mature egg from its developing follicle in the outer layer of the ovary. This usually occurs approximately 14 days preceding the next menstrual period (the 14th day of a 28-day cycle).

Ovulation induction: The administration of hormone medications (ovulation drugs) that stimulate the ovaries to ovulate.

Sperm: The male reproductive cells that fertilize a woman's egg. The sperm head carries genetic material (chromosomes), the midpiece produces energy for movement, and the long, thin tail wiggles to propel the sperm.

Surrogacy: In traditional surrogacy, a woman is inseminated with the sperm of a man who is not her partner in order to conceive and carry a child to be reared by the biologic (genetic) father and his partner. In this procedure the surrogate is genetically related to the child. The biologic father and his partner must usually adopt the child after its birth. Another type of surrogate is a gestational carrier, a woman who is implanted with the fertilized egg (embryo) of another couple in order to carry the pregnancy. The surrogate is not genetically related to the child in this case.

Surrogate: A traditional surrogate is a woman who is inseminated with the sperm of a man who is not her partner in order to conceive and carry a child to be reared by the biological (genetic) father and his partner. In this procedure the surrogate is genetically related to the child. The biologic father and his partner must usually adopt the child after its birth. Another type of surrogate is a gestational carrier. This process involves implanting a fertilized egg (embryo) into the surrogate's uterus. In this procedure the surrogate does not provide the egg and is therefore not biologically (genetically) related to the child.

Transvaginal ultrasound aspiration: An ultrasound-guided technique for egg retrieval. A long, thin needle is passed through the vagina into the ovarian follicle, and suction is applied to retrieve the egg. Also known as ultrasound guided egg aspiration and transvaginal egg retrieval.

References

1. Ryan G. Establishment of a clinical gestational carrier program: medical, ethical, legal and policy issues. Proc Obstet Gynecol, 2010;1(1):Article 8 [16p.]
2. Mundy L. Everything conceivable – how assisted reproduction is changing men, women, and the world. New York. Albert A Knopf, 2007.
3. ASRM. Third Party Reproduction. A guide for patients. Published by the American Society for Reproductive Medicine under the direction of the Patient Education Committee and the Publications Committee.
4. Department of Health. Brazier Report on Surrogacy, Published by Department of Health Press Office, London, 1998.
5. Utian WH, Goldfarb JM, Kiwi R, et al. Preliminary experience with in vitro fertilization—surrogate gestational pregnancy. Fertil Steril. 1989;52:633–8.
6. Cohen J. Jones H. Assisted reproduction. Rules and laws. International comparisons. Contracept Fertil Sex. 1999;27:I-VII.
7. Surrogacy Arrangements Act. Her Majesty's Stationary Office, London, 1985.
8. Human Fertilization and Embryology Act. 1990 can be found at www.parliament.uk
9. British Medical Association. Changing Conceptions of Motherhood. The Practice of Surrogacy in Britain. BMA Publications, London, 1996.
10. Brinsden PR, et al. Treatment by in vitro fertilization with surrogacy: experience of one British centre. BMJ. 2000;320:924–9.
11. Brinsden PR. Gestational surrogacy. Human Reproduction Update. 2003;9(5):483–91.
12. Fischer S, Gillman I. Surrogate motherhood: attachment, attitudes and social support. Psychiatry. 1991;54:13-20.
13. Golombok S, Murray C, Jadva V, et al. Families created through a surrogacy arrangement: parent child relationships in the first year of life. Dev Psychol. 2003.

14. Subramanian S. Wombs for Rent. Maclean's. 2007;2.

15. ICMR Guidelines on ART clinics available at www.icmr.nic.in

16. Guidelines for gamete and embryo donation: A Practice Committee report. Fertil Steril, 2008;90:530–44.

17. Guidelines on number of embryos transferred: ASRM Practice Committee. Fertil Steril, 2009;92:1518–9.

18. Recommendations for practices utilizing gestational carriers: An ASRM Practice Committee guideline. Fertil Steril. 2012;97:1301–8.

19. Maurice J. Promoting evidence based sexual and reproductive health care. Progress. 2005,71:1–8..

A Clinical Approach to Female Sexual Pain

Chapter 7

Shantanu Abhayankar

"The surgeon thinks of difficult coitus as a knife passed through muscles in spasm; the psychiatrist thinks of dyspareunia as a mental knot to be disentangled by analysis; the gynecologist who is weary of patching- poor and late patching—begins to think in terms of prevention through routine premarital examination and instruction."[1]

Introduction

Sexual medicine is a field infested with quacks, for want of physicians trained and willing to practice it and good research to support such practice. However, slowly and surely newer research has brought it into the ambit of modern, rational medicine and qualified doctors are rapidly replacing the quacks. An obstetrician-gynecologist often faces individuals/couples with sexual problems and the reactions range from awe to acute embarrassment. The person(s) seeking help are equally ill at ease. A good clinician should therefore be a good listener, be comfortable with the language used (which at times borders on the vulgar), be able to give adequate time, be non-judgmental and supportive.

Prevalence

Various studies have reported incidence of female sexual dysfunction between 6 to 27% prevalence.[2,3] Sporadic dyspareunia is estimated to be 4–8 fold higher.[4]

Problem of Classification

Women's sexual disorders have traditionally been classified according to the phases of the sexual response cycle; disorders of desire, arousal, orgasm, etc. This classification is now thought to be inadequate. Moreover disorders of sexual pain (Vaginismus and Dyspareunia) do not fit into any one 'phase' of the sexual response cycle. In fact the assumption that vaginismus and dyspareunia are two distinct entities has been challenged.[5-9] Both seem to have the following three components to varying extent.

- Problems of muscle tension, voluntary or involuntary; limited to the vaginal muscle or extending to the pelvic floor, at times involving the adductor muscles, back, jaw, etc.

- Fear of sexual pain associated with genital touching or coitus; or fear of intercourse for reasons other than pain.
- Tendency towards avoidance. Despite pain some women continue to accept and tolerate sexual touching or even intercourse while others rapidly guard their genitalia from any type of touch.
- With this background let us now dwell on what we know of vaginismus, dyspareunia and Vulvar Vestibulitis syndrome (VVS).

Definitions

Vaginismus

It is defined as an involuntary spasm of the pubococcygeus muscles in the female when coitus or insertion of a finger or object (e.g. speculum) in the vagina, is attempted.

An international committee has recently recommended the following definition;[10] 'The persistent or recurrent difficulties of the women to allow vaginal entry of the penis, a finger and/or any object, despite the women's expressed wish to do so. There is variable (phobic) avoidance, involuntary pelvic muscle contraction and anticipation/fear of experience of pain. Structural and other physical anomalies should be ruled out/addressed.'

This results in difficult, often impossible, penetration. Pain, burning at the introitus; and dyspareunia with forced intromission is reported. Commonly even a visual physical examination is refused and a lot of fuss made over separating the labia to look at the introitus.

Dyspareunia

Recurrent or persistent genital pain associated with sexual intercourse.[11] This can be subdivided into deep or superficial pain. Dyspareunia could be with or without VVS.

Vulvar Vestibulitis Syndrome

This includes painful penile vaginal intercourse or pain upon touching the vulvar vestibule and signs limited to variable vestibular erythema. (See under mucous membranes in sexual pain disorders as well.)

Neurobiology of the Pelvis

Readers are referred to textbooks of anatomy and physiology for a detailed review but a few points of clinical significance will be covered here.

Pelvic floor is now thought to be an integrated functional structure with varied disorders of micturition, defecation, sexual and genital pain; thought to be 'pelvic floor dysfunctions'. There is now evidence to show that the pelvic floor like some other muscle groups is indirectly innervated by the limbic system and therefore highly responsive to emotional stimuli and stress.[12-14]

The pelvis is innervated by the autonomic (sympathetic and parasympathetic), as well as somatic (sensory and motor) nerves. Odd as it may appear it is now known that the afferent sensory nerves of the pelvis carry efferent signals as well!! Electrical stimulation of the sensory nerves near the spinal cord leads to impulses towards the spinal cord (orthodromic) as well as towards the periphery (antidromic). The antidromic impulses produce vasodilatation, edema and hyperalgesia in the area of innervations. This is called neurogenic inflammation. This is an adaptive response in normal circumstances but can get maladaptive. This probably explains pain in interstitial cystitis, vulvodynia and many other painful conditions of the pelvis for which no cause has been discerned.

Neuropathic pain is typically characterized by spontaneous paresthesias, dysesthesias and evoked pain. Pain is experienced when impulses reach the brain via A delta or C fiber nociceptive afferents. Minor tissue injuries can cause reduction in the threshold for nociceptors resulting in "peripheral sensitization". This leads to responses to weak non-noxious stimuli – "allodynia". Further stimulation will lead to exaggerated pain response – "primary hyperalgesia". Allodynia can also occur because of abnormal signal amplification in the central nervous system called "central sensitization". Here the signals entering the CNS through non-nociceptive A – beta touch fibers evoke pain. The exact cause of increased descending excitatory signals and/or decreased inhibitory signals to allow this is unclear. Frequent success of therapies with tricyclic antidepressants, Venlafaxine, Carbamazepine or Gabapentin appears to support this theory.

Individual Psychological and Personality Characteristics in Women with Vaginismus

Women with vaginismus have been noted do to have higher rates comorbid anxiety disorders like agoraphobias without panic disorder and obsessive compulsive disorder. Personality traits suggest the presence of self-focused attention and negative self-evaluation.

Individual Psychological and Personality Characteristics in Women with Dyspareunia (and/or Vestibulitis)

In women with dyspareunia because of Vestibulitis, no definite trends have been noted apart from the fact that these women have increased anxiety and depressive disorders. Attention bias of hyper-vigilance for pain relation stimuli has been noted.

In those without Vestibulitis, signs of hostility, psychotic symptoms, erotophobia, negative/conservative attitude towards sex, sexual aversion are common. They have more problems with experiencing sexual arousal and relationship issues are common.

Mucous Membranes and Sexual Pain Disorders

Acute inflammation of the vulvovaginal mucous membrane is a common cause of dyspareunia. Often the cause is readily discernible; candidiasis, trichomoniasis, herpes being common.

In chronic vulvovaginal pain, it is difficult to pinpoint a cause. Iatrogenic inflammation because of self-treatment is a common cause that is often missed.

There are three main types of mucous membrane diseases; chronic vulvar dermatoses, vulvar vestibular syndrome, vulvodynias.

Chronic Vulvar Dermatosis

Lichen simplex, lichen sclerosus and lichen planus can cause severe sexual pain. Lichen simplex is the result of the itch-scratch cycle because of chronic scratching. Topical steroids and oral antihistaminic usually help.

Lichen sclerosis is a result of extreme thinning of the epidermis leading to parchment paper appearance of the skin. Topical steroids appear to be the treatment of choice.

Lichen planus gives rise to superficial ulcers with concomitant inflammation of the vaginal mucosa and profuse discharge. Often Behcet's syndrome like picture is seen with involvement of oral, esophageal mucosa. Topical steroids for a prolonged period, interleukin inhibitors and anti-inflammatory agents are the key to treatment.

Vulvar Vestibulitis Syndrome

The classical triad is Vulvar itching, burning and pain with sexual activity and even otherwise is complained of. Sitting or running too can be painful.

Vulvodynias (Syn: Dysesthetic Vulvodynia)

Intense burning sensation causing profound sexual and psychological distress is usually the presenting symptom. There are no positive findings at all. Culture, biopsies, etc. are negative. Topical treatment increases the pain. Oral tricyclic antidepressants or anticonvulsants offer a reduction in symptoms.

Common Etiologies

With the above background, the table below lists the **common causes** of sexual pain. Many of the conditions are commonly seen and sexual pain may or may not be the presenting compliant. The onus lies on the clinician to gently probe this aspect of the problem and help the patient open out and seek more specific treatment if need be.

Superficial

- VVS
- Atrophy
- Vulvitis, vulvovaginitis
- Interstitial cystitis
- Condylomata
- Dermatologic diseases
- Episiotomy neuroma
- Radiation

- Noninfectious inflammations
- Epithelial defects
- Scarring
- Size of penis
- Urethritis
- Anatomic variations
- Hymenal remnants
- Urethritis/cystitis.

Deep

- Estrogen deficiency
- Vaginitis
- Chronic PID
- Foreshortened vagina
- Endometriosis
- Vaginal septum
- Fixed inverted uterus
- Fibroid uterus
- Ovarian tumor
- Ovarian remnant syndrome
- Chronic abdominal pain
- Irritable bowel syndrome
- Hemorrhoids.

Clinical Approach to Sexual Pain

Clinicians are often perplexed about how exactly to go about asking details of sexual pain. Here is brief list of questions that will help.

Questions Qualifying the Pain

- Pain:
  - Where does it hurt? How would you describe the pain?
  - Is it with contact with introitus? With partial entry? Full entry? Deep thrusting? With ejaculation? After withdrawal? With subsequent micturation?
  - Does your body tense up on attempt at insertion by partner? What are your fears and feelings then?
  - How long does the pain last? Does touching elsewhere in the genital area cause pain? Does it hurt when you ride a two wheeler or wear tight clothes? Do other types of penetration hurt? (Tampons, fingers)
- Pelvic floor muscle tension:
  - Do you realize the sensation of pelvic floor muscle tension during sexual contact and/or in non-sexual situations?
- Arousal:
  - Do you feel subjectively aroused when sexually stimulated/dose your vagina feel sufficiently moist? Do you recognize the feeling of dying up?

- Consequences of the complaint:
  - What do you do when you experience pain during sexual contact? (continue/stop intercourse/continue to make love without intercourse)
  - Do you currently include intercourse or attempts at intercourse or do you use other ways to make love? If so, are you both comfortable with this arrangement?
  - What consequences does pain have on the rest of your relationship?
- Biomedical antecedents
  - When and how did the pain start? What tests have been done?

Educational Gynecological Sexological Examination

If conducted in a proper manner the examination of a patient with sexual pain in itself can be diagnostic as well as therapeutic.

An educational gynecological sexological examination is different than a routine one in following aspects.

It may not be the part of evaluation in the first consultation itself. The patient and the care provider are to decide the timing, nature and the persons present during this examination. As far as possible the participation of the sexual partner is encouraged.

There are three steps to be followed. Counseling about how and what is going to be done and about the anatomy of the genitals with the help of suitable diagrams/films, etc. Patient should be assured in advance that she has total control over the procedure and nothing will be done without her explicit consent. She is assured that during the examination her personal boundaries will be respected. She should also be told that the use of speculum or such other means for internal examination will not be used unless she permits it. The next is the examination proper where the patient is given a hand mirror and the examiner sees, points out, explores and examines the external genitalia while giving a running commentary about what is going on. Apart from seeking verbal approval for what is being done a close watch is kept for non-verbal signals from the patient and her partner. If all the findings are normal, it is important to specifically state so. The patient is asked to spread the vulva herself. The vulva is carefully inspected including the labia minora, majora, the crease between the clitoral hood and clitoris, the posterior fourchette, vestibule, hymen and hymenal edge. For women with introital dyspareunia areas of allodynia are explored using a cotton Q tip. The skin at the openings of the Skene's ducts must also be examined as it is frequently involved. A new instrument named Vulvalgesiometer is useful in quantifying the vulvovaginal pain. By bearing down or coughing the patient will be able to see the introitus getting larger. With good rapport and gentle technique an internal examination too may become possible. Some may even allow a transvaginal scan which is informative in deep dyspareunia.

Questionnaire Assessment of Patients with Sexual Pain

Questionnaires are the best way to save time, bypass embarrassment faced by the patient while narrating her complaints and get a quick overview of what is going to be said. Questionnaires administered before and after treatment can help in assessing the efficacy of treatment.

Many validated questionnaires are available in English; but in the Indian context they need to be translated and revalidated in the local language. Cultural ethos of the subcontinent needs to be considered while translating these questionnaires.

Here is the 'female sexual function index' (FSFI), which tests for several domains of female sexual dysfunction (and not just pain). The part provided here lists the questions with standard options. For scoring analysis protocols readers are advised to visit http://www.fsfiquestionnaire.com

Female Sexual Function Index

Subject Identifier .... Date..

Instructions: These questions ask about your sexual feelings and responses during the past 4 weeks. Please answer the following questions as honestly and clearly as possible. Your responses will be kept completely confidential. In answering these questions the following definitions apply:

Sexual activity can include caressing, foreplay, masturbation and vaginal intercourse.

Sexual intercourse is defined as penile penetration (entry) of the vagina.

Sexual stimulation includes situations like foreplay with a partner, self-stimulation (masturbation), or sexual fantasy.

Check Only One Box Per Question

Sexual desire or interest is a feeling that includes wanting to have a sexual experience, feeling receptive to a partner's sexual initiation, and thinking or fantasizing about having sex.

- Over the past 4 weeks, how often did you feel sexual desire or interest?
  - Almost always or always
  - Most times (more than half the time)
  - Sometimes (about half the time)
  - A few times (less than half the time)
  - Almost never or never
- Over the past 4 weeks, how would you rate your level (degree) of sexual desire or interest?
  - Very high
  - High
  - Moderate
  - Low
  - Very low or none at all

Sexual arousal is a feeling that includes both physical and mental aspects of sexual excitement. It may include feelings of warmth or tingling in the genitals, lubrication (wetness), or muscle contractions.

- Over the past 4 weeks, how often did you feel sexually aroused ("turned on") during sexual activity or intercourse?

- No sexual activity
- Almost always or always
- Most times (more than half the time)
- Sometimes (about half the time)
- A few times (less than half the time)
- Almost never or never
- Over the past 4 weeks, how would you rate your level of sexual arousal ("turn on") during sexual activity or intercourse?
  - No sexual activity
  - Very high
  - High
  - Moderate
  - Low
  - Very low or none at all
- Over the past 4 weeks, how confident were you about becoming sexually aroused during sexual activity or intercourse?
  - No sexual activity
  - Very high confidence
  - High confidence
  - Moderate confidence
  - Low confidence
  - Very low or no confidence
- Over the past 4 weeks, how often have you been satisfied with your arousal (excitement) during sexual activity or intercourse?
  - No sexual activity
  - Almost always or always
  - Most times (more than half the time)
  - Sometimes (about half the time)
  - A few times (less than half the time)
  - Almost never or never
- Over the past 4 weeks, how often did you become lubricated ("wet") during sexual activity or intercourse?
  - No sexual activity
  - Almost always or always
  - Most times (more than half the time)
  - Sometimes (about half the time)
  - A few times (less than half the time)
  - Almost never or never
- Over the past 4 weeks, how difficult was it to become lubricated ("wet") during sexual activity or intercourse?
  - No sexual activity
  - Extremely difficult or impossible
  - Very difficult
  - Difficult

- Slightly difficult
- Not difficult

■ Over the past 4 weeks, how often did you maintain your lubrication ("wetness") until completion of sexual activity or intercourse?
- No sexual activity
- Almost always or always
- Most times (more than half the time)
- Sometimes (about half the time)
- A few times (less than half the time)
- Almost never or never

■ Over the past 4 weeks, how difficult was it to maintain your lubrication ("wetness") until completion of sexual activity or intercourse?
- No sexual activity
- Extremely difficult or impossible
- Very difficult
- Difficult
- Slightly difficult
- Not difficult

■ Over the past 4 weeks, when you had sexual stimulation or intercourse, how often did you reach orgasm (climax)?
- No sexual activity
- Almost always or always
- Most times (more than half the time)
- Sometimes (about half the time)
- A few times (less than half the time)
- Almost never or never

■ Over the past 4 weeks, when you had sexual stimulation or intercourse, how difficult was it for you to reach orgasm (climax)?
- No sexual activity
- Extremely difficult or impossible
- Very difficult
- Difficult
- Slightly difficult
- Not difficult

■ Over the past 4 weeks, how satisfied were you with your ability to reach orgasm (climax) during sexual activity or intercourse?
- No sexual activity
- Very satisfied
- Moderately satisfied
- About equally satisfied and dissatisfied
- Moderately dissatisfied
- Very dissatisfied

■ Over the past 4 weeks, how satisfied have you been with the amount of emotional closeness during sexual activity between you and your partner?

- No sexual activity
- Very satisfied
- Moderately satisfied
- About equally satisfied and dissatisfied
- Moderately dissatisfied
- Very dissatisfied

- Over the past 4 weeks, how satisfied have you been with your sexual relationship with your partner?
  - Very satisfied
  - Moderately satisfied
  - About equally satisfied and dissatisfied
  - Moderately dissatisfied
  - Very dissatisfied
- Over the past 4 weeks, how satisfied have you been with your overall sexual life?
  - Very satisfied
  - Moderately satisfied
  - About equally satisfied and dissatisfied
  - Moderately dissatisfied
  - Very dissatisfied
- Over the past 4 weeks, how often did you experience discomfort or pain during vaginal penetration?
  - Did not attempt intercourse
  - Almost always or always
  - Most times (more than half the time)
  - Sometimes (about half the time)
  - A few times (less than half the time)
  - Almost never or never
- Over the past 4 weeks, how often did you experience discomfort or pain following vaginal penetration?
  - Did not attempt intercourse
  - Almost always or always
  - Most times (more than half the time)
  - Sometimes (about half the time)
  - A few times (less than half the time)
  - Almost never or never
- Over the past 4 weeks, how would you rate your level (degree) of discomfort or pain during or following vaginal penetration?
  - Did not attempt intercourse
  - Very high
  - High
  - Moderate
  - Low
  - Very low or none at all.

Treatment

Dyspareunia

Treatment varies as per the etiology. A lot of counseling is required for both the partners. This is not to suggest that the male partner is 'causing or aggravating' the problem but certainly to mean that 'he' too is affected by it.

Infective skin and mucosal lesions are best treated with appropriate antibiotics, antifungals and antiparasitic medications. Bacterial vaginosis is best approached with Ampicillin and stopping ritualistic cleaning of the genitalia that is often undertaken under the influence of modern day notions of 'hygiene and cleanliness'.

Pelvic infections are more difficult and the dyspareunia may be because of scarring, adhesions left behind by an infection treated long ago. Active infection needs appropriate antibiotic course. Chronic effects need to be diagnosed and tackled laparoscopically. Endometriosis is similarly dealt with medical/surgical management. A fixed inverted uterus, fibroids, ovarian tumors, ovarian remnant syndrome will all need appropriate surgical intervention.

Atrophy will best respond to local estrogen creams.

Condylomata accuminata will need Podophyllin application and/or cautery.

Many noninfectious inflammations will regress with mild steroids, like mometasone applied locally.

Scarring resulting from genital mutilation is difficult to treat and is thankfully not a problem in this part of the world. Scarring following radiation is equally difficult and needs serial dilatation and extreme perseverance.

The size of the penis is more of an imagined problem than real. Good foreplay, copious lubrication with water based jellies and gentle manner should take care of the problem; whether real or imagined.

Anatomic variations are mostly iatrogenic like those after hysterectomy, anterior/posterior repairs, sling operations for prolapse in young women or those for vault prolapse. Some adjustment in diameter and depth of the vagina happens over time with regular coitus. Avoiding coitus for the fear of pain will lead to atrophy and loss of elasticity which will compound the problem. Couples should be encouraged to have regular coital sex once the incisions have gained enough strength. This is usually after 2 to 3 months. Estrogen cream, lubricant jellies, good foreplay and gentle manner are stressed. Over correction during posterior colporrhaphy may at times change the direction of the vagina. Apart from dyspareunia, post void dribble also happens to be a complaint in such cases. Phenton's operation, wherein a vertical incision is places at 6 o'clock and sutured transversely is the surgery of choice.

Naturally occurring mismatch in size may be because of vaginal septum; that may be longitudinal or transverse (termed phimosis of the cervix); absent or rudimentary vagina or a tough hymen. Septum resection with vaginoplasty, Mc-Indoe's vaginoplasty and releasing incisions will take care of the respective conditions. Some improvization and surgical ingenuity will pay rich dividends.

Hymenal remnants, tags after episiotomy, episiotomy neuromas all need to be excised surgically.

Painful anal conditions may at times cause dyspareunia. Fissures, fistulae, hemorrhoids, helminthiasis and even irritable bowel syndrome may be cause and relevant management will bring relief.

Vaginismus

Every gynecologist should have a set of vaginal dilators. Even in routine obstetrics-gynecology practice there is a constant trickle of women who need this therapy and I am surprised as to how a great number of doctors practice without a set of this simple yet very useful instrument.

Relationship issues are identified and sorted out simultaneously with the treatment. An educational sexological gynecologic examination is the most crucial part. As elaborated earlier the anatomy is pointed out, with patient using the hand mirror to see her own genitalia and the husband present. The technique of coitus is described in detail with relevant models, charts, etc. Techniques of relaxing the muscles at will are thought. Yoga techniques are especially useful in this area. Best is to ask her to tighten the muscles first and then to let go on command.

Next would be to provide a set of plastic vaginal dilators. Fingers (her own, physician's or partner's), cervical dilators or even a set of candles with condoms may be used. Copious anesthetic lubricant jelly is used. Patients are initially amazed to see even the small dilator getting easily inside. Soon, they are convinced that little if any harm is possible and will readily accept bigger and bigger dilators. Next would be to let her use the dilators herself, then involve the partner too and finally give asset to be used just before coitus. The woman on top position (cowgirl position as it is called) is advisable with man asked not to thrust at all. Woman guides the penis in her vagina as she slowly sits over it. This allows her complete control over insertion. If relationships issues have been tackled the spontaneity of the act soon takes over.

Some surgical approaches are said to be useful in extreme cases, where all else fails. Many experts feel that the surgical approach is not useful at all since the condition is one of reflex spasm. The Fenton's approach is to place a longitudinal incision over the perineum at 6 O'clock and suture it horizontally, thus widening the introitus. Only recently Vishwaprakash et al have described a surgical technique of Z plasty of the bulbospongiosus muscle has been described.[14] This involves:

- developing flaps of the labia minora
- exposing the bulbospongiosus and lenghthening it with a Z plasty
- covering the defect with the flap.

Vishwaprakash is of the opinion that all midline scars will give rise to dyspareunia and hence the need for tackling the bulbocavernosus laterally and placing a flap to avoid scarring.

1. Define vaginismus.
2. What are the components common to vaginismus and dyspareunia?
3. Describe the modern view of the function and dysfunction of the pelvic floor.
4. What are the common causes of sexual pain?

5. Describe the concept of an 'educational gynecological sexological examination'.
6. What are the advantages and disadvantages of the questionnaire approach?
7. Discuss the investigations and management options in a patient with vestibular pain.
8. Describe the management of dyspareunia.

References

1. Dickinson RL. Human Sex Anatomy: A Topographical Hand Atlas. 2nd Ed London: Bailliere, Tindal and Cox, 1949.pp.102.
2. Laumann EO, Paik A, Rosen RC. Sexual dysfunction in the United States: Prevalence and predictors. JAMA. 1999;281:537–44.
3. Safarinejad MR. Female sexual dysfunction in a population-based study in Iran: prevalence and associated risk factors. Int J Impot Res. 2006;18:382–95.
4. Fugl-Meyer AR, Sjogren Fugl-Meyer K. Sexual disabilities, problems and satisfaction in 18–74 year-old Swedes. Scand J sexol. 1999;2:79–105.
5. Reissing Ed. Binik YM, Khalife S. Does vaginisums exist? A critical review of the literature. J Nerv Mental Dis. 1999;187(5):261–74.
6. Meana M, Bink YM, Khalife S, Cohen D. Dyspareunia .sexual dysfunction or pain syndrome? J Nerv Mental Dis. 1997;185(9):561–9.
7. Van Lankveld JJ, Brewaeys AM, Ter Kuile MM, Weijenborg PTHM. Difficulties in the differential diagnosis of vaginisums. Dyspareunia and mixed sexual pain disorder. J Psychosom Obstet Gynaecol. 1995;16(4):201–9.
8. Kruiff De MD, Ter Kuile MM, Weijenborg PTHM, Van Lankveld JJDM, Vaginisums and dyspareunia; is there a difference in clinical presentation? J Psychosom Obstet Gynaecol. 2000;21:149–55.
9. Basson R. Lifelong vaginisums; A clinical study of 60 consecutive cases. J Soc Gynecol Obstet. 1996;3:551–61.
10. Basson R, Leiblum S, Brotto L, Derogatis L, Fourcroy J, Fugl-Meyerk, et al. Definitions of women's sexual dysfunction reconsidered advocating expansion and revision. J Psychosom obstet Gynaecol. 2003;24:221.
11. Holstege G. The emotional motor system in relation to the supraspinal control of micturition and mating behavior. Behav Brain Res 1998;92;103–109.
12. Blok BFM, Sturms LM, Holstege G. A Pet Study on cortical and subcortical control of pelvic floor muscles. J comp neurol. 1997;389;535–44.
13. Blok BFM, Sturms LM, Holstege G. Brain activation during micturition in women. Brain 1998;121:2033–42.
14. Prakash V. Introduction to plastic, reconstructive and microsurgery of female genitalia. 1st ed. Peepee publishers and distributors (P) Ltd, 2005.pp.38–41

Domestic Violence Against Women—A Universal Challenge

8

Suchitra Dalvie

Introduction

Violence against women is a serious human rights abuse and public health issue. Many studies confirm that physical and sexual partner violence against women is widespread. The variation in prevalence within and between settings highlights that this violence in not inevitable, and must be addressed. It includes intimate partner violence but also street violence and institutionalized women (state violence) and that that is directed towards sex workers.

A WHO multi-country study found that between 15–71% of women reported experiencing physical and/or sexual violence by an intimate partner at some point in their lives (Fig. 8.1).[1] These forms of violence result in physical, mental, sexual and reproductive health and other health problems and may increase vulnerability to HIV.

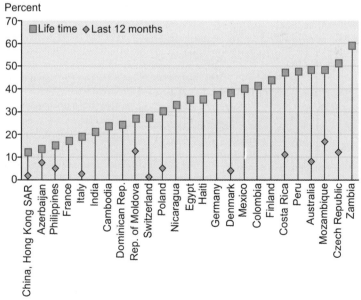

FIG. 8.1 Proportion of women experiencing physical violence (irrespective of the perpetrator) at least once in their lifetime and in the last 12 months, 1995-2006 (latest available) (*Courtesy:* http://unstats.un.org/unsd/demographic/products/Worldswomen/wwVaw2010.htm)

Risk Factors

Risk factors for being a perpetrator include low education, past exposure to child maltreatment or witnessing violence between parents, harmful use of alcohol, attitudes accepting of violence and gender inequality. Most of these are also risk factors for being a victim of intimate partner and sexual violence.

The magnitude of some of the most common and most severe forms of violence against women is immense: intimate partner violence; acid burning, dowry deaths, 'honor' killings, sexual abuse by non-intimate partners; trafficking, forced prostitution, exploitation of labor, and debt bondage of women and girls; physical and sexual violence against prostitutes; rape in war, sex selection, female infanticide and the deliberate neglect of girls. There are many potential perpetrators, including spouses and partners, parents, other family members, neighbors, and men in positions of power or influence. Most forms of violence are not unique incidents but are ongoing, and can even continue for decades. Due to the sensitivity of the subject, violence is almost universally under-reported. Nevertheless, the prevalence of such violence suggests that globally, millions of women are experiencing violence or living with its consequences (Fig. 8.2).[2]

Violence against women feeds off discrimination and also serves to reinforce it. When women are abused in custody, when they are raped by armed forces as

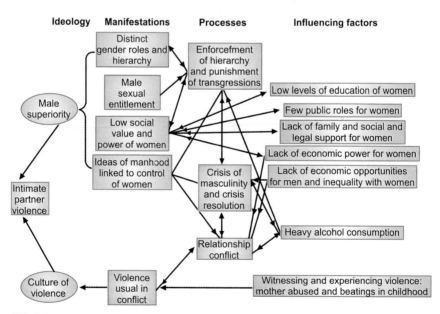

FIG. 8.2 Network of violence against women (*Courtesy:* Rachael Jewkes, Intimate partner violence: causes and prevention. The Lancet, Volume 359, Issue 9315, Pages 1423 -1429, 20 April 2002 doi:10.1016/S0140-6736(02)08357-5)

"spoils of war", or when they are terrorized by violence in the home, unequal power relations between men and women are both manifested and enforced.

Scope of the Problem

Around the world **at least one woman in every three** has been beaten, coerced into sex, or otherwise abused in her lifetime. Every year, violence in the home and the community devastates the lives of millions of women. **Gender-based violence kills and disables as many women between the ages of 15 and 44 as cancer, and its toll on women's health surpasses that of traffic accidents and malaria combined.**[3] Violence against women is rooted in a global culture of discrimination that denies women equal rights with men and that legitimizes the appropriation of women's bodies for individual gratification or political ends (Fig. 8.3).

The *WHO Multi-country study on women's health and domestic violence against women* in 10 developing countries found that, among women aged 15 to 49 years:

- Between 15% of women in Japan and 70% of women in Ethiopia and Peru reported physical and/or sexual violence by an intimate partner;
- Between 0.3–11.5% of women reported experiencing sexual violence by a non-partner;
- The first sexual experience for many women was reported as forced – 24% in rural Peru, 28% in Tanzania, 30% in rural Bangladesh, and 40% in South Africa.

Violence against women is compounded by discrimination on the grounds of race, ethnicity, sexual identity, social status, class and age. Such multiple forms of discrimination further restrict women's choices, increase their vulnerability to violence and make it even harder for women to obtain justice. Since institutionalized women are largely invisible to the public eye, little is done when the punishment of imprisonment is compounded with that of rape, sexual assault, groping during body searches and shackling during childbirth. Women are often coerced into providing sex for "favors" such as extra food or personal hygiene products, or to avoid punishment. There is little medical or psychological care available to inmates.

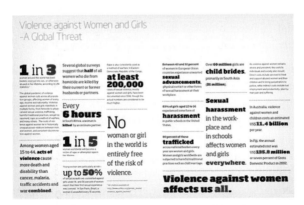

FIG. 8.3 Magnitude and effect of violence against women (*Courtesy:* http://www.unwomen.org/how-we-work/un-trust-fund/)

Though crimes in prison such as rape are prevalent, few perpetrators of violence against female inmates are ever held accountable.

Women's Rights are Human Rights[4]

The Universal Declaration of Human Rights states that "everyone is entitled to all the rights and freedoms set forth in this Declaration, without distinction of any kind, such as race, color, sex, language, religion, political or other opinion, national or social origin, property, birth or other status." (Article 2)

The Declaration on the Elimination of Violence Against Women states that "violence against women means any act of gender-based violence that results in, or is likely to result in, physical, sexual or psychological harm or suffering to women, including threats of such acts, coercion or arbitrary deprivation of liberty, whether occurring in public or in private life." (Article 1) It further asserts that states have an obligation to " exercise due diligence to prevent, investigate and, in accordance with national legislation, punish acts of violence against women, whether those acts are perpetrated by the State or by private persons." (Article 4-c)

The Convention on the Elimination of all forms of Discrimination Against Women (CEDAW), defines discrimination against women as any "distinction, exclusion or restriction made on the basis of sex which has the effect or purpose of impairing or nullifying the recognition, enjoyment or exercise by women, irrespective of their marital status, on the basis of equality between men and women, of human rights or fundamental freedoms in the political, economic, social, cultural, civil or any other field." (Article 1)

Intimate Partners and Sexual Violence

The United Nations **defines violence against women** as 'any act of gender-based violence that results in, or is likely to result in, physical, sexual or mental harm or suffering to women, including threats of such acts, coercion or arbitrary deprivation of liberty, whether occurring in public or in private life.[4]

Intimate partner violence refers to behavior in an intimate relationship that causes physical, sexual or psychological harm, including physical aggression, sexual coercion, psychological abuse and controlling behaviors.

Sexual violence is any sexual act, attempt to obtain a sexual act, unwanted sexual comments or advances, or acts to traffic, or otherwise directed against a person's sexuality using coercion, by any person regardless of their relationship to the victim, in any setting. It includes rape, defined as the physically forced or otherwise coerced penetration of the vulva or anus with a penis, other body part or object.

Health Consequences

Intimate partner and sexual violence have **serious short- and long-term physical, mental, sexual and reproductive health problems for victims and for their children**, and lead to high social and economic costs.

- Health effects can include headaches, back pain, abdominal pain, fibromyalgia, gastrointestinal disorders, limited mobility and poor overall health. In some cases, both fatal and non-fatal injuries can result.
- Intimate partner violence and sexual violence can lead to unintended pregnancies, gynecological problems, induced abortions and sexually transmitted infections, including HIV. Intimate partner violence in pregnancy also increases the likelihood of miscarriage, stillbirth, pre-term delivery and low birth weight.
- These forms of violence can lead to depression, post-traumatic stress disorder, sleep difficulties, eating disorders, emotional distress and suicide attempts.
- Sexual violence, particularly during childhood, can lead to increased smoking, drug and alcohol misuse and risky sexual behaviors in later life. It is also associated with perpetration of violence (for males) and being a victim of violence (for females).

Social and Economic Costs

The social and economic costs are enormous and have ripple effects throughout society. Women may suffer isolation, inability to work, loss of wages, lack of participation in regular activities and limited ability to care for themselves and their children.

Prevention

Currently, there are few interventions whose effectiveness has been scientifically proven. More resources are needed to strengthen the primary prevention of intimate partner and sexual violence, i.e. stopping it from happening in the first place.

The primary prevention strategy with the best evidence for effectiveness for intimate partner violence is **school-based programs for adolescents** to prevent violence within dating relationships. These, however, remain to be assessed for use in resource-poor settings. Evidence is emerging for the effectiveness of several other primary prevention strategies: those that combine microfinance with **gender equality training**; that promote **communication and relationship skills** within communities; that reduce access to, and the harmful use of alcohol; and that change cultural gender norms.

To achieve lasting change, it is important to **enact legislation and develop policies** that protect women; address discrimination against women and promote gender equality; and help to move the culture away from violence.

An appropriate **response from the health sector** can contribute in important ways to preventing the recurrence of violence and mitigating its consequences (secondary and tertiary prevention). Sensitization and education of health and other service providers is therefore another important strategy. To address fully the consequences of violence and the needs of victims/survivors requires a multi-sectoral response.[5]

WHO Response

The World Health Organization, in collaboration with a number of partners, is building the evidence base on the scope and types of intimate partner and sexual violence in different settings and supporting countries' efforts to document and measure this violence. This is central to understanding the magnitude and nature of the problem at a global level.

The WHO is also developing technical guidance for evidence-based intimate partner and sexual violence prevention and for strengthening the health sector responses to such violence. It is also disseminating information and supporting national efforts to advance women's rights and the prevention of and response to intimate partner and sexual violence against women; and collaborating with international agencies and organizations to reduce/eliminate intimate partner and sexual violence globally.

The WHO has recently published *Preventing intimate partner and sexual violence against women: taking action and generating evidence.*[13] This publication summarizes the existing evidence on strategies for primary prevention, identifying those that have been shown to be effective and those that seem promising or theoretically feasible.

Violence Against Women in Asia and India

Domestic spousal violence against women in developing countries like India is now beginning to be recognized as a widespread health problem impeding development and many studies are being conducted to assess the spread and impact of this problem.

In Bangladesh, 42% of 275 respondents had justified wife beating; in India, 51% of 13,078 male adolescents had supported wife beating; and in Nepal, 28% of 939 respondents had supported wife abuse. Individual-level factors, such as rural residency, low educational attainment, low economic status, being unemployed, and having a history of family violence, were positively associated with the justification of wife abuse. This multi-country study indicates a general trend of **male adolescents'** strong supportive attitude toward wife beating, and hence may suggest that policy makers can specifically target young groups of the population for various interventions for reducing violence against women.[6]

In another study from Bangladesh, about one-third of women were abused physically and/or sexually and about one third of their births in the last 5 years were unintended. Compared with women who did not suffer violence, women who were abused sexually had a 1.64-fold increased risk of unintended pregnancy. The prevalence of **unintended pregnancy** among those who experienced severe physical violence was 1.60 times higher than those who reported no abuse.[7]

A literature review from **Bangladesh** also suggests that spousal violence against women is high in Bangladesh.[8] The types of violence commonly committed are domestic violence, acid throwing, rape, trafficking and forced prostitution. Domestic violence is the most common form of violence and its prevalence is higher in rural areas. The majority of abused women remained silent about their experience because of the high acceptance of violence within society, fear of repercussion, tarnishing family honor and own reputation, jeopardizing children's future, and lack of an alternative place to stay. Interestingly, violence increased with membership of women in micro-credit organizations initially but tapered off as duration of involvement increased. The high acceptability of violence within society acts as a deterrent for legal redress.[9]

A series of in-depth interviews conducted in **Pakistan** showed that women tried to cope with violence by using various strategies, both emotion focused (e.g. use of religion, placating the husband, etc.) and problem focused (e.g. seeking support from formal institutions, etc.). However, the data also showed that few women opted for problem-focused strategies, such as seeking help from formal institutions, as these strategies could lead to overt confrontation with their husbands and may result in divorce, the outcome least desired by most of the Pakistani women.[10]

A literature survey for articles and reports on Intimate Partner Violence (IPV) in **Sri Lanka** indicates that the prevalence of IPV is high (40%). A common belief in Sri Lanka, even among medical students and police officers is that IPV is a personal matter that outsiders should not intervene. The laws against IPV identify the physical and psychological IPV, but not the sexual IPV. [11] Another study from Sri Lanka shows that lifetime prevalence of physical violence (34%), controlling behavior (30%), and emotional abuse (19%) was high and the prevalence of sexual violence was low (5%). Although living in a patriarchal society, low prevalence of child marriages and lack of dowry-related violence could be to Sri Lankan women's advantage relative to their Asian counterparts in preventing IPV.[12]

Studies suggest that in some ways **Indian** women are becoming more liberated, but others imply worsening conditions for Indian women, such as more violence against women. This increase in violence may be temporary, as India is in transition to a more modern society: There is evidence that some gender-based violence is a male response to increasingly "modern" attitudes among Indian women.[13]

A study for **South India** reveals that 36% and 50% of the participants report experiencing sexual and physical violence, respectively. The husband's characteristics found most significantly associated with their odds of experiencing sexual violence included the husbands' primary education, employment as drivers, alcohol consumption, and having multiple sex partners. Women's contribution to household income also increases their odds of experiencing sexual violence by almost two fold; however, if they are solely responsible for "all" household income, the relationship was found to be protective.[14]

Another study also found that women who were unemployed at one visit and began employment by the next visit had an 80% higher odd of violence, as compared to women who maintained their unemployed status. This would suggest that there are complex challenges for violence prevention.[15] Economic empowerment is not the sole protective factor. Economic empowerment, together with higher education and modified cultural norms against women, may protect women from IPV.[16]

Medical Complications Because of Violence Against Women

Intimate partner violence affected woman's physical and mental health, reduced sexual autonomy, increased risk for unintended pregnancy and multiple abortions. A study from India shows that the risk for sexual assault decreased by 59% or 70% for women contacting the police or applying for a protection order, respectively. However, the **quality of life** of IPV victims was found to be significantly impaired. Such women reported high levels of anxiety and depression that often led to alcohol and drug abuse. Violence on pregnant women significantly increased the risk for low birth weight infants, preterm delivery and neonatal death and also affected breastfeeding postpartum. Women preferred an active role to be played by health care providers in response to IPV disclosure.[17]

A study conducted in **rural India** showed that domestic violence affected 40–46% of the sample in Uttar Pradesh and 33–35% in Tamil Nadu and was widely accepted by women and by husbands. At least 27% of the sample reported pregnancy loss (including induced abortion), and 13% of the women who had a live birth experienced an infant death (16% from Uttar Pradesh and 10% from Tamil Nadu). Victims of domestic abuse were significantly more likely to experience fetal wastage or infant death regardless of religion or region of residence.[18]

Women who experienced physical violence during pregnancy were less likely to receive prenatal care, less likely to receive a home-visit from a health worker for a prenatal check-up, less likely to receive at least three prenatal care visits, and less likely to initiate prenatal care early in the pregnancy.[19]

Spousal violence is specifically associated as an independent risk factor for two adverse women's health outcomes—sexually transmitted infections (STIs) and attempted suicide. Public health and clinical programs targeting these outcomes must specifically address spousal violence.[20]

An analysis of data from India's 2006-2007 **National Family Health Survey-3** from the Central/Northern Indian state of **Uttar Pradesh** suggests that experiencing marital violence may have a negative impact on multiple aspects of women's reproductive health, including increased self-report of STI symptoms.[21]

Infant mortality was greater among infants whose mothers experienced IPV but this effect was significant only for girls. Child mortality was also greater among children whose mothers experienced IPV. Again, this effect was significant only for girls. An estimated 58,021 infant girl deaths and 89,264 girl child deaths were related to spousal violence against wives annually, or approximately 1.2 million female infant deaths and 1.8 million girl deaths in India between December 1985 and August 2005.[22]

Among married Indian women, physical violence combined with sexual violence from husbands was associated with an increased prevalence of HIV infection. Prevention of IPV may augment efforts to reduce the spread of HIV/AIDS.[23]

Findings provide the first empirical evidence that abused wives face increased HIV risk based both on the greater likelihood of HIV infection among abusive husbands and elevated HIV transmission within abusive relationships. Thus, IPV seems to function both as a risk marker and as a risk factor for HIV among women, indicating the need for interwoven efforts to prevent both men's sexual risk and IPV perpetration.[24]

A study from rural India highlights how violence is normalized, or considered acceptable, if women do not adhere to expected gender roles and how this impacts a woman's ability to use contraception and make fertility decisions in a context where being a wife implies obedience, limited mobility, sexual availability and high fertility.[25]

Economic Violence

Most studies on gender-based violence (GBV) focus on its physical, sexual, and psychological manifestations. There is however, also an economic violence experienced by women that also has consequences on health and development. Economic violence experienced included limited access to funds and credit; controlling access to health care, employment, education, including agricultural resources; excluding from financial decision making; and discriminatory traditional laws on inheritance, property rights and use of communal land. This results in deepening poverty and compromises educational attainment and developmental opportunities for women. It leads to physical violence, promotes sexual exploitation and the risk of contracting HIV infection, maternal morbidity and mortality and trafficking of women and girls. Economic abuse may continue even after the woman has left the abusive relationship.[26]

Role of the Law

Marriage in India is a voluntary union for life of one man and one woman to the exclusion of all others. However, the reality is that many women are ill-treated, harassed, killed or divorced for the simple reason that they do not get a dowry or do not get a sufficiently large one. To safeguard the interest of women against the cruelty they face within the four walls of their matrimonial home, the Indian Penal Code 1860 was amended in 1983 and section 498A was added. **Matrimonial Cruelty** in India is a cognizable, non-bailable and non-compoundable offence. Notwithstanding that the practice of demanding dowries was made illegal in India over 50 years ago, the (London) Times on 18 January 2012 reported that a study in 2007 concluded that "there is a dowry-related death in India every four hours". Official statistics in India show there were 8,391 dowry-related deaths in 2010, and there may well have been more.[27]

The **Dowry Prohibition Act in India** was passed in 1961 and amended in 1984 and 1986. The law was enacted in order to prevent "dowry deaths" or the murder of a wife by her husband.[28]

However, it is only recently that **domestic violence** has been considered a violation of the law. While legal and social changes over time have altered the criminal justice system s approach to domestic violence, there is much lacking in the responses of the police, and the prosecution of domestic violence.[29,30]

Role of Physician/Gynecologist

Screening

Abused women have an increased risk of cardiac, gastrointestinal, gynecologic, musculoskeletal, neurologic and psychological complaints. They also have a greater utilization of medical services and are more likely to access **outpatient primary care and specialty care, emergency departments and mental health and substance abuse services** than women without a history of partner violence. Most major US medical organizations recommend routine screening of all women for partner abuse. Offering abused women **empathy and validation along with referral** to local resources is encouraged. Physicians should also **document the abuse in the victim's medical record**.[31]

The primary healthcare institutions as well as private sector health services in India should **institutionalize the routine screening and treatment** for violence related injuries and trauma. Treatment records of this will also provide vital information to assess the situation to develop public health interventions, and to sensitive the concerned agencies to implement the laws related to violence against women.[32]

When women are asked what they would expect from the providers they suggested that providers should give a reason for why they are asking about IPV to reduce women's suspicions and minimize stigma, create an atmosphere of safety and support, and finally provide information, support and access to resources regardless of whether the woman discloses IPV (Fig. 8.4). They emphasized that

Medscape			
	IPV+	IPV-	
"Do you have daily contact with other people?"	63 (76.8%)	299 (92.9%)	P < 0.01
"Is there someone in your life that you can talk to about any problem?	58 (70.7%)	279 (86.7%)	P < 0.01
"Do you have someone to stay with in case of an emergency?"	58 (69.1%)	264 (82.5%)	P < 0.01
"Do you have a job outside the home?"	27 (32.9%)	174 (54.0%)	P < 0.01
"Do you usually have enough money to meet your needs?"	22 (26.8%)	152 (47.2%)	P < 0.01
Source: Western J Emerg Med © 2011 Western Journal of Emergency Medicine			

FIG. 8.4 The domestic violence questionnaire with psychometric properties for determining intimate sexual violence (*Courtesy:* http://www.medscape.org/viewarticle/741906_4)

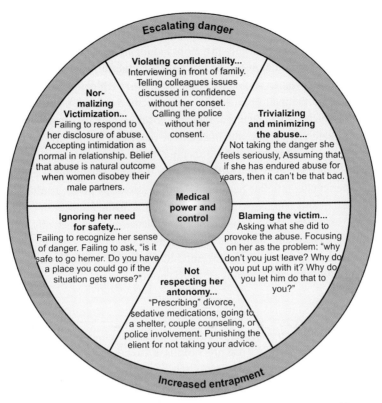

FIG. 8.5 Inadequacies in identifying and helping victims of violence (*Source: Developed by the domestic abuse intervention project, 202 East Superior Street Duluh Minnesota USA*)

a provider's asking about IPV is an opportunity to raise patient awareness of IPV, communicate compassion and provide information and not merely a screening test to diagnose a pathologic condition.[33]

In India, the questionnaires used currently are either too exhaustive or inadequate to assess domestic violence comprehensively. The Domestic Violence Questionnaire in Malayalam has adequate psychometric properties to identify intimate partner violence against women in the local population.[34]

However, studies have found that such screening can have both positive and negative consequences and that these depend on the behavior of the provider behavior. A better understanding of consequences can help providers tailor screening approaches and interventions for intimate partner violence (Fig. 8.5).[35]

Intimate partner violence (IPV) has consistently been found to afflict **one in twenty pregnant women** and is therefore considered a leading cause of physical injury, mental illness and adverse pregnancy outcome. A general antenatal screening policy should be advocated. **Gynecologists** do not receive any orientation or training in managing IPV as part of their medical education and hence, tend to largely underestimate the extent of the problem as well as feel insufficiently skilled to deal with it.[36] Thus the pre-service orientation and training of physicians is an important first step. The health services also need to ensure availability of screening tools, patient leaflets, formal referral pathways and physician feedback.[37]

Violence against women is not a private or family matter. The **FIGO Committee for the Study of Ethical Aspects of Human Reproduction** released statements to physicians treating women on this issue. **Physicians are ethically obliged** to inform themselves about the manifestations of violence and recognize cases, to treat the physical and psychological results of violence, to affirm to their patients that violent acts toward them are not acceptable and to advocate for social infrastructures to provide women the choice of seeking secure refuge and ongoing counseling.[38]

Health care providers in India are often the only institutional contact for women experiencing intimate partner violence, a pervasive public health problem with adverse health outcomes. A study revealed a distinct subset of 'physician champions' who responded to intimate partner violence more consistently, informed women of their rights and facilitated their utilization of support services. However, physician practices were mediated by individual attitudes and there was no system for a uniform training on screening or interventions.[39]

Conclusion

Violence against women is an all-pervasive phenomenon in India and across South Asia. Intimate partner violence and other forms of violence all have a serious impact on the health of the woman and her children.

The broader social costs are profound but difficult to quantify. Violence against women is likely to constrain poverty reduction efforts by reducing women's participation in productive employment. Violence also undermines efforts to improve women's access to education, with violence and the fear of violence contributing to lower school enrolment for girls. Domestic violence has also been shown to affect the welfare and education of children in the family.

Violence against women has been described as "perhaps the most shameful human rights violation and the most pervasive."

This violence can be prevented through long-term interventions involving education through schools, gender sensitization and implementation of relevant laws and policies. However, physicians, and gynecologists in particular are likely to be the first point of contact for these women and should be adequately equipped through training to be able to screen and manage them. The health system should provide appropriate support in terms of information material screening protocols, referral systems. Police referrals should be made judiciously and health care providers must document the injuries of the violence in a manner that is useful in court as evidence.

Any discussion with the women in our clinics about condom use, dual protection and abstinence after an abortion to prevent infection, adequate nutrition and rest during pregnancy and lactation, all would be rendered ineffectual unless we are able to see the client within the power dynamics of her own interpersonal relationships.

References

1. Ellsberg M, Jansen HA, Heise L, Watts CH, Garcia-Moreno C. Intimate partner violence and women's physical and mental health in the WHO multi-country study on women's health and domestic violence: an observational study. WHO Multi-country Study on Women's Health and Domestic Violence against Women Study Team. Lancet.2008;5;371(9619):1165–72.
2. Watts C, Zimmerman C. Violence against women: global scope and magnitude Lancet. 2002;359 (9313):1232–7.
3. UNFPA State of World Population 2005: The Promise of Equality. (UNFPA drew this figure from pg. 15 and 110 of the following report: UN Millennium Project Taking Action: Achieving Gender Equality and Empowering Women. Task Force on Education and Gender Equality. London and Sterling, Virginia: Earthscan. (2005a) 2005;65.
4. Fact sheet No. 239 Updated. September, 2011.
5. Krishnan S, Subbiah K, Khanum S, Chandra PS, Padian NS. An Intergenerational Women's Empowerment Intervention to Mitigate Domestic Violence: Results of a Pilot Study in Bengaluru, India, Violence Against Women, 2012. [Epub ahead of print]
6. Dalal K, Lee MS, Gifford M. Male adolescents' attitudes toward wife beating: a multi-country study in South Asia. Journal of Adolescent Health. 2012;50(5):437–42. Epub 2011 Dec 3.
7. Rahman M, Sasagawa T, Fujii R, Tomizawa H, Makinoda S. Intimate partner violence and unintended pregnancy among Bangladeshi women, Journal of Interpersonal Violence, 2012. [Epub ahead of print]
8. Johnston HB, Naved RT. Spousal violence in Bangladesh: a call for a public-health response. Journal of Health Population and Nutrition. 2008;26(3):366–77.
9. Wahed T, Bhuiya A. Battered bodies and shattered minds: violence against women in Bangladesh. Indian Journal of Medical Research. 2007;126(4):341–54.
10. Zakar R, Zakar MZ, Krämer A. Voices of strength and struggle: Women's coping strategies against spousal violence in Pakistan. Journal of Interpersonal Violence, 2012. [Epub ahead of print]
11. Jayatilleke AC, Poudel KC, Yasuoka J, Jayatilleke AU, Jimba M. Intimate partner violence in Sri Lanka. Bioscience Trends. 2010;4(3):90–5.
12. Jayasuriya V, Wijewardena K, Axemo P. Intimate partner violence against women in the capital province of Sri Lanka: prevalence, risk factors, and help seeking. Violence Against Women. 2011;17(8):1086–102. Epub 2011 Sep 1.
13. Simister J, Mehta PS. Gender-based violence in India: long-term trends. Journal of Interpersonal Violence. 2010;25(9):1594–611. Epub 2010 Jan 12.
14. Chibber KS, Krupp K, Padian N, Madhivanan P. Examining the determinants of sexual violence among young, married women in Southern India. Journal of Interpersonal Violence, 2012. [Epub ahead of print]
15. Krishnan S, Rocca CH, Hubbard AE, Subbiah K, Edmeades J, Padian NS. Do changes in spousal employment status lead to domestic violence? Insights from a prospective study in Bangalore, India. Social Science and Medicine. 2010;70(1):136–43. Epub 2009 Oct 14.
16. Dalal K. Does economic empowerment protect women from intimate partner violence? Journal of Injury and Violence Research. 2011;3(1):35–44.
17. Sarkar NN. The impact of intimate partner violence on women's reproductive health and pregnancy outcome. Journal of Obstetrics and Gynecology. 2008;28(3):266–71.
18. Jejeebhoy SJ. Associations between wife-beating and fetal and infant death: Impressions from a survey in rural India. Studies in Family Planning. 1998;29(3):300–8.
19. Koski AD, Stephenson R, Koenig MR. Physical violence by partner during pregnancy and use of prenatal care in rural India. Journal of Health Population and Nutrition, 2011;29(3):245–54.

20. Chowdhary N, Patel V. The effect of spousal violence on women's health: findings from the Stree Arogya Shodh in Goa, India. Journal of Postgraduate Medicine. 2008;54(4):306–12.

21. Sudha S, Morrison S. Marital violence and women's reproductive health care in Uttar Pradesh, India. Women's Health Issues. 2011;21(3):214–21.

22. Silverman JG, Decker MR, Cheng DM, Wirth K, Saggurti N, McCauley HL. Gender-based disparities in infant and child mortality based on maternal exposure to spousal violence: The heavy burden borne by Indian girls. Archives of Pediatric Adolescent Medicine. 2011;165(1):22–7.

23. Silverman JG, Decker MR, Saggurti N, Balaiah D, Raj A. Intimate partner violence and HIV infection among married Indian women. JAMA. 2008;13;300(6):703–10.

24. Decker MR, Seage GR 3rd, Hemenway D, Raj A, Saggurti N, Balaiah D. Intimate partner violence functions as both a risk marker and risk factor for women's HIV infection: findings from Indian husband-wife dyads. Journal of Acquired Immune Deficiency Syndromes. 2009;15;51(5):593–600.

25. Wilson-Williams L, Stephenson R, Juvekar S, Andes K. Domestic violence and contraceptive use in a rural Indian village. Violence Against Women. 2008; 14(10):1181–98.

26. Fawole OI. Economic violence to women and girls: Is it receiving the necessary attention? Trauma, Violence and Abuse. 2008;9(3):167–77. Epub 2008 May 21.

27. Shetty BS, Rao PP, Shetty AS. Legal terrorism in domestic violence - an Indian outlook. The Medico Legal Journal. 2012;80(Pt 1):33–8.

28. Agnes F. Marital murders – the Indian reality. Health for the Millions. 1993;1(1):18–21.

29. Erez E. Domestic violence and the criminal justice system: An overview. Online Journal of Issues in Nursing. 2002;7(1):4.

30. Danis FS. The criminalization of domestic violence: What social workers need to know. Social Work. 2003;48(2):237–46.

31. Gottlieb AS. Intimate partner violence: A clinical review of screening and intervention. Womens Health (London England). 2008;4(5):529–39.

32. Babu BV, Kar SK. Domestic violence against women in eastern India: A population-based study on prevalence and related issues. BMC Public Health. 2009;9:129.

33. Chang JC, Decker MR, Moracco KE, Martin SL, Petersen R, Frasier PY. Asking about intimate partner violence: Advice from female survivors to health care providers. Patient Education and Counselling. 2005;59(2):141–7.

34. Indu PV, Remadevi S, Vidhukumar K, Anilkumar TV, Subha N. Development and validation of the Domestic Violence Questionnaire in married women aged 18–55 years. Indian Journal of Psychiatry. 2011;53(3):218–23.

35. Chang JC, Decker M, Moracco KE, Martin SL, Petersen R, Frasier PY. What happens when health care providers ask about intimate partner violence? A description of consequences from the perspectives of female survivors. Journal of the American Medical Women's Association. 2003 Spring;58(2):76–81.

36. Gutmanis I, Beynon C, Tutty L, Wathen CN, MacMillan HL. Factors influencing identification of and response to intimate partner violence: a survey of physicians and nurses. BMC Public Health. 2007;7:12.

37. Roelens K, Verstraelen H, Van Egmond K, Temmerman M. A knowledge, attitudes, and practice survey among obstetrician-gynaecologists on intimate partner violence in Flanders, Belgium. BMC Public Health. 2006;6:238.

38. Schmuel E, Schenker JG. Violence against women: The physician's role. European Journal of Obstetrics Gynecology and Reproductive Biology. 1998;80(2):239–45.

39. Chibber KS, Krishnan S, Minkler M. Physician practices in response to intimate partner violence in southern India: Insights from a qualitative study. Women and Health. 2011;51(2):168–85.

Metabolic Disorders after Menopause

9

Chapter

Stamatina Iliodromiti, Mary Ann Lumsden

Introduction

For most Caucasian women living in the Western world, the menopause occurs at about the age of 50 years although this does vary with the ethnic group. Menopause is a universal and unavoidable stage in a woman's life that may in some instances be associated with unpleasant symptoms. Since menopause coincides with aging, it is associated with an increase in the risk of metabolic disorders that is more prevalent in older age, although the causal effect of the menopause itself is debatable. The increase in life-expectancy means that women live for a longer duration and may spend one-third of their life in the postmenopause, so it is important that we consider the health problems related to the menopause and identify modifiable factors that may improve women's health after menopause. Women after menopause lose the sex-derived protection against cardiovascular (CVD) events, and coronary heart disease (CHD) is the leading cause of mortality in both men and women with a higher prevalence in women.

The metabolic syndrome (MetS) is a cluster of risk factors that include central obesity, impaired glucose metabolism, adverse lipid profile and hypertension and overall increase the likelihood of developing diabetes type 2 and atherosclerotic events. It has various definitions, as shown in Table 9.1, including those of the International Diabetes Federation (IDF), the World Health Organization (WHO) and National Cholesterol Education Program Adult treatment Panel III (NCEP-ATPIII).

Menopause and Hyperlipidemia

The direct effect of menopause on lipid profile is difficult to assess because of the strong association between lipids and age. Previous studies suggested that menopausal transition is associated with raised total cholesterol and low density lipoprotein (LDL) (Peters et al, 1999; Bonithon-Kopp et al, 1990) but these studies were cross sectional in character and results must be interpreted with caution. A recent longitudinal and multiethnic study that followed 1,054 women over 9 years (Matthews et al, 2009) concluded that a significant increase in total cholesterol, LDL and apolipoprotein B (Apo B) occur within a year of the final menstrual

TABLE 9.1 Common definitions of metabolic syndrome

IDF	WHO	NCEP-ATPIII
		Three out of five
Central obesity (ethnic specific values) plus any two from the following	Insulin Resistance plus any two of the following	Central obesity waist ≥ 88 cm (women)
TGL (triglycerides) ≥ 150 mg/dL (1.7 mmol/L) or on treatment for this	TGL ≥ 1.7 mmol/L	TGL ≥ 1.7 mmol/L
HDL cholesterol < 50 mg/dL (1.29 mmol/L) (females) or on treatment for this	HDL < 1 mmol/ (females)	HDL < 1.30 mmol/L (females)
SBP ≥ 130 or DBP ≥ 85 mm Hg or on antihypertensive treatment	SBP ≥ 140 or DBP ≥ 90 mm Hg or on treatment	SBP ≥ 130 or DBP ≥ 85 mm Hg
(FPG) ≥ 100 mg/dL (5.6 mmol/L), or previously diagnosed type 2 diabetes	BMI ≥ 30 kg/m² or waist:hip > 0.85 (females)	FPG ≥ 6.1 mmol/L
	Urinary Albumin excretion rate ≥ 20 mg/min or albumin: creatinine ratio ≥	

IDF : International Diabetes Federation
SBP : Systolic blood pressure
DBP : Diastolic blood pressure
FPG : Fasting plasma glucose
HDL : High density lipoprotein
WHO : World health Organization
NCEP-ATPIII : National Cholesterol Education Program Adult treatment Panel III
Insulin resistance (WHO criteria) is identified by one of the following factors: a. Type 2 diabetes b. Impaired fasting glucose c. Impaired glucose tolerance or d. for those with normal fasting glucose levels, glucose uptake below the lowest quartile for the background population

period (FMP) irrespective of age, ethnicity, weight, weight gain or medications. The increase in lipoproteins was not linear, that would be suggestive of an age related effect, but it peaked during the early menopausal stage and thereafter it leveled off, but without returning to premenopausal levels. This study suggested early changes in lipid profile during the menopausal transition and highlighted the importance of close monitoring of the lipid profile and advocating preventive lifestyle modifications at this stage when indicated.

The Melbourne Women's Midlife health project followed up 150 women during the menopausal transition and demonstrated a substantial increase in high density lipoprotein (HDL) during the year preceding the FMP followed but a significant decline by the first year after FMP (Do et al 2000). Thus, the net change in HDL was minimal. Differences in other lipids over the menopausal transition were explained by the aging effect, modifications in activity levels, alcohol consumption and smoking habits. Although, this study had limitations because of its small sample size, it highlighted the critical stage of menopausal transition in lipid profile.

The studies investigating the role of the menopause on circulating lipids may seem contradictory, but all underpin the importance of menopausal transition in later cardiovascular health. Matthews et al followed up perimenopausal women for 20 years in relation to their risk of coronary calcification and concluded that baseline risk factors were strongly associated with later risk of calcification and this risk was independent of risk factors in late postmenopausal period (Matthews et al 2007). Therefore, it is important that clinicians target early premenopausal women with lifestyle modification rather than waiting until older age (Kuller et al 2001).

Menopause and Hypertension

The direct effect of menopause on blood pressure is challenging to clarify because of the coexistence of other risk factors of hypertension such as aging and obesity that coincide with the menopausal transition. The SWAN study followed women longitudinally over 9 years and showed that both diastolic and systolic blood pressure rise in a linear fashion along with advancing age and irrespective of the date of the FMP (Matthews et al 2009). An earlier cross sectional study that compared post with premenopausal women of similar age did not find a significant difference in systolic or diastolic blood pressure among both groups (Peters et al 1999). These findings were consistent with the Melbourne Women's Midlife health project, that despite of its small sample size, showed that the longitudinal change in diastolic blood pressure was independent of the menopausal transition (Do et al 2000).

The above clinical studies suggest that menopause per se is not a risk factor for hypertension, however, epidemiological papers show that women at a younger age have lower blood pressure than age matched men, whereas this reverses in older ages where blood pressure increases more rapidly in women than in men (Sjöberg et al 2004) studies have indicated that changes in the prevalence of hypertension, and overall cardiovascular risk profiles in postmenopausal women, might be due to ageing and not oestrogen deficiency. Undoubtedly, there is a strong multicolinearity between the two phenomena. Furthermore, hormone replacement therapy (HRT. In addition, the prevalence of hypertension is higher in menopausal women than in men of similar age and is reported in around 60% in women over 65 years of age (Taddei 2009). Several physiological mechanisms have been suggested in order to explain the above difference but none seem to tell the whole story. A combined model proposes that menopause alters the estrogen to androgen ratio and this subsequently causes changes in the sympathetic activity, the endothelin activity, angiotensin II and ω-hydroxylase activity and they all result in increased renal vascular resistance and hypertension (Yanes and Reckelhoff 2011).

Despite the debate regarding the causal effect of menopause in increasing blood pressure, the menopausal transition coincides with the rise in blood pressure. Since it is one of the main modifiable risk factors of cardiovascular disease, once again it is important to advocate effective preventative measures targeted in women of this age group.

Menopause and Diabetes

Several studies indicate that menopause, because of its physiological changes, may be associated with deterioration in glucose intolerance. Menopause is characterized by a relative hyperandrogenic state. Higher levels of endogenous androgens (higher testosterone and lower SHBG) (Burger et al 2000) are considered to increase the risk of diabetes type 2 in women (Ding et al 2012). In addition, menopause is associated with greater abdominal adiposity which has been shown to be linked with glucose intolerance.

However, menopause per se has not been proven to have a causal effect on the risk of diabetes in middle aged women. 949 women who had enrolled in the SWAN study, were followed up for 9 years regarding different parameters of the metabolic syndrome (Janssen et al 2008). This study showed that although the incidence of metabolic syndrome is progressively increasing during the menopausal transition starting 6 years prior the FMP and continuing for 6 years after it, this rise is independent of the blood sugar levels, which, surprisingly, show a small decrease over the above period (Janssen et al, 2008). The study concluded that the rise in metabolic syndrome remains after controlling for age and other traditional Cardiovascular disease (CVD) risk factors and is largely linked to the testosterone dominance. Therefore, the risk of diabetes is increasing after menopause secondary to the rise in metabolic syndrome, but menopause does not seem to have a direct effect on the blood sugar levels.

Consistent data were presented in the Diabetes Prevention program (DPP), a randomized trial that assessed metformin versus lifestyle modifications, and concluded that, after adjusting for age, menopause does not affect the risk of developing diabetes among women with glucose intolerance (C Kim et al 2011). Thus, menopause does not seem to affect the risk of diabetes in both women with and without high background risk.

Menopause and Endothelial Function

The metabolic syndrome causes impairment of endothelial function. Estrogens are believed to have vasodilatory effects through its activation of calcium channels on the blood vessel wall, stimulation of endothelium dependent vasodilatation and upregulation of prostacyclin synthesis. Early studies have shown that menopause decreases the endothelium dependent vasodilatation, as demonstrated by the decreased response to acetylcholine, that acts by stimulating nitric oxide release from vascular endothelium, to a greater degree than aging alone when compared to age matched men (Taddei et al 1996). In reverse, in individuals over 60 years of age, the decline in endothelial function is similar in both sexes. A similar study showed that the age related endothelial dysfunction in men starts 10 years earlier than in women and the effect of age is not evident in menstruating women (Celermajer et al, 1994).

Menopause and Obesity

The prevalence of obesity has increased sharply over the last two decades. One in three adults has a BMI > 30 kg/m² and over half of the remaining population in the developed world, is overweight. Globally, obesity is more common than under-nutrition and has been characterized as an epidemic of our era.

Cross sectional studies have shown that postmenopausal women accumulate more intra-abdominal fat than age matched premenopausal women. This is not only evident in westernized countries where urbanization can be blamed but in the South Asian Subcontinent too (Dasgupta et al 2012). More robust data were reported by Lovejoy et al, who assessed longitudinally, 156 middle aged healthy women over 4 years period (Lovejoy et al 2008). They found that all women gained subcutaneous fat along with advancing age but only women who went through menopause over the above period (n = 51) showed a significant increase in visceral fat, suggesting that the increase in intra-abdominal fat, that is associated with higher metabolic risk, is associated with menopausal transition.

Data suggest that body composition changes because of combined effect of chronological and ovarian aging. 543 women who participated in the SWAN study were followed over 6 years and showed a substantial increase in fat mass and decrease in skeletal mass (assessed by bioelectrical impendence analysis, BIA). These changes were associated both with advancing age and increasing levels of FSH (ovarian aging) (M Sowers et al 2007). In addition, waist circumference, which is an indirect way of assessing abdominal adiposity, was found to increase alongside. The rising trend was marked prior to FMP and plateaued within a year after FMP.

Interestingly, longitudinal data on non-obese peri and early menopausal women showed that menopausal transition was associated with a significant increase in body fat mass and visceral fat (assessed by DXA and CT retrospectively) but this was not associated with a simultaneous deterioration in metabolic risk factors (Abdulnour et al 2012). However, this conclusion resulted from a small study sample (n = 61) and referred to an overall healthy population with a baseline normal BMI, so the conclusions need to be tested in larger scale studies.

There are different theories explaining the tendency of aging women to gain weight and store more fat; sedentary lifestyle is common in midlife women and contributes to weight gain and increased BMI (Castelo-Branco et al 2003). Sex hormones are modulators of food intake and energy expenditure (Asarian and Geary 2006) their control by gonadal steroid hormones and their peripheral and central mediating mechanisms are reviewed. Adult female rats and mice as well as women eat less during the peri-ovulatory phase of the ovarian cycle (estrus in rats and mice, therefore, the rapid decrease of estrogens and the relative increase in androgens during menopausal transition could be responsible for the attenuated resting metabolic rate and the change in appetite in menopausal women. In addition, estrogen depletion inhibits the activity of lipoprotein lipase in femoral adipocytes and lipolysis in abdominal adipose tissue, predisposing to accumulation of abdominal fat (android-apple shaped) as opposed to gluteofemoral adipose tissue (gynoid-pear shaped) (Rebuffé-Scrive et al 1986).

The anecdotal belief that fewer hot flushes occur in menopausal, obese women has been questioned recently. It was thought to be because of the capacity of adipose tissue to aromatize androgen to estrogen. Recent studies suggest that women with higher BMI have increased frequency of hot flushes and indeed, midlife women with higher percentage of body fat have higher odds of reporting vasomotor symptoms (Thurston et al 2008). In particular, subcutaneous abdominal adiposity is associated with the frequency of hot flushes, regardless of ethnicity, favoring the thermoregulatory model of hot flushing and the insulating effect of adipose tissue (Thurston et al 2008). Conversely, this study did not show an association between intra-abdominal fat (visceral), that is related with metabolic disorders, and the severity of hot flushes.

Menopause and Coronary Heart Disease

Metabolic Syndrome is a risk factor for coronary heart disease (CHD) that is the leading cause of mortality worldwide accounting for around 12% of deaths. Despite the sex derived cardioprotection in women of reproductive age, CHD has a high incidence in midlife women with many adverse outcomes because of the aging effect. It was believed that ovarian failure and the subsequent decrease in endogenous estrogens was responsible for the gender difference in risk, but this has been questioned recently as the endogenous androgens seem to play a role too (Janssen et al 2008).

Cardiovascular risk is a cluster of modifiable and non-modifiable risks. The features of the metabolic syndrome, obesity, hypertension, lipid profile and glucose intolerance can be potentially modified, or at least their effects lessened, as has been discussed above. Lack or exercise (being sedentary), defined as spending less than 10% of daily activities on moderate or vigorous physical activity, contributes to increased cardiovascular risk. This may be attributed to reduced cardio-respiratory fitness, glycemia and subclinical coronary calcification in menopausal women (Gill et al, 2011) (Gabriel et al 2012), which are all, in addition, independent risk factors of CVD. The current guidelines about physical activity for adults, recommend 150 minutes per week of moderate intensity physical activity; however, these guidelines have resulted from research in Western Europe and North America and further research is needed before conclusions can be drawn for other ethnic groups.

Current practice, moves away from generic CVD risk factors towards individualized risk scores as several risk factors interact with each other and increase the CVD risk of each individual. The SCORE project, which at present only applies to European men and women, predicts the 10 year risk of CVD of each individual based on systolic blood pressure, gender, smoking status, age and cholesterol levels with good accuracy (AUC 0.71-084) (Conroy, 2003). Hence, it can be used in clinical practice and preventative measures can be suggested on high-risk individuals.

Metabolic Disorders and Vasomotor Symptoms

Hot flushes, although their incidence differ among different ethnic groups, affect a large proportion of menopausal women and are the main cause of women seeking medical advice and treatment (Freeman and Sherif 2007). Hot flushes tend to occur in perimenopausal and early postmenopausal period but one-third of women report symptoms that last up to 5 years after cessation of periods and in 20%, persist up to 15 years (Kronenberg, 1996)

Hot flushes have been linked, albeit inconsistently, with metabolic disorders. In the WHI (Women's Health Initiative) study, older postmenopausal women with moderate to severe hot flushes were at greater cardiovascular risk after prolonged hormonal use (Rossouw et al 2007). The links between hot flushes and CVD are not fully understood. The findings concerning vasomotor symptoms (VMS) and subclinical CVD, as has been highlighted above, are inconclusive. Some have suggested that VMS are related to inflammatory processes and altered hemostasis. FVIIc (factor VIIc), a protein of the coagulation cascade, and tPA (tissue plasminogen activator antigen), a protein related to fibrolysis directly secreted by the endothelium, were elevated in women with hot flushes after adjusting for covariates such as age and BMI (Thurston, El Khoudary et al 2011), whereas C-reactive protein) (CRP) was not statistically different after adjusting for covariates. This may highlight the importance of hemostatic mechanisms in the pathogenesis of hot flushes and potentially of cardiovascular risk. However, the results need to be interpreted with caution because inflammation and haemostasis are interrelated and obesity is linked with altered haemostatic factors.

In addition, both hot flushes and night sweats have been linked with insulin resistance. Women were followed up during menopausal transition and it was reported that VMS were associated with raised HOMA (homeostasis model assessment) index, a marker of insulin resistance, and to a lesser degree with fasting blood glucose (Thurston et al 2012). The difference in the HOMA index persisted after adjusting for covariates, whereas there was some interaction between fasting glucose and ethnicity, stage of menopause and obesity. The association between HOMA and VMS was pronounced in women who reported VMS for at least 6 or more days over 2 weeks, although this study did not assess VMS as a continuous variable resulting from a diary but as a categorical variable from a questionnaire that was completed retrospectively. Furthermore, the interactions between obesity and VMS and between obesity and insulin resistance may have biased the results towards a positive association between VMS and insulin resistance. Another study that was conducted in Korea, showed that among menopausal women, metabolic syndrome (assessed by the National Cholesterol Education Program Adult Treatment Panel III (NCEP-ATP III) criteria was more prevalent in women with VMS (measured again as a categorical variable based on the Menopausal Rating Scale) than in asymptomatic women (Lee et al, 2012).

Hot Flushes and Cardiovascular Disease Risk

The role of hot flushes in the risk of cardiovascular events was examined by the WHI-OS, a longitudinal observational study which assessed 78,249 menopausal women with no history of CVD. Women were categorized in four groups based on the timing of hot flushes with regards to menopause; one group consisted of non-flushers, the second of women with early vasomotor symptoms during menopausal transition that substituted thereafter, the third group of women with late vasomotor symptoms and the fourth one of women with persistent hot flushes. Interestingly, only women with hot flushes after the onset of menopause (late hot flushes) had a higher incidence of major CHD and all-causes mortality, which persisted after adjusting for co-variants (Szmuilowicz et al 2011).

More recently, vasomotor symptoms and in particular hot flushes have been examined as a surrogate marker of CVD and subclinical endothelial dysfunction but the results are conflicting. The SWAN heart, an ancillary arm to the SWAN that included 492 black and white women, concluded that women with any hot flushes have reduced flow mediated dilatation (FMD), greater calcification in the aorta (Thurston et al 2008) and greater carotid intima-media thickness (IMT) compared with age matched non-flushers (Thurston, Sutton-Tyrrell, et al 2011). Another study reproduced the findings that women with moderate to severe hot flushes had reduced endothelial function measured by FMD, whereas the IMT and the lipid profile were normal (Bechlioulis et al 2010). In reverse, Sassarini et al reported that menopausal women with severe hot flushes have increased endothelium dependent and independent vascular reactivity assessed by Laser Doppler Imaging with Iontophoresis (LDI) but an adverse lipid profile compared with non-flushers (Sassarini et al 2011). The above vascular response could be related to the peripheral thermoregulatory mechanisms and the need to lose heat during a hot flush. Alongside the above findings, Tuomikoski et al reported that women with a high flushing score had an increased vascular response to nitroglycerin assessed by means of pulse wave analysis. However, they did not find altered arterial stiffness between the groups and did not test other atherosclerotic factors (Tuomikoski et al 2009). These inconsistencies in the literature may be related with the methodological differences among the studies in measuring vascular response and assessing severity of hot flushes. Further studies are needed in order to underpin the effect of hot flushes in vascular reactivity by assessing simultaneously the micro and macro vascular bed. Undoubtedly, the evidence to date support that clinicians should not overlook the importance of hot flushes in the CVD risk stratification of middle aged women.

Menopause and Ethnicity

Although metabolic syndrome and type 2 diabetes are common in South Asian women of menopausal age, there are few studies about the prevalence of menopausal symptoms in South Asian women. The prevalence of hot flushes varies from in this group varying from 14 to 42% with marked differences between rural and urban populations (Freeman and Sherif 2007). A study conducted in South India reported that the most frequent menopausal symptoms were joint pains, backache, sleep disturbance and memory weakness rather than vasomotor (Bairy et al 2009). Interestingly, Indians who migrate away from South Asian subcontinent to the UK report the same prevalence of VMS as the background population and much higher from age matched women living in Delhi (Gupta et al 2006). However, the association with CVD risk has not been studied. There are very limited studies about the experience of menopause in African countries and the results are largely inconsistent among them, but the SWAN study suggested that African women living in Northern America have a high prevalence of hot flushes similar to White women living in the same urban areas (Avis et al 2001). The above regional differences in the experience of menopause can be explained because of differences between the studies in the way of assessing menopausal symptoms, recruiting participants (population based versus menopausal clinics) and in the baseline characteristics (e.g. BMI, menopausal stage, age) of the participants. Cultural differences and diverse awareness about health issues seem to play a role in the different reporting of symptoms.

Taking into consideration the reported differences in the prevalence of menopausal symptoms around the world along with the marked differences in the prevalence of metabolic syndrome among different ethnic groups, the potential associations between VMS and metabolic risk factors means it is essential that we aim towards ethnic specific research during menopausal transition.

Conclusion

Menopause is a critical stage at women's life course not only because of the related symptoms that come along and interfere with the women's quality of life, but because metabolic risk factors arise or amplify during menopausal transition. Although, the direct effect of menopause on these risks remains unclear, there is no doubt that menopause coincidences with the aging effect on women's health. During the menopausal transition, women are more likely to seek medical advice, hence clinicians should not only provide symptomatic treatment to somatic symptoms, but should show an interest in their future well-being too.

Bibliography

1. Abdulnour J, et al. The effect of the menopausal transition on body composition and cardiometabolic risk factors: a Montreal-Ottawa New Emerging Team group study. Menopause (New York, NY). 2012;19(7):760–7.
2. Asarian L, Geary N. Modulation of appetite by gonadal steroid hormones. Philosophical transactions of the Royal Society of London. Series B, Biological sciences. 2006;361(1471):1251–63.
3. Avis NE, et al. Is there a menopausal syndrome? Menopausal status and symptoms across racial/ethnic groups. Social science and medicine. 2001;(1982),52(3): 345–56.
4. Bairy L, et al. Prevalence of menopausal symptoms and quality of life after menopause in women from South India. The Australian and New Zealand journal of Obstetrics and Gynaecology. 2009;49(1):106–9.

5. Bechlioulis A, et al. Endothelial function, but not carotid intima-media thickness, is affected early in menopause and is associated with severity of hot flushes. The Journal of Clinical Endocrinology and Metabolism. 2010;95(3):1199–206.

6. Bonithon-Kopp C, et al. Menopause-related changes in lipoproteins and some other cardiovascular risk factors. International Journal of Epidemiology. 1990;19(1):42–8.

7. Burger HG, et al. A prospective longitudinal study of serum testosterone, dehydroepiandrosterone sulfate, and sex hormone-binding globulin levels through the menopause transition. The Journal of Clinical Endocrinology and Metabolism. 2000;85(8):2832–8.

8. Castelo-Branco C, et al. Age, menopause and hormone replacement therapy influences on cardiovascular risk factors in a cohort of middle-aged Chilean women. Maturitas. 2003;45(3):205–12.

9. Celermajer DS, et al. Aging is associated with endothelial dysfunction in healthy men years before the age-related decline in women. Journal of the American College of Cardiology. 1994;24(2):471–6.

10. Conroy R. Estimation of ten-year risk of fatal cardiovascular disease in Europe: the SCORE project. European Heart Journal. 2003;24(11):987–1003.

11. Dasgupta S, et al. Menopause versus aging: The predictor of obesity and metabolic aberrations among menopausal women of Karnataka, South India. Journal of Mid-life health. 2012;3(1):24–30.

12. Ding Eric L, Singa Yiqing, Malik VSL, Simin. Sex differences of endogenous sex hormones and risk of type 2 diabetes. JAMA. 2012;295(11):1288–99.

13. Do KA, et al. Longitudinal study of risk factors for coronary heart disease across the menopausal transition. American Journal of Epidemiology. 2000;151(6):584–93.

14. Freeman EW, Sherif K. Prevalence of hot flushes and night sweats around the world: a systematic review. Climacteric: The Journal of the International Menopause Society. 2007;10(3):197–214.

15. Gabriel KP, et al. Self-reported and accelerometer-derived physical activity levels and coronary artery calcification progression in older women: results from the Healthy Women Study. Menopause (New York NY), 2012.

16. Gill JMR, et al. Sitting time and waist circumference are associated with glycemia in UK South Asians: data from 1,228 adults screened for the PODOSA trial. Diabetes Care. 2011;34(5):1214–8.

17. Gupta P, Sturdee DW, Hunter MS. Mid-age health in women from the Indian subcontinent (MAHWIS): general health and the experience of menopause in women. Climacteric: The Journal of the International Menopause Society. 2006;9(1):13–22.

18. Janssen I, et al. Menopause and the metabolic syndrome. Arch Intern Med. 2008;168(14):1568–75.

19. Kim C, et al. Menopause and risk of diabetes in the Diabetes Prevention Program. Menopause (New York NY). 2011;18(8):857–68.

20. Kronenberg F. Hot flushes: phenomenology, quality of life, and search for treatment options. Experimental Gerontology. 1996;29(3-4):319–36.

21. Kuller LH, et al. Women's Healthy Lifestyle Project: A Randomized Clinical Trial : Results at 54 Months. Circulation. 2001;103(1):32–7.

22. Lee SW, et al. Association between menopausal symptoms and metabolic syndrome in postmenopausal women. Archives of Gynecology and Obstetrics, 2012;285(2):541–8.

23. Lovejoy JC, et al. Increased visceral fat and decreased energy expenditure during the menopausal transition. International journal of Obesity, 2005;32(6):949–58.

24. Matthews K, et al. Are changes in cardiovascular disease risk factors in midlife women due to chronological aging or to the menopausal transition? Journal of the American College of Cardiology. 2009;54(25):2366–73.

25. Matthews K, et al. Premenopausal risk factors for coronary and aortic calcification: a 20-year follow-up in the healthy women study. Preventive Medicine. 2007;45(4):302–8.
26. Peters HW, et al. Menopausal status and risk factors for cardiovascular disease. Journal of Internal Medicine. 1999;246(6):521–8.
27. Rebuffé-Scrive M, et al. Metabolism of mammary, abdominal, and femoral adipocytes in women before and after menopause. Metabolism: Clinical and Experimental. 1986;35(9):792–7.
28. Rossouw JE, et al. Postmenopausal hormone therapy and risk of cardiovascular disease by age and years since menopause. JAMA. 2007;297(13):1465–78.
29. Sassarini J, et al. Vascular function and cardiovascular risk factors in women with severe flushing. Clinical Endocrinology, 2011;74(1):97–103.
30. Sjöberg L, Kaaja R, Tuomilehto J. Epidemiology of postmenopausal hypertension. International Journal of clinical practice. Supplement, 2004;(139):4–12.
31. Sowers M, et al. Changes in body composition in women over six years at midlife: ovarian and chronological aging. The Journal of Clinical Endocrinology and Metabolism, 2007;92(3):895–901.
32. Szmuilowicz ED, et al. Vasomotor symptoms and cardiovascular events in postmenopausal women. Menopause (New York, NY). 2011;18(6):603–10.
33. Taddei S. Blood pressure through aging and menopause. Climacteric : The Journal of the International Menopause Society. 2009;12 Suppl 1:36–40.
34. Taddei S, et al. Menopause is associated with endothelial dysfunction in women. Hypertension. 1996;28(4):576–82.
35. Thurston RC, Sowers MaryFran R, et al. Abdominal adiposity and hot flushes among midlife women. Menopause (New York, NY). 2008;15(3):429–34.
36. Thurston RC, Sowers, Maryfran R, et al. Adiposity and reporting of vasomotor symptoms among midlife women: the study of women's health across the nation. American Journal of Epidemiology. 2008;167(1):78–85.
37. Thurston RC, El Khoudary SR, et al. Are vasomotor symptoms associated with alterations in hemostatic and inflammatory markers? Findings from the Study of Women's Health Across the Nation. Menopause (New York, NY). 2011;18(10):1044–51.
38. Thurston RC, Sutton-Tyrrell K, et al. Hot flushes and carotid intima media thickness among midlife women. Menopause (New York, NY). 2011;18(4):352–8.
39. Thurston RC, Sutton-Tyrrell K, et al. Hot flushes and subclinical cardiovascular disease: findings from the Study of Women's Health Across the Nation Heart Study. Circulation. 2008;118(12):1234–40.
40. Thurston RC, et al. Vasomotor symptoms and insulin resistance in the study of women's health across the nation. The Journal of Clinical Endocrinology and Metabolism. 2012;97(10):3487–94.
41. Tuomikoski P, et al. Evidence for a role of hot flushes in vascular function in recently postmenopausal women. Obstet Gynecol. 2009;113(4):902–8.
42. Yanes LL, Reckelhoff JF. Postmenopausal hypertension. American Journal of Hypertension. 2011;24(7):740–9.

Use of Mesh in Urogynecology

10

Chapter

Jay Iyer, Ajay Rane

Pelvic organ prolapse affects 1 out of every 9 women in their lifetimes, and about one-third of all women are likely to experience urinary incontinence in one form or the other. The management of prolapse has undergone a paradigm shift in recent times, and we are now able to offer our women minimally invasive and robust surgical management. Until about two decades ago, native tissue repair was the mainstay of treatment of pelvic organ prolapse. Our understanding of pelvic floor anatomy has changed dramatically since the description of "levels of pelvic organ support" by John Delancey. Fascial repairs, also known as native tissue repairs, traditionally address midline fascial defects, but are unable to treat paravaginal or lateral defects in the fascial hammock. These defects account for a significant proportion of cystoceles and a midline fascial plication is unlikely to completely 'fix' a paravaginal detachment from the 'white line'. A large enterocele is usually associated with vault descent and would be very difficult to manage surgically without achieving adequate level 1 support. Many of the treatments for pelvic organ prolapse offered today have been developed bearing in mind this renewed understanding of pelvic floor anatomy. We live in exciting times indeed!

Anatomy of the Pelvic Floor and the Functional Relationship to Pelvic Organ Prolapse

In order to fully understand the dynamics of mesh surgery, or indeed native tissue repair, it is important to have a brief overview of the functional anatomy of the pelvic floor. There has been a perennial 'tug-of-war' between the relative importance of the levator ani muscle complex and fascial-ligamentous supports in the maintenance of the pelvic organ support. The muscles of the pelvic diaphragm primarily form a basin or covering of the pelvic outlet and are often grouped together as the levator ani or levator sling (Fig. 10.1). Contained within this muscle diaphragm is the urogenital hiatus that distends to many times its diameter to allow vaginal childbirth. This potential weakness in the muscular pelvic floor is evolutionary and is one of the chief reasons why genital prolapse is almost exclusively a problem in bipeds.[1] The most medial portion and perhaps the most important part of the pelvic diaphragm is contributed by the puborectalis that borders the urogenital hiatus.[2-4] In

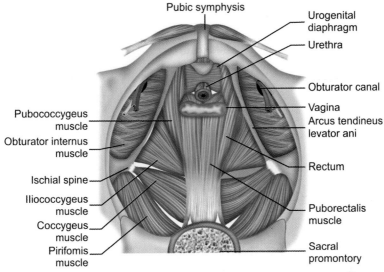

Pubic symphysis

Urogenital diaphragm

Urethra

Obturator canal

Pubococcygeus muscle

Obturator internus muscle

Vagina

Arcus tendineus levator ani

Ischial spine

Rectum

Iliococcygeus muscle

Coccygeus muscle

Puborectalis muscle

Pirifomis muscle

Sacral promontory

FIG. 10.1 The pelvic diaphragm viewed from above.(Adapted from Te Linde's Operative Gynecology. Editors: Rock, John A, Jones Howard W. Lippincott Williams and Wilkins. 10th Edition)

the standing patient, the puborectalis muscle is horizontal and can be palpated as a distinct band measuring 2 to 2.5 cm on each lateral side by running the examining finger under the urethra and along the ischiopubic ramus. If the muscle is intact then there will be just enough room to fit the palpating finger between the urethra medially and the insertion of the puborectalis muscle laterally. If there is no muscle palpable then this implies an avulsion injury on this side. It is possible to measure levator hiatus dimensions using 3D/4D transperineal ultrasound and predict the possiblity of pelvic organ prolapse and chance of recurrence.[5-8] Forming the bulk of the pelvic diaphragm, the pubococcygeus and iliococcygeus muscles cover the posterior and lateral portions of the pelvic outlet (Fig. 10.2) and are not thought to be active contributors to pelvic organ support.[2-4]

The iliococcygeus muscles, particularly at its insertion, provides a key landmark in the anatomy of pelvic organ support. The parietal fascia is thickened at these insertions which extend from the ischial spine to the pubic tubercles anteriorly. These lines of insertion are known as the arcus tendineus levator ani, inferior to which is a similar fascial thickening—the arcus tendineus fasciae pelvis (fascial arches) or white lines (Fig. 10.3).[9] These are key structures providing lateral attachment points for the pubocervical fascia and proximal rectovaginal septum.[10,11] The white line serves the function of laterally supporting the mid-vagina. These lateral fascial thickenings serve as the lateral attachments of the fascial hammock that supports the bladder, the rectum and the lateral vaginal walls.[9,10] Posterior to the iliococcygeus, the pelvic floor is covered by the coccygeus muscle and the closely associated sacrospinous ligament. These structures pass between the ischial spine and the coccyx. The midline confluence of the levator muscles forms a particularly strong band of connective tissue between the coccyx and anus known as the levator

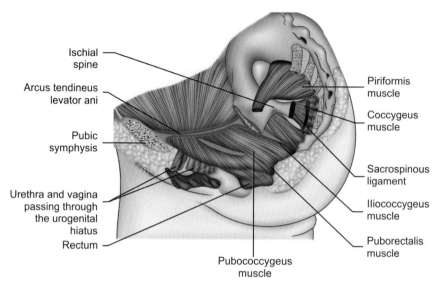

Ischial spine

Arcus tendineus levator ani

Pubic symphysis

Urethra and vagina passing through the urogenital hiatus

Rectum

Piriformis muscle

Coccygeus muscle

Sacrospinous ligament

Iliococcygeus muscle

Puborectalis muscle

Pubococcygeus muscle

FIG. 10.2 Muscles of the pelvic floor, lateral view. (Adapted from Te Linde's Operative Gynecology. Editors: Rock John A, Jones Howard W. Lippincott Williams and Wilkins. 10th Edition)

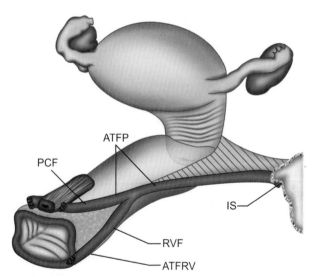

ATFP

PCF

IS

RVF

ATFRV

FIG. 10.3 The lateral attachments of the pubocervical fascia (PCF) and the rectovaginal fascia (RVF) to the pelvic sidewall. Also shown are the arcus tendineus fascia pelvis (ATFP), arcus tendineus fasciae rectovaginalis (ATFRV), and ischial spine (IS). (Adapted from Te Linde's Operative Gynecology. Editors: Rock John A Jones Howard W. Lippincott Williams and Wilkins. 10th Edition)

plate or sacrococcygeal raphe. This plate is oriented horizontally in the standing patient and prevents the prolapse of the vagina and the rectum that are suspended by the endopelvic fascia directly over it. The levator plates descend and the genital hiatus remains open during defecation. Chronic increases in intrabdominal pressure can change the normal horizontal axis of the proximal vagina to a vertical orientation and predisposes the central pelvic organs to prolapse.[12]

The connective tissues of the pelvis are collectively known as the endopelvic fascia, which in the main part is composed of fibroelastic connective tissue mixed with smooth muscle. These forms include loose areolar tissue capable of distention, neurovascular sheaths, septa and ligaments that support, suspend, and separate the pelvic organs, and dense skeletal muscle investments. These tissues connect to the central pelvic organs, chiefly to the cervix and upper vagina in the following arrangement:[2-4,9,10,13,14]

Anterior: The pericervical ring is located between the base of the bladder and the anterior cervix, where it connects with the pubocervical ligaments at the 11-o'clock and 1-o'clock positions and the proximal pubocervical septum centrally.

Lateral: Cardinal ligaments at the 3-o'clock and 9-o'clock positions.

Posterior: The pericervical ring is located between the rectum and the posterior cervix, where it connects with the uterosacral ligaments at the 5-o'clock and 7-o'clock positions and the proximal rectovaginal septum centrally.

The net effect of these structures is the suspension of the cervix in the posterior pelvis and the consequent placement of the vagina directly over the levator plate and away from direct exposure to the urogenital hiatus (see above).[12] In this position, intra-abdominal pressure from above closes the vaginal apex reducing a tendency toward prolapse. The normal vaginal axis is oriented posteriorly toward junction of third and fourth sacral vertebrae near the origin of the uterosacral ligaments. The pericervical ring marks the confluence of all structures constituting endopelvic connective tissue support. In other words, if the anatomical attachments to the pericervical ring are reconstituted, fascial repair or defect specific repair is more likely to succeed. In a post-hysterectomy patient, there is no known method to restore proximal anterior vaginal support. Therefore, procedures designed to either shorten the vagina or plicate the uterosacral-cardinal ligament complex are usually necessary to avoid the development of vault prolapse.[14]

The surgical goals for a reconstructive pelvic surgeon can be established by understanding the concepts of pelvic supports as described by John DeLancey.[9,10] In his biomechanical analysis of normal uterovaginal support by the deep endopelvic connective tissue, anatomic principles pertinent to pelvic organ prolapse are unified. (Fig. 10.4). DeLancey divided vaginal support into three levels (Fig. 10.5). Proximal vaginal level I support is attributed to suspension by the ligaments of the paracolpium. Damage to level I support results in uterovaginal prolapse, posthysterectomy vaginal prolapse and enterocele. The cause for level I support problems is necessarily at or above the level of the ischial spines. The primary load-bearing elements are the uterosacral ligaments and, to a lesser extent, the cardinal ligaments. This fact is consistent with cadaver observations made many years ago by Mengert showing that prolapse occurred only after 85% of the integrity of the paracolpium was severed.[15] Midvaginal level II support is because of lateral attachment of the fascial septa to the pelvic sidewalls. The septa attach to the arcus

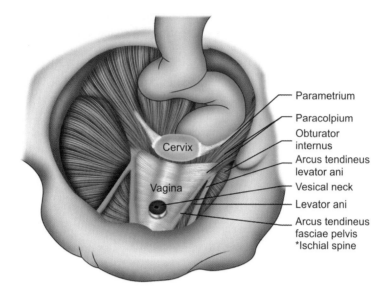

FIG. 10.4 Three-dimensional view of the endopelvic fascia. Notice the location of the cervix in the proximal anterior vaginal segment. (Adapted from DeLancey JO. Anatomic aspects of vaginal eversion after hysterectomy. Am J Obstet Gynecol. 1992;166:1717.)

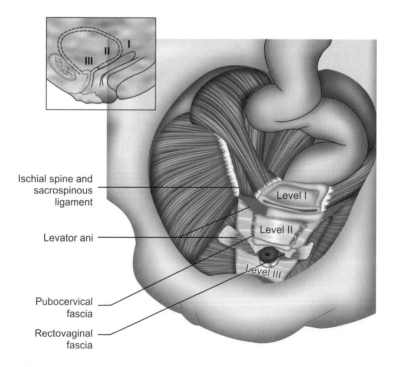

FIG. 10.5 The endopelvic fascia of a posthysterectomy patient divided into DeLancey's biomechanical levels: level I proximal suspension; level II lateral attachment; level III distal fusion. (Adapted from DeLancey JO. Anatomic aspects of vaginal eversion after hysterectomy. Am J Obstet Gynecol. 1992;166:1717.)

tendineus fascia pelvis and the arcus tendineus fasciae rectovaginalis.[10,11] Damage at this level results in paravaginal and pararectal defects. Level III support is attributed to fusion to the urogenital diaphragm anteriorly and to the proximal perineum posteriorly. Damage at these sites results in urinary incontinence anteriorly and in perineal body deficits posteriorly. Cystocele and rectocele are defects within the fabric of the pubocervical and rectovaginal septa.[2-4, 9-11]

Why did Pelvic Floor Surgeons Feel the Need for Mesh?

The foregoing discussion of functional pelvic floor anatomy has highlighted the importance of fascial and ligamentous supports and the interrelationships of pelvic organ support. A well-supported bladder in the anterior compartment of the pelvis is dependent on the competently supported middle compartment, i.e. cervix/vaginal vault. Similarly the rectum in the posterior compartment relies on the support from the other pelvic organs. The current concept of pelvic floor support is predicated on the arcus-to-arcus support based on John DeLancey's work highlighted above.[9]

The recently introduced needle driven mesh devices were developed with the aim of recreating a two- or four-point fixation mimicking the hammock-like arrangement of pelvic organ supports. PERIGEE was the first needle driven mesh device developed for the management of large and recurrent cystoceles. This device has two set of needles that traverses the obturator foramen through 2 separate entry points on each side and utilizes the fixation points inferior to the sacrospinous ligaments (on the ilieococcygeus fascia/muscle) and the obturator internus muscles, close to the white line. As a result, the prolapsed bladder is suspended at four points like a hammock. A similar device called the APOGEE was developed to treat complex rectoenteroceles and vault prolapse.

In recent years market forces and safety concerns raised by the USFDA, forced manufacturers to search for alternatives.[16,17] The second generation of mesh kits used a single vaginal incision for both dissecting the prolapse and introducing the mesh device. This obviates the need to use 'blind' needle passes in the obturator foramen reducing the complication rates. The Anterior Elevate is a mesh kit used for the treatment of cystocele and the Posterior Elevate device developed for managing rectoenteroceles. Second generation kits especially the Anterior Elevate represents an improvement over the PERIGEE because it provides better level 1 support.

Surgical Technique

Stepwise Approach to Any Type of Vaginal Repair Surgery

We recommend the use of hydrodissection in all cases of vaginal repair surgery. This, in our unit, involves use of Marcaine (0.5%) with 1 in 100,000 Epinephrine a volume of 20 milliliters (mL) diluted with 20 mL of normal saline. Hydrodissection, in our opinion, allows the surgeon to get in the right surgical plane in a bloodless manner (Fig. 10.6). Not only does it help in developing the natural, relatively avascular tissue planes in the pelvic floor, it also facilitates proper mesh placement, reduces the incidence of visceral or neurovascular damage and is of immense benefit in

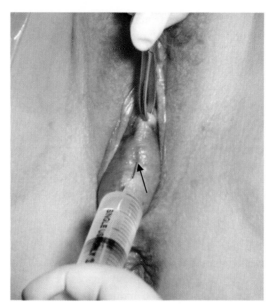

FIG. 10.6 Single point infiltration with no bleeding

carrying the dissection through the full thickness of the vagina.[18] Follow the 'gray bubble'(Vincent Lucente, personal communication) that is the appearance created by the infiltrated fluid as it dissects the fascia off the viscus and that helps define the correct plane of dissection (Fig. 10.7). Sharp and blunt dissection is carried out in this plane, that lies between the fascia and the serosa of the prolapsing viscus and not between the vagina and the fascia. Dissection in the latter plane leads to 'vaginal skinning' and deeper dissection ensues the placement of mesh on the viscus-fascia interface rather than superficial fascial-vaginal skin plane.

Full thickness dissection also allows access to the obturator membrane and the sacrospinous ligament and bladder base in the vesicovaginal space. The tissue planes between the viscus and the lateral pelvic wall can usually be developed efficiently with a combination of blunt and sharp dissection. These techniques ensure that the mesh lies directly abutting the prolapsing viscus, reducing the chance of mesh erosion and the prolapse (M Cosson, personal communication).[18] Robust anchorage is essential to the success of mesh replacement surgery. The sacrospinous ligament is an accessible and sturdy anchor, is relatively avascular, has a fixed anatomic location with well-circumscribed boundaries and is identifiable even in obese women.[19,20]

The mesh supports the bladder in a tension free manner and the final result is often (Figs 10.8 and 10.9) "visually unpleasing", as if the prolapse has not been reduced at all—an indirect indicator of appropriate mesh tensioning (Fig. 10.10).[18] It is important to avoid excision of the vaginal skin as the vagina usually remodels to the normal dimensions in 6–8 weeks time.[21,22]

Every needle, every Kit is different and surgeons should familiarize themselves with all nuances. It also requires a detailed knowledge of anatomical safety—

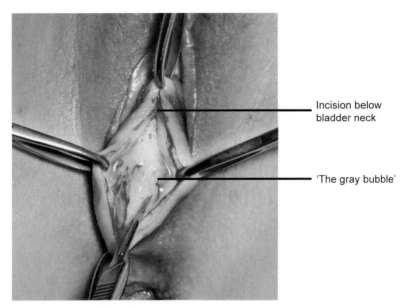

Incision below
bladder neck

'The gray bubble'

FIG. 10.7 Plane of dissection

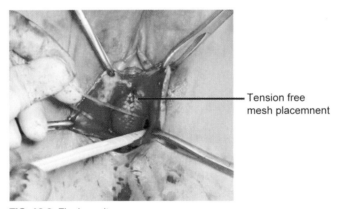

Tension free
mesh placemnent

FIG. 10.8 Final result

preferably demonstrated on cadavers first. It is important to appreciate directional reversals of the needle tips with respect to the handles and spatial relationships in the three dimensions of pelvic anatomy. A good understanding of anatomy and biomechanics of each device is key to preventing major visceral and vascular injuries.[18, 23] Unfortunately there have been very few robust randomized controlled trials or case controlled studies done to address the pros and cons of this relatively new technology.[24-27] The proliferation of different types of synthetic and biologic meshes without comprehending their individual biodynamics could lead to delayed complications.[16, 17, 26, 27]

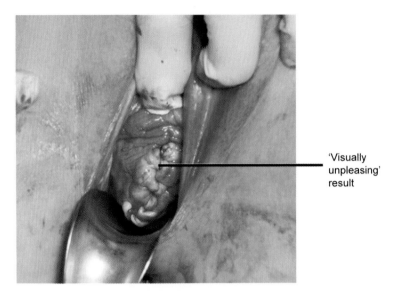

'Visually unpleasing' result

FIG. 10.9 Final view often unpleasant

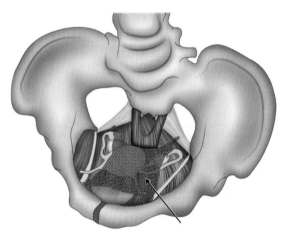

FIG. 10.10 Mesh under the bladder

Perigee^{tm} (American Medical Systems, MN)

This is the first generation mesh device that is the precursor of all the current devices in use. This procedure involved two needle passes through each obturator foramen in their path towards the vaginal dissection; the superior (pink) needle passing through the obturator internus muscle along the white line and the inferior (gray) needle piercing the levator ani 1 cm cranial to the ischial spine for optimal arcus-to-arcus support. The mesh is threaded through the needles at the vaginal incision and pulled back along the trajectory they have passed through. The mesh is then placed on the dissected bladder and gently tensioned.

Anterior Elevate (American Medical Systems, MN)

Following the warning by the FDA in 2008,[16,17] it became important to devise a mesh implantation system that avoided the obturator foramen while maintaining the success rates of the transobturator procedure. The Anterior Elevate™ transvaginal mesh replacement system was born out this concept. It involves the passage of anchors into the sacrospinous ligament that provide surrogate anchorage for the mesh threaded through it. The system also provides for two additional anchors interwoven into the mesh that deploy in the obturator internus muscle (Fig. 10.10).

Uphold™ (Boston Scientific, MA)

This mesh kit utilizes suture anchorage to the sacrospinous ligament instead of anchors. The ethibond sutures attached to mesh arms are tacked in place by means of the Capio device which is a needle driven system that delivers the suture to the appropriate location in the ligament and also retrieves the suture on its return journey. The mesh arms are then pulled through the sacrospinous ligament providing robust anchorage which provides level 1 support and some level 2 support. Its predecessor Pinnacle™ has been withdrawn from the market recently.

Prosima™ (Johnson and Johnson, NJ)

This mesh kit also involves the intravaginal introduction of mesh that is 'tucked' in to the sacrospinous ligament using a metal carrier device and then held in place by means of inflatable balloon that remains in the vagina for two weeks. At the end of two weeks it is expected that the mesh will 'stick in place'. This product has also been withdrawn from the market voluntarily by the manufacturer.

So far studies have shown very little difference in clinical outcomes between these various devices. Having said that most studies do not use imaging like 3D/4D ultrasound to observe meshes over a period of time.[6,7] It is useful to think of mesh as a medication that needs to be used in the 'correct dose'-, so trim the mesh to meet individual requirements (L Brubaker, personal communication). It is vital that replacement mesh surgery be performed per protocol established by the manufacturer as any deviations from the accepted technique can cause untold damage to the woman besides being medicolegally indefensible. The introduction of newer meshes that are lighter, softer and less dense have made a discernible change in patient outcomes in a few studies.

Tips and Pearls

The most important lessons we have learnt in our unit over the last 9 years of mesh usage are:
- Proper patient selection – avoiding use of mesh in small prolapses, appropriate patient counseling before surgery
- Hydrodissection and full thickness dissection as mentioned before

- Gentle tissue handling
- Avoidance of excessive traction to the mesh
- Avoidance of vaginal trimming.

Mesh surgery requires a 'leap of faith' especially for those surgeons that are used to traditional fascial surgery. For one the end result is often disappointing and 'visually unpleasing'; this is good way of preventing complications arising from placing the mesh under too much tension. The vagina is 'an innocent victim of prolapse'; in fact it is the viscus behind the bulging vagina that is prolapsing.

Postoperative Orders and Management

In our patients the use of local anesthetic for hydrodissection has reduced the need for postoperative narcotic analgesia to less than 3%. We advise the use of intraoperative antibiotics like cephalosporins and metronidazole. We also routinely prescribe antibiotics for 5 days postsurgery. Pain relief is achieved by a diclofenac suppository postsurgery and oral ibuprofen, codeine and paracetamol. Patients using codeine are advised to use stool softeners like lactulose.

All patients undergo a trial of void postsurgery and a post void residual bladder volume (PVRBV) of <100 mL is our cut-off. We do not routinely use vaginal packing. Our patients are sent home, if they are pain free, not bleeding excessively and have passed their trial of void, with access to a 24-hour hotline number. A nurse calls all patients the next day and performs a visual analog score for pain, bleeding and bladder function with appropriate referral as necessary. Using this protocol we have managed to perform day surgery for over 92% of our patients.

Change in Practice Following the FDA Notifications

In light of recent developments in the use of mesh by untrained or inadequately trained surgeons and the consequent complications we offer all our patients-two documents based on the issues raised by the USFDA.

Patient Document 1: Use of Mesh in Pelvic Organ Prolapse by the Transvaginal Route

- Recently the FDA has issued a notice regarding the use of mesh transvaginally for the treatment of vaginal prolapse.
- Our unit has been in the forefront of teaching, innovation and training in such procedures.
- Professor Rane is the inventor of Perigee one of the first such devices to be used since 2004. He is a certified Urogynecologist from the Royal Australian College Of Obstetricians and Gynecologists and has received specialized training in the use of mesh for prolapse. He has trained more than 400 surgeons worldwide in these techniques.
- Our unit has followed up patients for more than 5 years and more than 2000 such procedures have been done in this unit since 2004 with minimal complications.

- We continue to audit our practice annually and have invited external auditors as well from time to time.
- Since 2004 our mesh erosion rate has reduced from 11% to less than 2%. This is a phenomenon when a part of the mesh protrudes of the vagina after surgery and may require another minor operation to remove that part.
- Mesh in our unit is predominantly used in the anterior compartment (85%) where the bladder is prolapsed. As compared to traditional repair techniques this method has a far less recurrence rate (25% vs 5% approximately) in our hands.
- Once mesh is inserted for treatment, it remains in your body permanently. In less than 4% of patients mesh can cause pain during intercourse and rarely more than one operation is required to remove the mesh. This may not resolve symptoms completely.
- Occasionally during these procedures, as with any other surgical operation, including non-mesh repairs, there can be trauma to blood vessels, bowel and bladder.
- We are happy to discuss the benefits and risks of nonsurgical options, non-mesh options, surgical mesh placed abdominally and the likely success and failure rates of all these alternatives.
- We will as always provide you with detailed information about the product being used.

Patient Document 2: Questions that Patients Need to Ask

1. Be aware of the risks associated with surgical mesh for transvaginal repair of pelvic organ prolapse (POP). Know that having a mesh surgery may put you at risk for needing additional surgery because of mesh-related complications.
2. In a small number of patients, repeat surgery may not resolve complications.
3. Ask your surgeon about all POP treatment options, including surgical repair with or without mesh and nonsurgical options, and understand why your surgeon may be recommending treatment of POP with mesh.
4. In addition, ask your surgeon these questions before you agree to have surgery in which surgical mesh is used.
   - Are you planning to use mesh in my surgery?
   - Why do you think I am a good candidate for surgical mesh?
   - Why is surgical mesh being chosen for my repair?
   - What are the alternatives to transvaginal surgical mesh repair for POP, including nonsurgical options?
   - What are the pros and cons of using surgical mesh in my particular case? How likely is it that my repair could be successfully performed without using surgical mesh?
   - Will my partner be able to feel the surgical mesh during sexual intercourse? What if the surgical mesh erodes through my vaginal wall?
   - If surgical mesh is to be used, how often have you implanted this particular product? What results have your other patients had with this product?
   - What can I expect to feel after surgery and for how long?

- Which specific side effects should I report to you after the surgery?
- What if the mesh surgery does not correct my problem?
- If I develop a complication, will you treat it or will I be referred to a specialist experienced with surgical mesh complications?
- If I have a complication related to the surgical mesh, how likely is it that the surgical mesh could be removed and what could be the consequences?
- If a surgical mesh is to be used, is there patient information that comes with the product, and can I have a copy?

The Future of Mesh in Urogynecology

The introduction of the use of mesh in pelvic organ prolapse has undoubtedly improved our ability to offer our patients robust and long lasting treatments. The "Great Mesh Debate" has been occasioned by indiscriminate use of mesh, by inadequately trained surgeons, resulting in avoidable complications. The aggressive marketing tactics pursued by the mesh manufacturers has also contributed to this problem and they may well have "killed the goose that laid the golden egg". This is a pity because the concept of mesh replacement surgery is based on robust anatomic and biomechanical principles and has the potential to do far more good than harm. The responsible use of mesh in appropriately selected patients by suitably trained surgeons is the only way forward!

References

1. Bump RC, Norton PA. Epidemiology and natural history of pelvic floor dysfunction. Obstet Gynecol Clin North Am, 1998;25:723.
2. Wei JT, DLJ. Functional anatomy of the pelvic floor and lower urinary tract. Clinical Obstetrics and Gynecology. 2008;47(1):3–17.
3. Hollinshead WH, Rosse C. Textbook of Anatomy. 4th ed. Philadelphia: Harper and Row, 1985.
4. Retzy SS, Rogers RM, Richardson AC. Anatomy of female pelvic support. In: Brubaker LT, Saclarides TJ, eds. The Female Pelvic Floor: Disorders of Function and Support. Philadelphia: FA Davis, 1996;3.
5. Dietz HP, Shek C. Levator avulsion and grading of pelvic floor muscle strength. Int Urogynecol J. 2008;19(5):633–6.
6. Dietz HP, Lekskulchai O. Ultrasound assessment of pelvic organ prolapse: the relationship between prolapse severity and symptoms. Ultrasound in Obstetrics and Gynecology. 2007;29:688–91.
7. Barry C, Dietz HP. The use of Ultrasound in the evaluation of pelvic organ prolapse. Reviews in Gynaecological and Perinatal Medicine, 2005;5(3):182–95.
8. Dietz HP, Lanzarone V. Levator trauma after vaginal delivery. Obstet Gynecol. 2005;106:707.
9. DeLancey JO. Anatomy and biomechanics of genital prolapse. Clin Obstet Gynecol. 1993;36:897.
10. DeLancey JO. Structural anatomy of the posterior pelvic compartment as it relates to rectocele. Am J Obstet Gynecol. 1999;180:815.

11. Leffler KS, Thompson JR, Cundiff GW. Attachment of the rectovaginal septum to the pelvic sidewall. Am J Obstet Gynecol. 2001;185:41.

12. Nichols DH, Milley PS, Randall CL. Significance of restoration of normal vaginal depth and axis. Obstet Gynecol. 1970;36:251.

13. Buller JL, Thompson JR, Cundiff GW. Uterosacral ligament: description of anatomic relationships to optimize surgical safety. Obstet Gynecol. 2001;97:873.

14. Barber MD, Visco AG, Weidner AC, et al. Bilateral uterosacral ligament vaginal vault suspension with site-specific endopelvic fascia defect repair for treatment of pelvic organ prolapse. Am J Obstet Gynecol. 2000;183:1402.

15. Mengert WF. Mechanics of uterine support and position. Am J Obstet Gynecol. 1936;31:775.

16. FDA Public Health Notification: Serious Complications Associated with Transvaginal Placement of Surgical Mesh in Repair of Pelvic Organ Prolapse and Stress Urinary Incontinence. Date Issued:October 20, 2008.

17. FDA Safety Communication: UPDATE on Serious Complications Associated with Transvaginal Placement of Surgical Mesh for Pelvic Organ Prolapse Date Issued: July 13, 2011.

18. Muffly TM, Barber MD. Insertion and removal of vaginal mesh for pelvic organ prolapse. Clinical Obstetrics and Gynecology. 2010;53(1):99–114.

19. Cespedes RD, Anterior approach bilateral sacrospinous ligament fixation for vaginal vault prolapse. Urology. 2000;4(56(6Supp)):70-5Gynaecology. 2011.

20. Rane A, Frazer M, Jain A, Kannan, Iyer J. The sacrospinous ligament conveniently effective or effectively convenient? J Obstet Gynaecol. 2011;31(5):366–70.

21. Alperin M, Moalli PA, Remodeling of vaginal connective tissue in patients with prolapse. Current Opinion in Obstetrics and Gynecology. 2006;18(5)8:544–50.

22. Kannan K, McConnell A, McLeod M, Rane A. Microscopic alterations of vaginal tissue in women with pelvic organ prolapse. J Obstet Gynaecol. 2011;31(3):250–3.

23. Moore RD, Miklos JR, Vaginal mesh kits for pelvic organ prolapse, friend or foe: a comprehensive review. Scientific World Journal. 2009;9:163–89.

24. Davila GW, Drutz H, Deprest J. Clinical implications of the biology of grafts: conclusions of the 2005 IUGA Grafts Roundtable. International Journal of Urogynecology and Pelvic Floor Dysfunction. 2006;17 Suppl 1:S51–5.

25. Galloway NT. Words of wisdom. Re: the perils of commercially driven surgical innovation. European Urology. 2010;58(1):179.

26. Ostergard DR. Lessons from the past: directions for the future. Do new marketed surgical procedures and grafts produce ethical, personal liability, and legal concerns for physicians? International Journal of Urogynecology and Pelvic Floor Dysfunction. 2007;18(6):591–8.

27. Ostergard DR. Vaginal mesh grafts and the Food and Drug Administration. International Journal of Urogynecology and Pelvic Floor Dysfunction. 2010;21:1181–3.

Intrapartum Fetal Monitoring towards Improved Perinatal Outcome

11

Chapter

Niraj Yanamandra, Sabaratnam Arulkumaran

Introduction

Monitoring the fetus for its well-being is among the most important aspects of labor management. Over the decades there have been several encouraging developments and inventions in obstetrics that have led to safer intrapartum care and has significantly contributed towards reducing perinatal morbidity and mortality. There is no doubt that fetal death in labor is less common now compared to 1960s, when electronic fetal monitoring (EFM) was introduced in clinical practice. It is, however, difficult to know how much of the improvement is due to more intense monitoring of fetal condition in labor and how much may be attributed to spontaneous improvement in the natural history of reproduction.

Fetal asphyxia could cause long-term neurological damage expressed as cerebral palsy, mental retardation or both and in some cases can even cause fetal death. The aim of intrapartum fetal surveillance is to detect fetal hypoxia prior to the development of asphyxia and it's serious consequences.

The value of any fetal monitoring system during labor is usually expressed by its ability to predict that fetus is hypoxic or acidotic. The ideal fetal surveillance would have a high sensitivity (detect all fetuses with developing hypoxia) and a high specificity (be reassuring about all fetuses with no hypoxia). The test should also be easy to perform, not interfere with labor progress, and have a high acceptability to women. Unfortunately the ideal monitoring technique does not currently exist.

Various tools for intrapartum fetal surveillance are available and based on the resources available. This may range from intermittent auscultation through to continuous electronic fetal monitoring using cardiotocograph (CTG) to the most sophisticated ST wave analysis. Because of its cost-effectiveness, the fact that it is noninvasive and does not need any significant level of training, intermittent auscultation (IA) remains the most common modes of fetal surveillance, especially in developing countries, although it should be used as a screening tool rather than a diagnostic test of fetal health.

Prognosis

The hope that fetal heart rate (FHR) monitoring will abolish cerebral palsy has proven to be an unmeasurable and unrealistic goal. Because of the rarity of cerebral palsy, the hope that FHR monitoring may lead to a measurable decrease in this condition is also unrealistic. It is also difficult to establish what fetal and neonatal morbidity can be avoided using FHR monitoring.

A fetus suffering from hypoxia initially compensates by producing energy through anaerobic metabolism. At some stage, the fetus becomes decompensated and basic cellular functions fail, with risks of permanent morbidity or mortality. How long a fetus can survive on anaerobic metabolism differs because metabolic reserves differ. An increasing body of evidence has clarified brain-damaging mechanisms. Neuronal loss occurs in two phases: initially, during the primary hypoxic event and later during the reperfusion/reoxygenation phase. Intrapartum diagnostic tools should aim for detecting fetal hypoxemia/hypoxia when the fetus is still compensated. This may be achieved by assessment of biochemical data such as pH, lactate and oxygen saturation, with the aim of prophylactic intervention before the fetus becomes decompensated. The measurement of cord blood levels of oxygen free radicals and excitatory amino acids at the time of birth may prove to be helpful in determining the risk of brain damage and evaluating the effect of prophylactic treatments to prevent or ameliorate brain injury from hypoxia (Nordstrom and Arulkumaran, 1998).

Conditions such as fetal infection and anemia can affect fetal ability to cope with labor adversely. Fetal infection not only reduces the reserve to cope with hypoxia but may also cause certain fetal heart rate changes. A fetus with anemia either acute or chronic is at greater risk of hypoxia and also has a very reduced reserve to cope with hypoxia as hemoglobin acts as a buffer in metabolic acidosis.

In labor, fetus is exposed to intermittent episodes of relative hypoxia. With each contraction there is a relative decrease in uterine blood flow, placental perfusion and gas exchange. The fit, mature fetus with abundant stores of glycogen is able to withstand this hypoxia for a prolonged period of time without developing serious oxygen debt and hypoxia. On the contrary a fetus who is exposed to chronic hypoxia/ malnutrition is already on the brink of hypoxia and has little reserve to withstand the acidotic process of labor.

Fetal surveillance in labor can be:
- Clinical surveillance
  - *Maternal history*: to assess for risk factors, e.g. IUGR, oligohydramnios
  - *Meconium in liquor*
  - *Intermittent auscultation (IA); Admission test*
- Biophysical
  - *Continuous electronic fetal monitoring (CEFM)*
  - *Analysis of ST segment of the fetal ECG (STAN) used in combination with CTG*
  - *Fetal oximetry*
- Biochemical
  - *Fetal blood sampling (FBS) for pH and base-excess*
  - *FBS for lactate.*

Clinical Surveillance

Clinical surveillance should help as a screening method in identifying babies who are particularly at high risk of developing intrapartum hypoxia. Monitoring should pay particular attention to the presence of fetal growth restriction, pregnancy complications and amount and color of amniotic fluid in those with ruptured membranes.

Maternal History

The presence of risk factors for pathologies that may increase the risk of fetal hypoxia should be considered.

Risk Assessment

- Increased risk of cord compression—breech, oligohydramnios, strong uterine contractions especially in induced labors
- Reduced retroplacental pool of blood as in cases of suspected fetal growth restriction, pre-eclampsia, antepartum or intrapartum hemorrhage
- Reduced fetal reserve—Prematurity, fetal infection, fetal anemia, multiple pregnancy, growth restriction
- Increased risk of severe acute hypoxic event, e.g. scar rupture during vaginal birth after cesarean section.

Meconium in Liquor

Majority of labors complicated by meconium stained liquor (MSL) have normal outcomes, but the presence of MSL increases the risk of a number of adverse neonatal outcomes. The risk of poor outcome increases with the grade of meconium seen in the liquor. The presence of meconium may be regarded as a warning sign of a possibility of pre-existing hypoxia, which may deteriorate during the course of labor, particularly if prolonged.

The risk includes meconium aspiration syndrome that can be a life-threatening condition. Among infants with meconium aspiration, there is a risk of about 20% for cerebral palsy or global developmental delay.

Intermittent Auscultation

If the woman has no risk factors (low risk) and there is no meconium in amniotic fluid then intermittent auscultation should be recommended. If this is acceptable to the woman, it is recommended that the operator listen for one minute soon after a contraction using a pinnard stethoscope or a hand-held Doppler machine. This should be done every 15 minutes in first stage of labor and every 5 minutes in the second stage of labor. Intermittent auscultation is compatible with excellent outcome in experienced hands and particularly when used judiciously.

In favorable circumstances, in a well-grown fetus with adequate liquor volume, IA can be just as effective as EFM in preventing fetal or neonatal death from asphyxia in labor (MacDonald et al, 1985).

Continuous electronic fetal monitoring should be commenced if any of the following occur:

- Baseline abnormality
- Any audible deceleration (variable or late)
- New meconium staining of the liquor is observed
- A new risk factor develops during the course of labor (such as oxytocin therapy or intrapartum hemorrhage.

Shortfalls with Intermittent Auscultation

In labors lasting more than 5 hours from time of admission, IA may not be as effective as EFM in preventing hypoxic ischemic encephalopathy (HIE). It is also not helpful in pregnancies with either antenatal or intrapartum risk factors.

Admission Test

This includes performing a CTG on admission to labor ward and may be appropriate for all women who present in labor. This can be used as a screening tool to identify those who need further tests of fetal surveillance.

In low and high-risk groups, admission test may have specificity as high as (94.7%) and a negative predictive value up to 81.8% in predicting fetal distress (when a reactive trace is compared with a nonreactive trace) and in identifying the compromised fetus thereby helping in reducing the neonatal morbidity and mortality by early intervention (Khandelwal et al 2010).

It may have a role in obstetric units with a heavy workload (>10,000 deliveries/ year) with limited resources to help in 'Triaging' fetuses. In developed countries with good antenatal care, such fetuses may have been picked up by serial ultrasound or Doppler scans, alleviating the need for an admission CTG (Arulkumaran, 2008).

Shortfalls with Admission Test

Although, it may provide a 'snap-shot' view of fetal well-being at the time of admission, it does not identify those fetuses that would subsequently develop intrapartum hypoxia if the labor is longer than two to four hours, if there would be acute events or the use of oxytocin.

Biophysical Methods of Fetal Surveillance

These include methods such as Continuous Electronic Fetal Monitoring (CEFM), Fetal ECG monitoring and Fetal Pulse Oximetry (FPO).

Continuous Electronic Fetal Monitoring (CEFM)

Continous electronic fetal monitoring (CEFM) is a screening tool that is used to assess fetal well-being during labor and to identify the possibility of asphyxia. It was first developed in the 1950s and became commercially available in the 1960s.

Current techniques rely predominantly on the use of electronic fetal monitoring through the use of CTG. This technique allows detection and analysis of the fetal heart rate (FHR) and a semi-quantitative analysis of myometrial activity and contractions. The interpretation of data collected depends on the relationship between the two traces. During labor, EFM is used to assure fetal well-being because the inexplicable interplay of antenatal complications, inadequate placental perfusion and intrapartum events can lead to adverse outcomes (ACOG, 2009).

This technology when it was introduced was widely embraced as an undoubted 'good thing', which would lead to better outcomes and reduce the incidence of conditions such as cerebral palsy that were postulated to be largely because of episodes of intrapartum cerebral ischemia. Clinicians originally anticipated that FHR monitoring would solve two problems. First, it would serve as a screening test for severe asphyxia (asphyxia severe enough to cause neurologic damage or fetal death). Second, FHR monitoring would allow recognition of early asphyxia so that timely obstetric intervention could avoid asphyxia-induced brain damage or death in the newborn. Unfortunately, subsequent evidence has not borne out this optimism.

Abnormality of the CTG sometimes severe enough to be described as a pathological trace is commonly termed 'fetal distress', although many fetuses with such traces may not have hypoxia and metabolic acidosis. In current practice, the events are appropriately termed 'pathological CTG trace' or 'acidotic pH' rather than 'fetal distress'. Accurate interpretation of CTG is essential, and it is important to recognize a fetus that shows a pathological CTG in labor that may imply possible hypoxia and birth asphyxia. Considering the wider clinical picture in interpreting the CTG, and taking timely and appropriate action based on the findings, may help prevent birth asphyxia (Chandraharan and Arulkumaran, 2007).

Reassuring patterns require no specific action. Non-reassuring patterns occur in about 15% of labors monitored by CTG and may prompt clinical actions ranging from simple maneuvers, such as a change of maternal position, through to expedited birth of the baby (vacuum, forceps, cesarean section). Fetal heart rate patterns suggestive of progressive hypoxia are progressive tachycardia, progressive bradycardia, loss of variability and widening and deepening of decelerations. Abnormal patterns usually prompt expedited birth with the aim of preventing or minimizing hypoxia in the fetus. The positive predictive value of CTG for adverse outcome is low and the negative predictive value high (Umstad, 1993), although this is improving with computerized interpretation of CTGs (Strachan et al, 2001).

Cardiotocography is associated with low specificity for fetal acidosis and poor perinatal outcome leading to unnecessary operative deliveries. Randomized controlled trials of FHR monitoring have shown that there is a marginal advantage for electronic FHR monitoring over intermittent auscultation (MacDonald et al, 1985, Vintzileos et al, 1995, Thacker et al, 1995). Some limitations for the randomized controlled trials were that there were no standard criteria for FHR interpretation, no standard treatment protocols for non-reassuring FHR patterns, and no standard care for neonatal resuscitation or successive neonatal intensive treatment (Parer and King, 2000).

Mahomed et al (Mahomed et al, 1994) compared the abilities of intermittent electronic monitoring, a hand held Doppler ultrasound monitor, and the Pinard stethoscope to detect abnormalities in fetal heart rate and their contribution to mode of delivery and fetal outcome. The ultrasound monitor was better at detecting abnormalities in fetal heart rate than the Pinard stethoscope and was associated with lower neonatal morbidity and mortality and perinatal outcome was no worse than that achieved with electronic monitoring. Doppler ultrasound monitoring should therefore be promoted in developing countries where electronic monitoring is not feasible. They concluded that the abnormalities in fetal heart rate were more reliably detected by Doppler ultrasonography than with Pinard stethoscope and its use resulted in good perinatal outcome.

Compared with IA, EFM is associated with a significantly increased likelihood of operative vaginal delivery, overall cesarean delivery, as well as with non-reassuring fetal heart rate tracing or fetal acidosis. Although the use of EFM and intrapartum interventions significantly decreases the rate of neonatal seizures, its use is not associated with a significantly lower rate of cerebral palsy or of neonatal death (ACOG, 2009). Cochrane review (Alfirevic et al, 2006) reported that EFM was associated with 1 additional cesarean delivery for every 58 women monitored continuously and 661 women would have EFM during labor to prevent 1 neonatal seizure.

Shortfalls of Electronic Fetal Monitoring Using Cardiotocography

The major drawbacks of EFM relate not so much to the technique itself but more to the difficulties in reading and interpreting the FHR tracings that is partly because of the many factors that may affect the FHR and its variability and the lack of consensus among obstetricians on how to read and interpret FHR tracings. Although extensively used in developed countries, the complexity of the monitoring equipment, however, makes it susceptible to technical and mechanical failures. The costs of the equipment, its maintenance and replacement may be prohibitive, particularly in developing countries with scarce resources. Extensive investment in this equipment by such countries is clearly impractical and often impossible. Fetal heart rate monitoring with less expensive and sophisticated technology may well be just as effective. Thus, while a normal CTG usually indicates reassuring fetal status, a non-reassuring or abnormal CTG does not necessarily equate with 'suspected fetal compromise'.

Cardiotocography has very high sensitivity and is capable of excluding intrapartum hypoxia, if all the features are in the 'reassuring' category. However, the 'trade-off' is that the CTG has a high false positive rate. Hence, it is a poor predictor of fetal hypoxia and metabolic acidosis. Even with significant abnormalities in the CTG, the risk of fetal acidosis in fetal blood sampling could be only 50%. As CTG changes often are not specific for hypoxia, there might be a tendency for the staff to neglect abnormal traces.

Fetal ECG for Intrapartum Fetal Monitoring

Fetal ECG waveform analysis as an adjunct to electronic fetal monitoring (EFM) has developed over the last 3 decades. From a multitude of potential parameters,

ST waveform analysis has been documented to provide the information required to shift EFM from a screening device to a diagnostic tool that meets the standards of evidence-based medicine. With more accurate identification of fetal hypoxia and reduction of unnecessary intervention rates, incorporation of ST waveform analysis (STAN) of fetal electrocardiography into cardiotocography has improved the standard of intrapartum fetal monitoring.

The fetal electrocardiogram (FECG) is continuously recordable and reflects the oxygenation and cellular metabolism of the myocardium and the cardiac conduction fibers. It is therefore of potential use in the detection of changes in acid-base status STAN allows detailed assessment of both fetal heart rate and ST waveform during delivery after a standard fetal scalp electrode has been applied. Cardiotocography along with ST analysis provides accurate information about intrapartum hypoxia similar to that obtained by scalp-pH (Luttkus et al, 2004). The ST waveform of the fetal electrocardiogram (ECG) provides continuous information on the ability of the fetal heart muscle to respond to the stress of labor. An elevation of the ST segment and T wave, quantified by the ratio between the T wave and QRS amplitudes (T/QRS), identifies fetal heart muscle responding to hypoxia by a surge of stress hormones (catecholamines), that leads to utilization of glycogen stored in the heart (an extra source of energy). An ST segment depression can indicate a situation where the heart is not fully able to respond. The ST waveform changes are identified automatically and clinical action should be taken strictly according to the guidelines that are based on extensive research (Rosen et al, 2004).

Compared with conventional cardiotocography, ST analysis shows a non-significant reduction in metabolic acidosis. ST analysis significantly reduces the incidence of additional fetal blood sampling, operative vaginal deliveries and total operative deliveries. For other outcomes, no differences in effect are seen between ST analysis and conventional cardiotocography. The additional use of ST analysis for intrapartum monitoring reduces the incidence of operative vaginal deliveries and the need for fetal blood sampling but does not reduce the incidence of metabolic acidosis at birth (Becker et al, 2012). The timing of CTG and ST changes relates to the level of acidosis at birth (Noren et al, 2007).

Combined CTG and ST changes are a more specific sign of hypoxia than CTG changes alone, and thereby not easily neglected. Furthermore, the 'log function' of the monitoring system alerts the staff more distinctly than changes in the CTG trace alone (Rosen et al, 2004).

Shortfalls of Fetal ECG

Factors such as poor signal quality, difficulties in CTG interpretation, failure to comply with STAN clinical guidelines and deterioration of the CTG without ECG alert are among a few pitfalls that prevent severe metabolic acidosis being eradicated completely using this method (Noren et al, 2007, Doria et al, 2007).

Fetal Pulse Oximetry

Pulse oximetry was introduced in 1980s. It measures oxyhemoglobin and deoxyhemoglobin in arterial blood using alternating pulses of red and near-infrared light. It has had a significant impact on patient care in a variety of settings.

In obstetrics, it was expected to improve the accuracy of the evaluation of fetal well-being during labor. Fetal pulse oximetry has been advocated as a means of improving the specificity of cardiotocography in intrapartum fetal surveillance (Yam et al, 2000). Because intrapartum fetal asphyxia has generally been viewed to occur via hypoxemia, the use of fetal pulse oximetry in obstetrics was thought to be a logical extension in identifying those fetuses that may benefit from further intervention and as an adjunct to rather than replacement of the CTG monitor.

This method has two potential advantages over conventional fetal heart rate monitoring (East et al, 2004):

- It directly measures the proportion of hemoglobin that is carrying oxygen: thus, oxygenation, the primary variable underlying the tissue damaging effects of hypoxia/ischemia is being monitored
- It relies on an established, safe, noninvasive, widely used technology found in every modern intensive care unit and operating theater.

The electrode is placed during a vaginal examination to attach to the top of the fetal head by suction or clip, lie against the fetal temple or cheek, or to lie along the fetal back. The sensor remains in situ and fetal pulse oximetry values are recorded for approximately 81% of the monitoring time.

One of the most important questions that several studies tried to address was the 'critical threshold of fetal arterial oxygen saturation above which acidemia does not occur'. Clinical observations of thousands of cases and published studies, suggest that a critical threshold of 30% would be appropriate for clinical use, a threshold used in the American RCT and subsequently approved by the US Food and Drug Administration (FDA) (Dildy et al, 1996, Seelbach-Gobel et al, 1999). There is limited support for the use of fetal pulse oximetry when used in the presence of a nonreassuring CTG, to reduce caesarean section for non-reassuring fetal status.

Shortfalls of Fetal Pulse Oximetry

There have been several controversies surrounding the use of FPO in clinical use. The American College of Obstetricians and Gynaecologists (ACOG, 2001) had three main concerns regarding this technology:

- Signal registration time
- Possible false negative readings
- Lack of proven cost benefit.

There are concerns that its introduction could further escalate the cost of medical care without necessarily improving clinical outcome. One other criticism about FPO is based on the fact that 'Fetal brain injury is because of ischemia, not hypoxemia'. This theory would suggest that normally oxygenated blood could perfuse the skin of the presenting part while the brain suffers ischemic damage, thus raising concerns about it's use in fetal surveillance in labor.

Biochemical Means of Fetal Surveillance

Biochemical tests for intrapartum fetal assessment includes obtaining fetal scalp blood for pH and base excess or lactate measurement. Contrary to screening tests such as IA, CTG, fetal ECG or oximetry, biochemical tests are diagnostic tests.

Saling, in 1962 introduced the method of collecting fetal scalp blood and analyzing the pH as an indicator of hypoxia. Through a vaginal amnioscope, a capillary blood sample is taken from a small incision on the fetal scalp and analyzed for indices of fetal acid-base status. The procedure is best performed in the left lateral position as the lithotomy position may lead to supine hypotension in the mother, producing further fetal acid-base compromise. Arbitrarily, a pH < 7.20 was chosen as cut-off value to recommend intervention.

FBS is employed to reduce the false positive rate of the CTG. This approach helps in identifying hypoxic fetuses, that actually need an intervention and to avoid unnecessary intervention to those fetuses that are not subjected to a hypoxic insult.

Fetal Blood Sampling

Fetal blood sampling (FBS) is an intrusive and uncomfortable assessment to obtain a sample of blood from fetal scalp for biochemical analysis. Appropriate verbal consent should be obtained from the woman. It should be performed with the woman in left lateral position as lithotomy position increases maternal postural hypotension. If a fetal blood sample cannot be achieved because of early cervical dilatation or the level of the fetal head is high, then delivery rather than fetal blood sampling is appropriate (Table 11.1).

Contraindications for FBS include:

- Maternal HIV
- Hepatitis B or C infection
- Known maternal immunothrombocytopenia
- Possible fetal bleeding disorder
- Non-recovering prolonged deceleration (bradycardia) or pre-terminal CTG pattern (absent variability with recurrent decelerations).

Unless delivery is imminent, pathological CTG with meconium liquor should be considered as a contraindication to performing FBS.

TABLE 11.1 Interpretation and management of FBS results (scalp pH)

Normal (> 7.25)	Sampling should be repeated no more than 60 minutes later if the CTG remains suspicious/pathological, or sooner, if there are further abnormalities
Borderline (7.21–7.24)	Sampling should be repeated no more than 30 minutes later if the CTG remains pathological, or sooner, if there are further abnormalities
Abnormal (< 7.20)	Prompt delivery should be conducted

pH and Base Excess

During active labor, the integrity of uteroplacental circulation and the frequency and intensity of uterine activity influence the fetal acid-base status. If the uteroplacental circulation or fetus is compromised or uterine activity is excessive, there is an initial reduction in oxygen supply and an accumulation of CO_2 (respiratory acidosis). If the negative influence persists, anaerobic respiration ensues, resulting in accumulation of lactic and pyruvic acids (metabolic acidosis). The speed of development of metabolic acidosis depends on the particular insult and the ability of the fetus to compensate.

An indication for an FBS is a suspicious or a pathological fetal heart rate trace. The analysis of pH is complicated, however, and needs a relatively large amount of blood (30–50 µL), and sampling failure rates of 11–20% have been reported (Tuffnell et al, 2006, Westgren et al, 1998). Estimation of pH alone does not discriminate between respiratory and metabolic acidemia, the latter being associated with neonatal morbidity (Low et al, 1994).

The results should be interpreted taking into account the previous pH measurement, the rate of progress in labor and the clinical features of the woman and baby. It is important to evaluate both the pH and the base excess (BE) as the base excess will provide an idea of the degree of depletion of the buffering system. This will in turn indicate the degree of metabolic acidosis. Although, the use of fetal blood sampling may reduce operative delivery rates, there is no evidence to suggest that it confers any improvement to the overall neonatal outcome (Bix et al, 2005).

In more recent years, respiratory acidemia (CO_2 accumulation) has been confirmed as being harmless to the fetus, whereas metabolic acidemia (lactacidemia) is associated with neonatal morbidity (Low et al, 1994, Goldaber et al, 1991). In blood from the cord artery, acidemia is usually regarded as pH, 7.10 – 7.00 and metabolic acidemia is present when the base deficit (BD) is > 8 mmol/L (moderate) or > 12 mmol/L (severe). These BD values are often also applied to FBS but are not evaluated in clinical trials.

A pH value < 7.0 in umbilical arterial blood is associated with (but not predictive of) neurologic and other organ damage (Low et al, 1994, Goldaber et al, 1991). It occurs in about 3 per 1000 births. Newer evidence is accumulating that some morbidity is seen in fetuses with an umbilical arterial pH between 7.0 and 7.1. Although morbidity seen after pH values in this range is generally not catastrophic or permanent, it is costly and distressing in that the newborn may have a supplemental oxygen requirement, intravenous lines, and admission to the neonatal intensive care nursery. Therefore, an umbilical arterial blood pH of < 7.1 should be avoided if possible. A pH of < 7.1 is at about the 2.5th percentile, and therefore this gives us a more substantial target population of fetuses that could benefit from FHR monitoring (Parer and King, 2000) (Table 11.2).

Fetal Blood Lactate Measurements

This is less well validated than pH and is less widely used but requires a small sample of fetal blood. Lactate is present in different concentrations in the different blood

	pH	Lactate (mmol/L)
Normal	> 7.25	< 4.2
Pre-acidemia/Pre-lactemia	7.20 – 7.25	4.2 – 4.8
Acidemia/Lactemia	< 7.20	> 4.8

TABLE 11.2 Clinical guidelines for FBS pH and Lactate

compartments; concentrations are highest in plasma, lower in hemolyzed blood and lowest in whole blood (with intact erythrocytes). Both maternal and fetal lactate concentrations increase with the duration of active bearing-down. It is estimated that fetal lactate increases by 1 mmol/L for every 30 minutes of pushing; the corresponding value for the woman is 2 mmol/L per 30 minutes (Nordstrom et al, 2001). It can also be performed reliably in the presence of caput succedaneum.

A lactate concentration of 4.8 mmol/L should be taken as cut-off value for intervention (Kruger et al, 1999). One of the main advantages of fetal blood lactate over pH is that because of the small sampling volume (5μL) needed, sampling failure has almost been abolished for lactate analysis. Lactate analysis of a blood sample collected in a glass capillary or stored in a clamped cord should be carried out within 10 minutes of sampling/clamping because lactate increases linearly with time.

Shortfalls of Fetal Blood Sampling

The effectiveness of FBS in clinical practice has been questioned. The decision to obtain an FBS depends on the interpretation of the CTG. If the level of CTG interpretation is suboptimal, the value by monitoring with FBS is limited. Intervention should occur with high lactate measurements, even if the pH measurement is normal. As far as the lactate measurement is concerned, two possible sources of 'falsely' measured high lactate concentrations are amniotic fluid contamination and delay between sampling and analysis >10 minutes.

Summary

The performance of fetal monitoring depends on the ability of the staff to interpret recordings and to manage the cases according to specific guidelines. Intrapartum hypoxia is thought to contribute to the incidence of cerebral palsy, seizures and mental retardation. Long-term neurological complications such as learning difficulties and motor impairments may be due to causes other than birth asphyxia. Electronic fetal monitoring has a high false positive rate whereas fetal blood sampling, which is an invasive procedure, only allows an intermittent assessment. In modern obstetrics, fetal electrocardiogram waveform analysis and the intermittent measurement of lactate levels by fetal blood sampling seem to be the most reliable methods of establishing fetal well-being in labor.

Bibliography

1. ACOG. Fetal pulse oximetry. Obstetrics and Gynecology. 2001;98:523–24.
2. ACOG. Intrapartum fetal heart rate monitoring: nomenclature, interpretation and general management principles. Washington. 2009.
3. Alfirevic Z, Devane D, Gyte GM. Continuous cardiotocography (CTG) as a form of electronic fetal monitoring (EFM) for fetal assessment during labor. Cochrane database of systematic reviews, CD006066, 2006.
4. Becker JH, Bax L, Amer-Wahlin I, Ojala K, Vayssiere C, Westerhuis ME, et al. ST analysis of the fetal electrocardiogram in intrapartum fetal monitoring: a meta-analysis. Obstetrics and gynecology. 2012;119:145–54.
5. Bix E, Reiner LM, Klovning A, Oian P. Prognostic value of the labor admission test and its effectiveness compared with auscultation only: a systematic review. BJOG: An International Journal of Obstetrics and Gynaecology. 2005;112:1595–604.
6. Chandraharan E, Arulkumaran S. Prevention of birth asphyxia: responding appropriately to cardiotocograph (CTG) traces. Best practice and research. Clinical Obstetrics and Gynaecology. 2007;21:609–24.
7. Chandraharan E and Arulkumaran S. Electronic fetal heart rate monitoring in current and future practice. The Journal of Obstetrics and Gynecology of India. 2008;58:121–30.
8. Dildy GA, Thorp JA, Yeast JD, Clark SL. The relationship between oxygen saturation and pH in umbilical blood: implications for intrapartum fetal oxygen saturation monitoring. American Journal of Obstetrics and Gynecology. 1996;175:682–7.
9. Doria V, Papageorghiou A, Gustafsson A, Ugwumadu A, Farrer K and Arulkumaran S. Review of the first 1502 cases of ECG-ST waveform analysis during labor in a teaching hospital. BJOG: An International Journal of Obstetrics and Gynaecology. 2007;114:1202–7.
10. East CE, Chan FY, Colditz PB. Fetal pulse oximetry for fetal assessment in labor. Cochrane database of systematic reviews, CD004075, 2004.
11. Goldaber KG, Gilstrap LC, Leveno KJ, Dax JS, Mcintire DD. Pathologic fetal acidemia. Obstetrics and Gynecology. 1991;78:1103–7.
12. Khandelwal S, Dhanraj M, Khandelwal A. Admission test as precursor of perinatal outcome: a prospective study. Archives of Gynecology and Obstetrics, 2010;282:377-82.
13. Kruger K, Hallberg B, Blennow M, Kublickas M, Westgren M. Predictive value of fetal scalp blood lactate concentration and pH as markers of neurologic disability. American journal of Obstetrics and Gynecology. 1999;181:1072–8.
14. Low JA, Panagiotopoulos C, Derrick, EJ. Newborn complications after intrapartum asphyxia with metabolic acidosis in the term fetus. American Journal of Obstetrics and Gynecology. 1994;170:1081–7.
15. Luttkus AK, Noren H, Stupin JH, Blad S, Arulkumaran S, Erkkola R, et al. Fetal scalp pH and ST analysis of the fetal ECG as an adjunct to CTG. A multi-center, observational study. Journal of Perinatal Medicine. 2004;32:486–94.
16. Macdonald D, Grant A, Sheridan-Pereira M, Boylan P, Chalmers I. The Dublin randomized controlled trial of intrapartum fetal heart rate monitoring. American Journal of Obstetrics and Gynecology. 1985;152:524–39.
17. Mahomed K, Nyoni R, Mulambo T, Kasule J and Jacobus E. Randomised controlled trial of intrapartum fetal heart rate monitoring. BMJ. 1994;308:497–500.
18. Nordstrom L, Achanna S, Naka K, Arulkumaran S. Fetal and maternal lactate increase during active second stage of labor. BJOG: An International Journal of Obstetrics and Gynaecology. 2001;108:263–8.

19. Nordstrom L, Arulkumaran S. Intrapartum fetal hypoxia and biochemical markers: a review. Obstetrical and Gynecological Survey. 1998;53:645–57.
20. Noren H, Luttkus AK, Stupin JH, Blad S, Arulkumaran S, Erkkola R, et al. Fetal scalp pH and ST analysis of the fetal ECG as an adjunct to cardiotocography to predict fetal acidosis in labor–a multi-center, case controlled study. Journal of Perinatal Medicine. 2007;35:408–14.
21. Paper JT and KING T. Fetal heart rate monitoring: is it salvageable? American Journal of Obstetrics and Gynecology. 2000;182:982–7.
22. Rosen KG, Amer-Wahlin I, Luzietti R, Noren H. Fetal ECG waveform analysis. Best practice and research. Clinical Obstetrics and Gynaecology. 2004;18:485–514.
23. Seelbach-Gobel B, Heupel M, Kuhnert M, Butterwegge M. The prediction of fetal acidosis by means of intrapartum fetal pulse oximetry. American Journal of Obstetrics and Gynecology. 1999;180:73–81.
24. Strachan BK, Sahota DS, Van Wijngaarden WJ, James DK, Chang AM. Computerised analysis of the fetal heart rate and relation to acidaemia at delivery.BJOG: An International Journal of Obstetrics and Gynaecology. 2001;108:848–52.
25. Thacker SB, Stroup DF, Peterson HB. Efficacy and safety of intrapartum electronic fetal monitoring: an update. Obstetrics and Gynecology. 1995;86:613–20.
26. Tuffnell D, Haw WL, Wilkinson K. How long does a fetal scalp blood sample take? BJOG : An International Journal of Obstetrics and Gynaecology. 2006;113:332–4.
27. Umstad MP. The predictive value of abnormal fetal heart rate patterns in early labor.The Australian and New Zealand Journal of Obstetrics and Gynaecology. 1993;33:145–9.
28. Vintzileos AM, Nochimson DJ, Guzman ER, Knuppel RA, Lake M, Schifrin BS. Intrapartum electronic fetal heart rate monitoring versus intermittent auscultation: a meta-analysis. Obstetrics and Gynecology. 1995;85:149–55.
29. Westgren M, Kruger K, Grunevald C, Kublickas M, Naka K, Wolff K, et al. Lactate compared with pH analysis at fetal scalp blood sampling: a prospective randomised study. British Journal of Obstetrics and Gynaecology. 1998;105:29–33.
30. Yam J, Chua S, Arulkumaran S. Intrapartum fetal pulse oximetry. Part I: Principles and technical issues. Obstetrical and Gynecological Survey. 2000;55:163–72.

Gestational Diabetes Mellitus—A Growing Concern

12

Chapter

Sujata Mishra

Diabetes mellitus is one of the most common medical disorders complicating pregnancy with incidence of about 7%.[1] The pregnant women with diabetes may either be a case of pre-gestational diabetes, where diabetes antedated the pregnancy, or may have gestational diabetes mellitus (GDM) which is defined as carbohydrate intolerance (hyperglycemia) of variable severity with onset or first recognition during the present pregnancy.[2] The definition applies irrespective of whether or not insulin is used for treatment or the condition persists after pregnancy. It does not exclude the possibility that glucose intolerance may have antedated the present pregnancy.[3]

The overall incidence of GDM that was earlier said to be 3-6%, has steadily increased over time to 15% in the Indian subcontinent.[4] This remains a major cause of perinatal morbidity and mortality, as well as maternal morbidity. Hence screening for GDM, diagnosis and management are the tripods for curbing the rising trend of the diabetic population globally.

Gestational Diabetes Mellitus Pathogenesis

Pregnancy per se is a state of physiological insulin resistance that is beneficial to the baby in terms of increases transplacental transfer of glucose to the developing fetus. This results in a sluggish first phase insulin release and excessive resistance to action of insulin on glucose utilization because of placental hormones (Placental lactogen, progesterone, prolactin and cortisol). A woman with normal glucose tolerance is associated with a 200% to 250% increase in her insulin secretion to maintain euglycemia above the insulin resistance and thereby maintains her glycemic levels. A pregnant woman, who is not able to increase her insulin secretion to overcome insulin resistance that occurs even during normal pregnancy, develops gestational diabetes. It has been observed that women with gestational diabetes have a significantly lower insulin response at 30 and 60 minutes after oral glucose compared to normal pregnant women. Insulin resistance plays an important role mainly in the fasting state of the mother to ensure that the fetus receives an adequate supply of glucose by switching the maternal metabolism from carbohydrates to lipids. In the fed state, insulin secretion has to be augmented to revert back to the maternal metabolism to utilize carbohydrates.

Etiopathogenesis of Gestational Diabetes Mellitus Possible Explanations

The possible mechanisms leading to Gestational diabetes are as mentioned in Table 12.1:[5]

TABLE 12.1

Autoimmune destruction of the beta cells of the:
Impaired beta cell function
Increased insulin degradation

Decreased tissue sensitivity to insulin
  * Impaired insulin – insulin receptor binding
  * Impaired intracellular insulin signaling

Screening and Diagnosis

Gestational diabetes is not only associated with an increase in maternal and perinatal morbidity and mortality; it also increases the likelihood of subsequent diabetes in the mother.[6]

In a quest to curb this rising trend, several groups, as mentioned in Table 12.2 have suggested various screening tests and criterion to diagnose gestational diabetes.

TABLE 12.2

• American Diabetes Association (ADA) • Canadian Diabetes in Pregnancy Study Group (CANDIPS) • National Diabetes Data group (NDDG) (USA and Europe) • Australasian Criteria	• Japan Diabetes Association • German Diabetes Association • Diabetes, UK (NICE Guidelines)

A comparative analysis of the criteria of some of the groups has been depicted in a tabular form (Table 12.3).

The diagnostic criteria for GDM were based on the long-term effects on the mother and only in the past decades has the association between OGTT thresholds and neonatal outcomes been investigated. The original O' Sullivan criteria was

TABLE 12.3 Criteria for diagnosis of gestational diabetes with a 75-g oral glucose load [mg/dL (mmol/L)]

	WHO	European Association for Study of Diabetes	Fourth International Workshop on GDM	Australasian Criteria
Fasting	Not advocated	-	95 (5.3)	99 (5.5)
1 h	-	-	180 (10.0)	-
2 h	140 (7.8)	162 (9.0)	155 (8.6)	144 (8.0)

1. Two or more of the venous plasma concentrations must be met or exceeded for a positive diagnosis.
2. The test should be performed in the morning after an 8 to 14 hours fast and after at least 3 days of unrestricted diet and physical activity.

based on the risk for developing type 2 diabetes rather than the risk for adverse outcome during pregnancy. In 1964, O' Sullivan and Mahan reported the results of a study of a 3-h oral 100-g glucose tolerance test (OGTT) in 752 healthy pregnant women. Norms were established for whole blood during fasting, 1-h, 2-h, and 3-h *(Fasting–90 mg/dL, 1-h 165 mg/dL, 2-h 145 mg/dL, 3-h 125 mg/dL).*[8] values after glucose ingestion. These studies used venous whole blood samples. Later, a group of 1,013 women undergoing the OGTT during pregnancy were followed up and the incidence of adult onset diabetes in this populationwas determined.[9] After several years of follow-up, the cumulative incidence rate was 29% for women exhibiting OGTT values greater than two standard deviations during pregnancy. O'Sullivan and Mahan suggested that pregnant women exhibiting this degree of carbohydrate intolerance during pregnancy be designated as gestational diabetes. Following a shift to measurement of plasma venous samples, the National Diabetes Data Group (NDDG) in 1979 recommended conversion by an upward adjustment of 15% to account for the difference in sample measurements.[10] Recent studies report that the risk for subsequent diabetes may be as high as 15–30% after 2 years of follow-up.[11]

It is noteworthy that all of these criteria were validated based on predictive value of subsequent risk of diabetes in the mother and not specifically to determine maternal or fetal risk during pregnancy.[12]

World Health Organization Diagnostic Criterion[13]

In centers, where WHO criterion of impaired glucose tolerance is in use to identify women with gestational diabetes, a higher proportion of pregnancies are diagnosed as abnormal in comparison to use of other criteria. WHO proposed that using a 2-h 75-g Oral Glucose Tolerant Test (OGTT) with a threshold plasma glucose concentration of greater than 7.8 mmol/L (140 mg/dL) at 120 minutes is similar to that of impaired glucose tolerance in the non pregnant state.[13] The fasting plasma glucose is not favored as a screening procedure. The drawbacks were that the WHO criterion was not tailored specifically for use during pregnancy, nor were the thresholds set, for detection of either maternal or fetal complications.

American Diabetes Association Criterion-Evolution

The current diagnostic criteria for gestational diabetes in the United States was derived from the work of O' Sullivan and Mahan. The National Diabetes Data Group (NDDG) accepted and then converted the O' Sullivan criterion by applying a factor of 1.14 to convert whole blood to plasma thus creating glucose thresholds known as the NDDG criteria.

Carpenter and Coustan suggested an additional modification of the original O'Sullivan criteria which incorporated the change in the substrate and method used. Performance of either the 75-g 2-hour or the 100-g 3-hour oral glucose tolerance test evaluates the fasting (between 8 and 14 hours) glucose level and the value at 1 and 2 hours after the glucose load. The 100-g test includes an additional glucose assessment at 3-hours. Normal values based on Carpenter and Coustan criteria include a fasting plasma glucose level of 95 mg/dL or less (5.3 mmol/L); 1 hour, 180 mg/dL or less (10.0 mmol/L); 2 hour 155 mg/dL or less (8.6 mmol/L); and for the 100-g load 3 hour 140 mg/dL or less (7.8 mmol/L).[14]

Normal values based on NDDG criteria include a fasting plasma glucose level of 105 mg/dL or less (5.8 mmol/L); 1 hour, 190 mg/dL or less (10.5 mmol/L); 2 hour, 165 mg/dL or less (9.2 mmol/L); and 3 hour 145g/dL or less (8.0 mol/L). In tests, two or more of the venous plasma concentrations must be exceeded to be positive.[3]

ADA Diagnostic Criteria

The Fourth International Workshop on Gestational Diabetes supported by the American Diabetes Association (ADA), and the American College of Obstetricians and Gynecologists (ACOG) recommended that both the Carpenter-Coustan and NDDG criteria be used for diagnosis of GDM in either a one or a two-step approach.[14]

One-Step Approach

The Conference consensus statement further recommended that the 75-gm load (popular in Europe) be used in the diagnosis of GDM using the threshold suggested by the Carpenter-Coustan criteria (fasting 95 mg/dL, 1-h 180 mg/dL, 2-h 155 mg/dL). This recommendation eliminated the 3-h sample and used two or more abnormal values for diagnosis. The result was a one-step approach in which the OGTT is performed without prior plasma or serum glucose screening Table 12.4.[15]

Two-Step Approach

This approach recommends universal or selective screening with an initial 50-gm oral glucose load (GCT). The glucose thresholds that are used as positive test results are still not universally accepted and range from 130 mg/dL to 140 mg/dL. A positive screening result should be followed by the traditional OGTT as recommended by the NDDG or Carpenter-Coustan criteria (C and C) (Table 12.5).

The Consensus statement, raised questions about universal versus. selective screening. Two recent major studies attempted to determine the lowest threshold for GDM diagnosis: Hyperglycemia and Adverse Pregnancy Outcome (HAPO) Study[16] and the NICHD mild hyperglycemia study.[17]

TABLE 12.4 One-Step Approach for Diagnosis

• Perform OGTT without prior plasma or serum glucose screening • May be cost effective in high-risk patients • Diagnosis of GDM with a 75-g oral glucose load		
Fasting	mg/dL	mg/dL
	95	5.3
1-h	180	10.0
2-h	155	8.6

TABLE 12.5 Two-step approach of diagnosis

- Initial 50-g oral glucose load (GCT)
- Perform a diagnostic OGTT for women exceeding the glucose threshold value on the GCT
- Diagnosis of GDM with 100-g oral glucose load

	Carpenter-Coustar	NDDG
Fasting	95	105
1-h	180	190
2-h	155	165
3-h	140	145

Landon MB, Spong TE, Gabbe ST, et al: 2002. A planned randomized clinical trial of treatment for mild gestational diabetes mellitus. J Mat- Fetal & Neonatal Med 11(4): 226- 31.

Hyperglycemia and Adverse Pregnancy Outcome (HAPO) Study

This study was a 7-year prospective observational study that enrolled over 23,000 non-diabetic pregnant women in nine countries. It aimed to establish the diagnostic criteria for gestational diabetes and to clarify the accurate glucose threshold of maternal hyperglycemia and related adverse perinatal outcomes. At entry into the study, each participant underwent a 75 g oral glucose tolerance test, with plasma glucose levels measured fasting and 1 and 2 h (Mean Fasting 81 mg/dL, 1- h 134 mg/dL, 2- h 111 mg/dL) after ingestion.[17]

HAPO reported that the neonatal birth weights and the rates of primary cesarean section increased with increasing plasma glucose levels, even among normal nondiabetic pregnancies. The frequency of primary cesarean sections was 13% among women with fasting glucose < 75 mg/dL compared with 26.3% among women with fasting glucose >100 mg/dL. In addition, hypoglycemia occurred in 37% of neonates with the highest cord serum c-peptide values. This study also highlighted that, the mean fasting and postprandial glucose concentrations were lower than the current criteria for diagnosis of gestational diabetes (Table 12.6).

International Association of Diabetes and Pregnancy Study Groups (IADPSG) Recommendations

Screen for undiagnosed type 2 diabetes at the first prenatal visit in those with risk factors, using standard diagnostic criteria.

TABLE 12.6 HAPO and ADA diagnostic criteria for gestational diabetes

	HAPO (mean glucose level)	American Diabetes Association Criteria	
		Gestational diabetes	Type 2 diabetes
Fasting plasma glucose	81 mg/dL	>95 mg/dL	>126 mg/dL
2-h (75 g or 100g OGTT)	111 mg/dL	>155 mg/dL	>200 mg/dL

TABLE 12.7 Screening for and diagnosis of GDM

Perform a 75-g OGTT, with plasma glucose measurement fasting and at 1 and 2 h, at 24–28 weeks of gestation in women not previously diagnosed with overt diabetes
The OGTT should be performed in the morning after an overnight fast of at least 8 h
The diagnosis of GDM is made when any of the following plasma glucose value is exceeded: • Fasting—92 mg/dL (5.1 mmol/L) • 1 h—180 mg/dL (10.0 mmol/L) • 2 h—153 mg/dL (8.5 mmol/L)

Fasting plasma glucose level ≥ 92 mg/dL (5.1 mmol/L) or random plasma glucose level ≥ 200 mg/dl or HbA1c ≥ 6.5%, the pregnant woman is likely to be a pre-diabetic. If found normal in the first visit, screening has to be done between 24-28th weeks of gestation.

In healthy pregnant women, screen for GDM at 24–28 weeks of gestation, using a 75-g 2-hOGTT and the diagnostic cut points in Table 12.7.

Screen women with GDM for persistent diabetes 6–12 weeks postpartum.

Women with a history of GDM should have lifelong screening for the development of diabetes or prediabetes at least every 3 years.

The group recommended that all women not known to have diabetes undergo a 75-g OGTT at 24–28 weeks of gestation. Additionally, the group developed diagnostic cut points for the fasting, 1-h, and 2-h plasma glucose measurements that conveyed an odds ratio for adverse outcomes of at least 1.75 compared with the mean glucose levels in the HAPO study. Current screening and diagnostic strategies, based on the IADPSG statement,[18] are outlined in Table 12.7.

Pharmacotherapy

Historically, insulin has been the therapeutic agent of choice for controlling hyperglycemia in pregnant women. The need for multiple daily injections, potential for hypoglycemia, and increase in appetite and weight make this therapeutic option cumbersome for many pregnant women.[19]

Among the oral hypoglycemic agents, Glibenclamide and Metformin are the two drugs that have been extensively studied for management of GDM. The added risk of these drugs in the pregnant state are determined by the transplacental passage, association with fetal anomalies, potential for maternal adverse effects; and the safety of the medications during breastfeeding.

Glibenclamide (Category C in Pregnancy)

It is a second-generation oral sulfonylurea, that acts by enhancing the release of insulin from the pancreatic beta cells in normal and diabetic patients. The overall incidence of adverse effects ranges from 3.2 to 4.1%. While 1–5% os cases may have hypoglycemia with Glibenclamide , the most common adverse effects are gastrointestinal (nausea, vomiting, dyspepsia) and dermatologic (pruritus, urticaria, erythema, and maculopapular eruptions). Though elevations of liver function tests have been reported, the incidence of jaundice is rare.[20]

Following oral administration, it is well absorbed and independent of food intake. It is metabolized by the liver and time to peak concentration is 2–3 hours with a half-life of 7–10 hours. The initial dose of Glibenclamide is 2.5 mg once or twice a day and can be increased after titration with blood glucose values up to a maximum of 20 mg/day. Care should be taken that no more than 7.5 mg should be taken at each time. Prescribing glibenclamide rather than insulin during pregnancy may increase patient compliance and overall maternal and neonatal outcome. Unlike other sulfonylureas, there is substantial evidence demonstrating the lack of transplacental passage of glibenclamide to the fetus[21] suggesting insignificant fetal exposure with this drug and its safety in pregnancy.[22] Possible explanations for such lack of placental transport include the extensive plasma protein binding and short elimination half-life.[23] Lim in 1997 first reported that there was no difference in pregnancy outcomes of women using this drug for gestational diabetes.[24]

Langer in his study compared glibenclamide with insulin in the treatment of gestational diabetes.[25] The daily blood glucose concentrations and glycosylated hemoglobin values were similar between patients on glibenclamide and insulin. There were no differences in the infants who were large for gestational age or with macrosomia, lung complications, hypoglycemia, admission to the neonatal intensive care unit, or fetal anomalies. Also, the cord insulin concentrations were similar between the groups. Glibenclamide was not detected in the cord serum of infants of mothers administered the drug. Langer concluded that glibenclamide was a clinically effective alternative to insulin therapy in women with gestational diabetes.[26] Glibenclamide was found to be significantly less costly than insulin. To assess the comparative effectiveness of glibenclamide versus insulin, Nicoloson et al, did a meta- analysis of the RCTs of glibenclamide versus insulin in the treatment of GDM.

Three randomized controlled trials including a total of 478 participants were conducted in India, the United States, Brazil, Australia and New Zealand. The observations there of showed no differences in the glycemic control of the fasting and 2-hour postprandial plasma glucose. There were similar rates of cesarean delivery and newborn birth weights between the groups. Dhulkotia el al, also did a systematic review and meta-analysis to compare OHAs versus insulin in the management of gestational diabetes and concluded that there were no differences in glycemic control or pregnancy outcomes when OHAs were compared with insulin.[27] Conway, in an observational trial to examine factors predicting failure of glibenclamide treatment in gestational diabetes, found that among women with high FPG levels greater than or equal to 110 mg%/dL, 24% failed to respond to glibenclamide.[28]

Metformin (Category B Medication in Pregnancy)

Metformin is a biguanide that improves insulin sensitivity and reduces both fasting and postprandial plasma glucose. It functions by decreasing hepatic glucose output by inhibition of gluconeogenesis and enhances peripheral glucose uptake in the muscles and adipose tissues. It also decreases intestinal glucose absorption and increases insulin sensitivity. It is metabolized by the CYP 450 pathway with a half-life of 6 hours and is excreted in urine. Metformin is available in 250 mg, 500 mg, 850 mg and 1000 mg tablets in both regular-release and extended-release forms. The usual starting dose is 500–1000 mg/day that can be increased gradually to a maximum dose of 2500 mg/day.

Coetzee and colleagues did the first studies on metformin during the 1970s. Women with insulin-independent diabetes were prospectively followed throughout gestation; 22 women received metformin compared with 42 women who received insulin. The perinatal mortality rate was same for both. There were no cases of maternal hypoglycemia or lactic acidosis with metformin. In addition, metformin use in the first trimester was not associated with congenital anomalies.[29] In a follow-up study, Coetzee was able to achieve glycemic control in women on metformin within 24 hours compared with 2–3 weeks for insulin.[29] In 2000, Hellmuth and colleagues[30] performed a cohort study of type 2 DM pregnant women on metformin versus glibenclamide versus insulin. Their findings suggest concern for the use of metformin because of the increased rate of pre-eclampsia (32% metformin vs 7% glibenclamide vs 10% insulin) and intrauterine fetal death (8% vs 0% vs 2.3%,) respectively. However, this study has become controversial with critics claiming that women in the study were not well matched. In contrast, in a series of 90 women with polycystic ovarian syndrome (PCOS) who conceived on 1.5–2.5 g/day of metformin and continued metformin in pregnancy, metformin was not associated with pre-eclampsia in pregnancy (5.2% metformin vs 3.6% no metformin).[30]

Other studies have been conducted primarily in women with PCOS treated for infertility. In an observation trial of 72 women who conceived on 2.5 g/day of metformin, there was a higher live birth rate in those who received metformin compared with those without metformin (75% vs 34%). The spontaneous abortion rate was lower with metformin (17% vs 62%). There were no cases of lactic acidosis, fetal anomalies, or maternal or neonatal hypoglycemia.[31] The neonates whose mothers received metformin were also followed prospectively, and they displayed normal weight and social and motor skill at 6 months. At 18 months, there were no differences in height, weight, motor, or social skills between the neonatal groups.[31] Another's study involving PCOS women who conceived on metformin showed a lower rate of developing gestational diabetes later in pregnancy (3% metformin vs 31% no metformin).[32]

An Australian study (Metformin in Gestational diabetes—MiG study) conducted by Rowan and colleagues included 751 women (371 received metformin, and 378 received insulin) who were randomized between 20 and 33 weeks of pregnancy[33] (25). The metformin failure rate was 7.4% in which a second diabetic agent was needed to maintain controlled glucose levels. Although there was no difference in mean fasting blood glucose levels between groups, those on metformin had lower 2-hour postprandial glucose levels. There was no difference in the rate of pre-eclampsia. Infants of women randomized to metformin experienced a lower rate of hypoglycemia compared with insulin (insulin 8.1% vs metformin 3.3%, P = 0.008). There was no difference in any other perinatal outcome. The risk from metformin in pregnancy includes the potential for neonatal hypoglycemia. Metformin has been found to have a maternal-to-fetal transfer rate of 10–16%[34](26) Neonatal hypoglycemia is always a concern postnatally. In those, who did develop neonatal hypoglycemia, it was determined that this outcome was related to maternal hyperglycemia at the time of delivery[35]27. There were no cases of neonatal lactic acidosis.

Hypoglycemia related to metformin may occur in 0–21% of pregnant women[36] (28). The frequently observed gastrointestinal adverse effects include diarrhea, flatulence, nausea, and vomiting, with the incidence ranging from 2 to 63%[35] (27). These are the reasons why metformin is started at a low dose and increased gradually.

In breastfed infants whose mothers are on metformin, the mean infant exposure to drug is less than 1% of the weight-normalized maternal dose that is much below the 10% level of concern for breastfeeding[37] (29). Based on these findings, metformin use by breastfeeding mothers is considered to be absolutely safe.

Other OHA's

Drug	Status
Alpha-glucosidase inhibitor, thiazolidin-ediones, glinides, and glucagon-like DPP4 inhibitor agonists	Considered experimental during pregnancy
Alpha-glucosidase inhibitor (Acarbose)	– Delays the absorption of carbohydrate in the gut – Zarate has done a small study with 6 different pregnant women, showing efficacy of acarbose in blood sugar control without any complications. No systematic review available – Too early to comment on efficacy and safety of
Glitazones	– Cause of growth retardation and fetal death in animal – Not recommended in pregnancy
Glinides have	Not been approved for use in pregnancy
DPP4 inhibitors	Have not been approved for use in pregnancy

Although recent evidences show promising finding in safety and efficacy of some OHA's in treating pregnant diabetics, larger clinical studies will be needed to ensure safety and efficacy of these drugs in pregnancy. As of date no oral hypoglycemic agents have been endorsed for use in GDM by any decision making body for routine use.

Insulin

Regular and NPH (neutral protamine Hagedorn) insulin are routinely used in diabetic pregnancy with different regimens. McCance et al have demonstrated in a spin-off study that there is minimal and no increase in insulin antibodies during pregnancy for either insulin aspart or human long-acting insulin, and that there is no appreciable transplacental transfer of either insulins.[38]

Insulin antibodies are not associated with fetal birth weight. A similar low immunogenicity of insulin aspart as well as the comparator drug short-acting human insulin was observed in a small randomized trial in gestational diabetes by Pettitt et al.[39]

No randomized trials have been performed with insulin lispro or the newest one, insulin glulisine.

The long-acting analog insulins glargine and detemir are not registered for use in pregnancy. Presently glargine is classified as Pregnancy Category C according to the FDA.

At of now, the short-acting insulin analogs are the drugs of choice in pregnancy over human short-acting ones, with insulin aspart being the only one studied in a randomized trial. The situation is less-clear regarding the new long-acting insulin analogs glargine or detemir and new rapid acting analog glulisine.

Dosage: During pregnancy, the dose of insulin is adjusted to the glucose profile. The most efficient method to achieve optimal glycemic control is to mimic physiologic insulin levels through frequent administration. This entails intensive insulin treatment with delivery of basal, background insulin, and bolus insulin doses with each meal or large snack. Basal insulin is approximately 50% to 60% of the total daily insulin requirement; the remaining insulin would then be divided into injections of short-acting insulin is either administered as MDI injection therapy or subcutaneous insulin infusion with an externally worn pump (CSII). Target levels set by the American Diabetes Association are a fasting glucose level between 60 and 90 mg% and postprandial levels at 2 hour after beginning the meal between 100 and 120 mg%.[40] Insulin dose generally increases at mid-gestation and can increase even three to four times the preconceptional dose. After 32 weeks of pregnancy, some patients show a decrease in insulin requirement. This has no clinical meaning and does not indicate endangered fetoplacental unit.

At minimum, women with prepregnancy diabetes require three to four injections per day or the continuous insulin pump for optimal glucose control during pregnancy. Traditional types of insulin used for treatment of diabetes in pregnancy have been regular human and (NPH). Although these types of insulin have been widely used, their insulin profiles do not mimic the in vivo state as well as newer insulins and insulin analog. Use of the newer very-short-acting insulins, lispro and aspart, better mimic postprandial insulin secretion and thus return the glucose level to normal more quickly than the traditional short-acting regular insulin. Dosing regimens vary according to insulins used and delivery systems. NPH and regular insulin can be dosed in three injections per day. Two-thirds of the total daily dose is given in the morning in a ratio of 2:1 NPH to regular insulin. At supper, one-sixth of the total daily dose is given as regular insulin and one-sixth of the total daily dose is given at bedtime as NPH. Insulin lispro or aspart and NPH and can be administered in four injections per day. NPH is dosed as 2/3 of the total daily dose. Of the 2/3 daily dose of NPH, 2/3 is given in the morning, and 1/3 at bedtime.

Continuous Glucose Monitoring

Self-measurement of blood glucose levels (SMBG) by finger stick measurement is the mainstay of glucose monitoring. This technique has revolutionized self-management of patients during the 1980s but has some drawbacks. It gives, generally, a snapshot image of the glucose profile, is performed mostly six to eight times (all premeals, 2 h postmeals and 2 am) a day maximally is painful and can be logistically difficult. Kerssen et al have shown that at least 10 SMBG are necessary to obtain a reasonable idea of the profile.[41] Continuous glucose monitoring is a new technique, enabling to obtain a almost continuous glucose profile. With this technique, a needle impregnated with a glucose-dependent enzyme is inserted in the subcutis. The enzyme interacts with the glucose in the interstitial glucose, generating a current proportional to the glucose concentration. This current is translated to a glucose value every one to five minutes (depending on the device) that can be read at a later date after uploading this sensor device (off-line). Recently, the on-line sensor has been developed that provides direct reading of the actual glucose value. With real-time continuous glucose monitoring (RTCGM) alarm thresholds can be set for the device to alert the individual when glucose values fall outside these limits. Dynamic thresholds can also be set, alerting when change of glucose levels fall outside the pre-set range. There is little experience with continuous glucose monitoring in pregnancy with the exception of the study by Murphy et al.[42]

In this study, 71 patients with either type 1 or type 2 diabetes were randomized to off-line repetitive continuous glucose monitoring or standard care. Patients in the intervention group received extensive counseling; those in the control group did not, potentially introducing a bias increasing the contrast between the two groups. With repetitive offline continuous glucose monitoring, HbA1c initially fell comparable to the control group but, in contrast, did not increase in the third trimester as HbA1c did in the control group. The incidence of macrosomia was significantly lower with off-line continuous glucose monitoring: median birth weight centile 69 versus 93 (p = 0.02), macrosomia (> 90th percentile) 35 vs 60% p < 0.05).

Labor and Delivery

The practical endocrine aspects of labor and delivery are limited. In this context, it is wise to keep the maternal glucose level between 70–120 mg%. Neonatal hypoglycemia occurs more frequently with higher maternal levels. In practice, one can give a glucose 5% solution to the woman in labor to prevent maternal hypoglycemia (e.g., 500–1000 ml every 24 h) and either add a fixed amount of short-acting (human of analogue) insulin (8 U) to 500 mL of the intravenous solution, or, alternatively, measure glucose levels every hour or every two hours and increase glucose infusion with hypoglycemia or inject low dose short-acting analog) insulin with hyperglycemia (>140 mg%). After delivery, insulin requirement falls sharply and it is prudent to decrease the insulin dose to 25–40% of the pre-delivery dose to prevent hypoglycemia. This is the more important in women after a cesarean section that does not eat or are not allowed to eat for hours to days. Breastfeeding that should be stimulated as much as possible, does lead to even lower insulin requirements and insulin dose should be decreased further if necessary to prevent hypoglycemia. Hypoglycemia unawareness may occur in this setting. The period of acceptable lesser control may extend for a number of months. Insulin analogs can be safely used in lactation.[43]

KEY POINTS
- HbA1c is a reasonable parameter of glycemic control but does not capture the complexity of the glucose profile fully.
- Hypoglycemia is frequent in the preparation for and during pregnancy; repetitive hypoglycemia can induce reversible hypoglycemia unawareness.
- Analog short-acting insulin aspart and lispro are considered safe in pregnancy; no definite information is available on analog long-acting insulins.
- Continuous subcutaneous insulin infusion (CSII, insulin pump) is a good treatment option but adequate trials with adequate endpoints are lacking, making the decision in this option an individual one.
- The place of forms of continuous glucose monitoring techniques need to be established.

Fetal Monitoring

Fetal monitoring is essential in both GDM and pregestational diabetes. The frequency and type of testing depends upon the severity of glucose intolerance, associated medical complications, and patient compliance.

The ACOG recommends the need of antenatal fetal monitoring in patients with pregestational diabetes, gestational diabetes with poor glycemic control and patients with other obstetrical complications.[52]

Twice weekly NST should be started at a gestational age of 32 weeks. In patients with IUGR and pre-eclampsia, testing should be started at 28 weeks of gestation.

Gestational diabetics controlled on diet alone, can be managed by fetal kick counting only starting at 32 weeks POG. NST is optional and it can be started any time between 32 – 40 weeks of gestation. Patients on oral hypoglycemic drugs and/or insulin should be managed with twice-weekly biophysical profile from 32 weeks onwards. Presence of IUGR, pre-eclampsia and oligohydramnios necessitates starting these tests at 28 weeks POG.

Poor glycemic control in mother leads to fetal hyperglycemia, that stimulates fetal pancreas for increased insulin release. This leads to fetal macrosomia. Macrosomia is associated with antenatal and intrapartum complications. ACOG recommends elective cesarean section in patients with GDM and estimated fetal weight > 4500g.[52]

The USG is poor predictor of detecting fetal macrosomia and there is little data to support elective LSCS on basis of USG finding. To avoid the antenatal and intrapartum complications of fetal macrosomia, induction is advised at 38–38.5 weeks POG.

Prolongation of pregnancy beyond 38 weeks increases the risk of macrosomia without reducing the cesarean section rates. Therefore, it is advisable to induce the patients with diabetes at 38 completed weeks POG.[53]

Patients controlled on diet only with no other complication can be managed by expectant management until term.

Puerperal and Neonatal Care

Irrespective of the women being a pregestational diabetic or gestational diabetic, appropriate puerperal and neonatal care is mandatory. It should be designed to tackle both, the immediate consequences and the long-term effects of the diabetic state. Following delivery, the insulin sensitivity returns to the normal state within

Method	Analysis
Fetal kick counting	Perception and counting of the fetal movements is the simplest, subjective, and least expensive method for monitoring fetal well being in second half of pregnancy. It is said to correlate directly with the ultrasonographic confirmation of fetal movements. The "count 10 method' is the most commonly used one. Patient is instructed to lie on her lateral (preferably left) side and is advised to concentrate on fetal movements. Perception of ten movements in 2 h is reassuring. Borderline variations in maternal blood glucose levels do not affect the fetal gross body movements, breathing, heart rate, and Doppler velocimetry.
Fetal non stress test (NST)	NST is started at the gestational age of 32 weeks in diabetic women and done on a twice weekly basis. It should be started at 28 weeks in patients with hypertension, renal disease and IUGR. The negative predictive value of NST is 90%, but the positive predictive value varies from 50–70%. False positive rate of NST varies from 45–70% thus increasing the possibility of unnecessary and sometimes preterm delivery of a normal fetus. The test can better rule out rather than predicting fetal compromise.
Biophysical profile	Biophysical profile helps in prediction of acute and chronic tissue hypoxia. The parameters of Biophysical profile (BPP) include NST, fetal gross body movements, fetal tone, breathing movements, and amniotic fluid index detected on ultrasound. Amniotic fluid volume indicates the chronic fetal perfusion and oligohydramnios in absence of any other cause is indicator of chronic fetal hypoxia. Each parameter of BPP is given score of 0 or 2 depending upon the finding. The term "modified BPP" is used when only NST and amniotic fluid volume are done. Sometimes NST is omitted and score of 8 is considered as normal. Twice weekly NST and amniotic fluid index assessment can be used to prevent stillbirth in diabetic pregnancy.[44] In a study of 15,482 women who were identified as high risk were monitored by antenatal tests. The false negative rate of modified BPP (NST and Amniotic fluid index) was 0.8/1000. Sixty percent of patients delivered because of abnormal test had no evidence of short or long-term fetal compromise. The false negative rate of modified BPP was lower than non stress test and was comparable with false negative rate of complete BPP and Contraction Stress test.[45] Johnson and Lange[46] reported on the use of twice-weekly BPP in 50 insulin-dependent and 188 gestational diabetic pregnancies. No stillbirths were reported; abnormal BPP rate was only 3.3%, and of the eight women whose last BPP was abnormal, three had significant neonatal morbidity. Thus, the BPP used twice weekly appears to be an adequate test with few unnecessary interventions.
Ultrasonography	Ultrasonography is an important component of antenatal fetal monitoring in patients with gestational diabetes and pregestational diabetes. Women with uncontrolled pregestational diabetes have 4–8 times more risk of major congenital anomalies in the fetus.[47] A detailed level II scan in second trimester is essential to rule out congenital anomalies in the fetus. Most commonly involved systems are cardiovascular and central nervous systems. Fetal echo is also recommended in all patients with pregestational diabetes or GDM diagnosed in first trimester. In the third trimester too, ultrasonography plays an important role for assessment for fetal growth and well-being. The main drawback of ultrasonography is the limited sensitivity to

Contd...

Contd...

Method	Analysis
	detect macrosomia. The sensitivity of ultrasonography for weight estimation in third trimester varies from 24–97% and specificity varies form 82–98%.[48] Another method to predict weight in a macrosomic baby is serial abdominal circumference estimation.[49] Miller et al introduced another formula to detect fetal macrosomia. The difference between fetal abdominal circumference and biparietal diameter is calculated, if it is ≥ 2.6 cm is diagnostic of macrosomia.[50] Macrosomia occurs in 88% of pregnancies if estimated fetal weight and abdominal circumference both exceed 90th percentile.[51] USG also helps in amniotic fluid assessment and dynamic fetal assessment by biophysical profile and Doppler studies. Intrauterine growth retardation (IUGR, fetal weight less than 10th percentile) is also seen in patients with advanced pregestational diabetes with vascular complications.
Contraction stress test	This test has been used for a long time to detect fetal distress. As the test evaluates the fetal heart response to uterine contractions, it can also diagnose a chronic condition and placental perfusion. The test is performed weekly and has high negative predictive value. There are some limitations of the test. The false positive rate of test is 50–60%. It results in unnecessary preterm delivery of a normal fetus. Overall, the test is more expensive, less convenient, and less efficient than NST. So it is not used widely, these days for fetal surveillance.
Doppler velocimetry	Doppler studies are important, especially in patients with pregestational diabetes. These patients develop vascular complications because of long standing diabetes. They are more prone to develop intrauterine growth restriction, pre-eclampsia, and further decreased placental perfusion. Doppler changes are calculated in terms of increased systolic diastolic ratio (S/D ratio). With increasing fetal compromise, there occurs increased S/D ratio, absent diastolic flow and ultimately reversal of diastolic flow. Absent end diastolic flow necessitates daily Doppler, anytime reversal of diastolic flow indicates the need of immediate termination of pregnancy.

minutes in women with gestational diabetes. Blood glucose monitoring of the baby should be commenced, using accurate method, at 2–4 hours after birth. If the woman was only on diet control, random blood glucose is tested the day after the birth and four blood glucose levels (fasting and 2 hours postmeals for three meals) done one day prior to discharge. I`the levels are within the normal range, blood glucose monitoring is not required further. The patient is advised regarding the diet and lifestyle modification factors (planned physical activity, weight control, smoking cessation) and called for review after 6 weeks following delivery.

At 6 weeks postpartum, glucose metabolism in women who have been diagnosed with GDM may return to normal, or there may be ongoing impaired glucose regulation (IGT or impaired fasting glycemia) or frank diabetes (including pre-existing type 1 or type 2 diabetes that was unrecognized before pregnancy).[1] Medical nutrition therapy (MNT) and, if necessary, pharmacological therapy should be continued to maintain good glycemic control and provide sufficient calories for lactation and infant well being.

According to ADA 2011, screening for diabetes should be done at 6–12 weeks postpartum according to the OGTT criteria for non-pregnant women using a two-hour 75-gram oral glucose tolerance test. Because women with GDM are at a considerably increased risk of developing diabetes later, lifelong screening for diabetes should be performed at least every 3 years. At the time of this review, the ADA has endorsed the use of the hemoglobin A1c as a diabetes screen, and no studies have examined its diagnostic properties compared with other glucose screens in the postpartum GDM population. The longer-term risks for babies born to mothers with GDM include a doubling of the risk of developing childhood obesity and an increased risk of the child developing T2DM in adult life.

Postpartum management should focus on both shorts and long-term goals: Maternal-infant well being, healthy nutrition, breastfeeding, provision of appropriate contraception, and need for preconception care in future pregnancy.

Prevention and Assessment of Neonatal Hypoglycemia

Clinical hypoglycemia in the newborn is a complication of GDM, but in studies that enroll participants, closer monitoring than in general settings leads to relatively infrequent incidence of hypoglycemia.

In HAPO,[54] only (2.1%) infants had clinical hypoglycemia. In ACHOIS,[55] the prevalence of clinical hypoglycemia was 7% in GDM receiving intervention and 5% in GDM not receiving intervention, a non-significant difference.

Glycemia monitoring is recommended for newborns of mothers with GDM treated with insulin or in whom the birth weight is < 10th or > 90th percentile. In the absence of clinical signs, glycemia monitoring must start only after the first feed or just before the second. The presence of clinical signs indicates that glycemia monitoring should be started earlier.

Blood glucose monitoring should be commenced, using accurate method, at 2–4 hours after birth.[4]Observational data indicate that testing blood glucose within the first 2 h of life is very likely to yield low values. It is recommended that hypoglycemia readings identified with glucose test strips be confirmed by laboratory measurement.[56]

Assessment of Other Complications

The newborn should receive the usual monitoring for neonatal jaundice. Complete blood count for polycythemia is indicated according to the clinical signs. Blood tests for hypocalcemia and hypomagnesemia should be carried out for babies with clinical signs.

Babies of women with diabetes should have an echocardiogram performed if they show clinical signs associated with congenital heart disease or cardiomyopathy, including heart murmur.

Breastfeeding

All women, including those with prior GDM, should be actively encouraged to exclusively breastfeed to the greatest extent possible during the first year of the infant.

Apart from all the potential benefits of breastfeeding, benefits particularly related to women with GDM/PGDM are that it encourages weight loss, is associated with better glucose tolerance and reduced incidence of future metabolic syndrome.[57,58]

Breastfeeding is associated with a lower risk of overweight and obesity during childhood and adolescence in the general population, but whether breastfeeding has the same protective effects among women with GDM has not been studied.[59]

Breastfeeding has been suggested to reduce the incidence of T2DM, the metabolic syndrome and cardiovascular disease. It appears to reduce the risk of premenopausal breast cancer and ovarian cancer.[60]

Contraception or Pregnancy Planning

Contraceptive options should be tailored to individual lifestyle and preference. The NICE postnatal care guideline[37] recommends that contraception should be discussed within the first week of birth.[61]

Barrier Methods

Barrier methods are well-suited for women with prior GDM because of their lack of systemic side effects or influence on glucose tolerance. Use of condoms should be encouraged in all women who appear at risk for sexually transmitted diseases and human immunodeficiency virus.

The Intrauterine Device

The 2009 WHO Medical Eligibility Criteria for Contraceptive Use does not consider prior GDM/PGDM as a contraindication to IUD prescription. Both copper and LNG-IUDs can be used safely and without any specific restrictions in women with a history of GDM and may be continued if they develop diabetes.

Limited evidence on the use of the LNG-IUD among women with insulin- or non-insulin-dependent diabetes suggests that these methods have little effect on short-term or long-term diabetes control (e.g. HbA1c levels), hemostatic markers or lipid profile.

Hormonal Contraceptives

Hormones have been reported to influence glucose and fat metabolism andcoagulation.

Combination Oral Contraceptives

Existing evidence supports the prescription of low-dose combination oral Contraceptions (COCs) in women with a history of GDM, containing the lowest dose of ethinyl estradiol and the lowest dose/potency progestin. When coexisting hypertension or other cardiovascular risk factors are present, non-estrogen method of contraception should be considered. It is to be avoided in diabetic women who smoke, are older (> 35 years), or have hypertension or diabetes-related vascular complications.

Short-term controlled trials failed to demonstrate any decrease in glucose tolerance or adverse effects on lipid metabolism but found a slight decrease in insulin sensitivity that do not lead to development of diabetes.

Progesterone only Oral Contraceptives (POCs)

Progestins do not increase coagulation factors or BP. Their shortcomings are irregular bleeding and the need to be taken daily at strict time intervals. They are well suited for women with T1 DM where estrogen-containing methods are contraindicated and for women with prior GDM, who have several cardiovascular risk factors.[62]

In the Latino population of breastfeeding women, the use of POC's (e.g. 0.35 mg/day norethindrone) and long-acting injectable depot medroxyprogesterone acetate (150 mg every 3 months) was associated with a two- to threefold increase in diabetes risk. DMPA should be used with caution in breastfeeding women and those with elevated triglyceride levels (>150 mg/dL). Close attention should be paid to weight gain, that also has been demonstrated to increase the risk of subsequent diabetes. The WHO, however, feels that the limited evidence is inconsistent regarding the development of non-insulin-dependent diabetes among users of POCs with a history of gestational diabetes. History of GDM is Category 1 (WHO) for POC use.

Progestin-only pills may be used in nonlactating women, especially when contraindications for oral contraceptive use (e.g. hypertension) are present.

Implanon is also a Suitable Contraceptive Option for Diabetic Women

Only few studies have focused specifically on women with a history of GDM; they have not demonstrated significant glucose metabolism impairment with hormonal contraception, whether combined oral or progestogen only. The presence of obesity, hypertension, or dyslipidemia should steer the selection towards a contraception method without cardiovascular effects. In these situations, the intrauterine device (IUD) is the recommended method.[63]

According to the Cochrane review (2009), until properly designed trials showing no influence of hormonal contraceptives have been conducted.

The Cu-IUD appears to be the safest choice of contraceptive in patients with DM. LNG-IUD might be safe to use as well, since no effects on glucose or lipid metabolism were observed.[64]

Lastly, operative sterilization is an excellent choice for women who have decided that they no longer are interested in childbearing. This option should be offered to parous women, especially those delivering by cesarean section, where the sterilization can be performed during the surgical procedure.

Long-term Risks for Baby

The longer-term risks for babies born to mothers with GDM include a doubling of the risk of developing childhood obesity and an increased risk of the child developing T2DM in adult life. Genetic predisposition for type 2 DM and obesity may also be inherited from one or both parents by offspring of GDM mothers.

There is also evidence that the children of mothers with GDM have a worse attention span, perform less well in tests of motor function and have increased risk of language impairment. The extent to which strict control of maternal GDM or postnatal modification in diet, such as breastfeeding or bottle-feeding modifies childhood risks is unknown.

A study has found that children of GDM mothers who were breastfed for >3 months had a 45% decrease in rates of being overweight (BMI > 90th percentile) at 2–8 years compared with those who were bottle-fed.[65]

Diabetes Prevention

The diagnosis of GDM identifies women at high risk for diabetes. While the risk of recurrence of GDM varies from 30% to 84%, published studies show that 35–60% of these women develop T2DM within 10 years. Thus, accurate diagnosis of glucose abnormalities permits the initiation of strategies for primary prevention of diabetes, a primary goal of follow-up care.

Factors associated with a higher risk of T2D following gestational diabetes:
- Overweight (Waist circumference and BMI are the strongest anthropometric measures associated with development of type 2 diabetes in women with GDM)
- Diagnosis of GDM prior to 24 weeks gestation
- High glucose values in diagnostic OGTT
- The requirement for insulin
- Neonatal hypoglycemia, and GDM in more than one pregnancy
- HDL cholesterol < 50 mg/dL and age > 35 years have been identified as predictors.[66] The risk for the occurrence of the metabolic syndrome increases by 2 to 5-fold and that of cardiovascular disorders, by around 1.7-fold.

Cases of decreased gestational glucose tolerance during pregnancy (not amounting as GDM) are at an increased risk of developing T2DM by a factor of 2 to 3.[67]

The progression of IGT to T2D following GDM can be prevented/delayed by lifestyle changes and use of metformin or thiazolidinediones (troglitazone and pioglitazone). Currently, however, medications are not recommended for the prevention of diabetes amongst women with recent GDM. The use of Troglitazone in Prevention of Diabetes Study found that randomization to a thiazolidinedione was associated with a decreased risk of diabetes among women with recent GDM, but the trial was discontinued because the side effects of troglitazone, and the drug was subsequently withdrawn from the market.

Metformin may offer a reasonable alternative for women with histories of GDM who have impaired glucose tolerance and who are overweight.

Cardiovascular Disease Risk Factor Assessment

A history of GDM increases the subsequent risk of cardiovascular problems 1.7-fold. A history of moderate hyperglycemia during pregnancy increases cardiovascular risk by 1.2-fold.[68]

It has been observed that a substantial number of women with prior GDM share many characteristics with subjects that have the metabolic syndrome (e.g., glucose intolerance, insulin resistance, central obesity, elevated triglycerides, and low HDL cholesterol) and inflammatory markers (e.g. high-sensitivity C-reactive proteinhs (CRP) and interleukin-6).

As specific strategies for women with GDM have not been established, standards creening guidelines for CVD risk factor assessment should be followed at the times that glucose metabolism is evaluated.[69]

Several studies on lipids in women with previous GDM, show in Asia, total cholesterol, LDL cholesterol, and triglycerides were significantly higher, and HDL cholesterol was significantly lower in women with prior GDM versus control subjects after adjustment for age, BMI, and smoking. On the other hand, standard lipoprotein concentrations were not different in women with prior GDM compared with controls.[24]

Lifestyle Modification

Majority of women with histories of GDM are overweight or obese, have sedentary lifestyles, and consume few vegetables and fruits. In contrast, weight targets of < 25 kg/m², physical activity of ≥ 2.5 hours/week of moderate aerobic activity or 75 minutes/week of vigorous intensity aerobic activity or an equivalent,[70] along with consumption of five or more servings of fruits and vegetables per day, are recommended.[71] Similarly, in the immediate postpartum period,caloric restriction as well as physical activity is mandatory to reduce/maintain standard weight.

Women with diabetes should be reminded of the importance of contraception and the need for pre-conception care when planning future pregnancies. Those with prior GDM should be educated about the chances of recurrence (30–84%) of GDM in next pregnancy.

References

1. Witkop CT, Neale D, Wilson LM, Bass EB, Nicholson WK. Active compared with expectant delivery management in women with gestational diabetes: a systematic review. Obstet Gynecol. 2009;113(1):206–17.
2. Metzger BE. Proceedings of the third international workshop-conference on gestational diabetes mellitus. Diabetes. 1991;40:1–201.
3. Seshiah V. Handbook on Diabetes Mellitus. Diabetes and Pregnancy. New Delhi and Chennai, All India Publishers and Distributors. 2009;281.
4. Beischer NA, Oats, JN, Henry OA, Sheedy MT, Walstab JE, Incidence and severity of gestational diabetes mellitus according to country of birth in women living in Austraila. Diabetes. 1991;40Suppl2:35–8.
5. Seshiah V. Handbook on Diabetes Mellitus. Diabetes and Pregnancy. New Delhi and Chennai, All India Publishers and Distributors. 2009;281.
6. Ronald Kahn C, Gordon C Weir, George L King, Alan M Jacobson, Alan C Moses, Robert J Smith. Diabetes Mellitus. Fourteenth edition. Lippincott Williams and Wilkins. 2005;1042.
7. Derek Le Roith, Simeon I Taylor, Jerrold M Olefsky. Diabetes Mellitus: A Fundamental and clinical text. Lippincott Williams and Wilkins. 2000;884.
8. Venkataraman S, Seshiah V, Manjula N, et al. The need to revise O' Sullivan and Mahan's criteria for gestational diabetes mellitus. International J Diab Dev. Countries. 1991;11:5–6.

9. O' Sullivan JB, Mahan CM. Criteria for the oral glucose test in pregnancy. Diabetes. 1964;13:278–84.

10. National Diabetes Data Group. Classification and diagnosis of diabetes mellitus and other categories of glucose intolerance. Diabetes. 1979;18:1039–57.

11. Metzger BD, Bybee DE, Freinkel M. Gestational diabetes mellitus: Correlations between the phenotypic and genotypic characteristics of the mother and abnormal glucose tolerance during first year postpartum. Diabetes. 1985;34:111–5.

12. Swinn RA, Wareham NJ, Gregory R, et al. Excessive secretion of insulin precursors characterizes and predicts gestational diabetes. Diabetes. 1995;44:911–5.

13. Alberti K, Zimmett P. WHO consultation, Definition, diagnosis and classification of diabetes mellitus and its complications. Diabetes Med. 1998;15:539–53.

14. Carpenter MW, Coustan DR. Criteria for screening tests for gestational diabetes. Am J Obstet Gynecol. 1982;638–41.

15. Oded Langer. The Diabetes in pregnancy Dilemma. British Library Cataloging in Publication. 2006;453–4.

16. HAPO Study Cooperative Research Group. The hyperglycemia and adverse pregnancy outcome study. Int J Gynecol Obstet. 2002;78:69.

17. HAPO Study Cooperative Research Group. Hyperglycemia and adverse pregnancy outcome. The New England J of Medicine. 2008;358:1991–2000.

18. Metzger BE, Gabbe SG, Persson B, et al. International association of diabetes and pregnancy study groups recommendations on the diagnosis and classification of hyperglycemia in pregnancy. Diabetes Care. 2010;33:676–82.

19. Norman RJ, Wang JX, Hague W. Should we continue or stop insulin sensitizing drugs during pregnancy? Curr Opin Obstet Gynecol. 2004;16:245–50.

20. Anjalakishi C, Balaji V, Balaji MS, Seshiah V, A prospective study comparing insulin and glibenclamide in gestational diabetes mellitus in Asian Indian women. Diabetes Res Clin Paract. 2007;76:474–5.

21. Elliott BD, Langer O, Schenker S, Johnson RF. Insignificant transfer of glyburide occurs across the human placenta. AM J Obster Gynecol. 1991;165:807–12.

22. Elliott BD, Schenker S, Langer O, Johnson R, Prihoda T. Comparative placental transport of oral hypoglycemic agents in humans: A model of human placental drug transfer. AM J Obstet Gynecol. 1994;171:653–60.

23. Garcia-Bournissen F, Feg DS, Koren G. Maternal-fetal transport of hypoglycaemic drugs. Clin Pharmacokinet. 2003;42:303–13.

24. Lim JM, Tayob Y, O Brien PM, Shaw RW. A comparison between the pregnancy outcome of women with gestation diabetes treated with glibenclamide and those treated with insulin. Med J Malaysia. 1997;52:377–81.

25. Langer O, Conway DL, Berkus MD, Xenakis EM, Gonzales O, A comparison of glyburide and insuin in women with gestational diabetes mellitus. N Engl J Med, 2000;343:1134–8.

26. Nicholson W, Bolen S, Witkop CT, Neale D, Wilson L, Bass E. Benefits and risks of oral diabetes agents compared with insulin in women with gestational diabetes: A Systematic review. Obstet Gynecol. 2009;113:193–205.

27. Dhulkotia JS, Ola B, Fraser R, Farrell T. Oral hypoglycemic agents vs insulin in management of gestational diabetes: A systematic review and metaanalysis. AM J Obstet Gynecol. 2010;203:457,e1–9.

28. Conway D, Gonzales O, Skiver D. Use of glyburide for the treatment of gestational diabetes : The San Antonio experience. Obstet Gynecol Surv. 2004;59:491–3.

29. Cotezee EJ, Jackson WP. Oral hypoglycaemics in the first trimester and fetal outcome. S afr Med J. 1984;65:635–7.

30. Hellmuth E, Dammn P, Molsted-Pedersen L. Oral Hypoglycaemic agents in 118 diabetic pregnancies. Diabe Med. 2000;17:507–11.

31. Glueck CJ, Bornovali S, Pranikoff J, Goldenberg N, Dharashivkar S, Wang P. Metformin, preeclampsia, and pregnancy outcomes in women with polycystic ovary syndrome. Diabet Med. 2004;21:829–36.

32. Glueck CJ, Wang P, Kobayashi S, Phillips H, Sieve-Smith L. Metformin therapy throughout pregnancy reduces the development of gestational diabetes in women with polycystic ovary syndrome. Fertil Steril. 2002;77:520–5.

33. Rowan JA, Hague WM, Gao W, Battin MR, Moore MP; MiG Trial Investigatiors. Metformin versus insulin for the treatment of gestational diabetes. N Engl J Med. 2008;358:2003–15.

34. Nanovskaya TN, N, Nekhayeva IA, Patrikeeva SL, Hankins GD, Ahmed MS. Transfer of metformin across the dually perfused human placental lobule. AM J Obstet Gynecol. 2006;195:1081–5.

35. Glueck CJ, Goldenberg N, Streicher P, Wang P. Metformin and gestatonal diabetes. Curr Diab Rep. 2003;3-303–12.

36. Bolen S, Feldman L, Vassy J, Wilson L, Yeh HC, Marinopoulos S, et al. Systematic review. Comparative effectiveness and safety of oral medications for type 2 diabetes mellitus. Ann Intern Med. 2007;147:386–99.

37. Asche CV, McAdam-Marx C, Shane-McWhorter L, Sheng X, Plauschinant CA, Association between oral antidiabetic use, adverse events and outcomes in patients with type 2 diabetes. Diabetes Obes Metab. 2008;10-638–45.

38. McCance DR, Damm P, Mathiesen ER et al. Evaluation of insulin antibodies and placental transfer of insulin aspart in pregnant women with type 1 diabetes mellitus. Diabetologia. 2008;51:2141–3.

39. Pettitt D, Ospina P, Howard C et al. Efficacy, safety and lack of immunogenicity of insulin apsart versus regular insulin for women with gestational diabetes. Diabet Med. 2007;24:1129–35.

40. Kitzmiller JL, Block JM, Catalano FM, et al. Managing pre-existing diabetes for pregnancy. Diabetes Care. 2008;31:1060–79.

41. Kerssen A, de Valk HW, Visser GHA. Do HbA1c levels and the self monitoring of glucose levels adequately reflect glycaemic control during pregnancy in women with type 1 diabetes? Diabetologia 2006;49:25–8.

42. Murphy HR, Rayman G, Lewis K et al. Effectiveness of continuous glucose monitoring in pregnant women with diabetes: randomised clinical trial. BMJ. 2008;337:a1680. doi:10.1136/bmj.a1680

43. Harold W de Valk, Gerard HA Visser. Insulin during pregnancy, labour and delivery. Best Practice and Research Clinical Obstetrics and Gynaecology. 25 (2011)65–76.

44. Kjos SL, Leung A, Henry OA, Victor MR, Paul RH, Medearis AL. Antepartum surveillance in diabetic pregnancies: predictors of fetal distress in labor. Am J Obstet Gynecol. 1995;173:1532–9.

45. Miller DA, Rabello YA, Paul RH. The modified biophysical profile: antepartum testing in the 1990. Am J Obstet Gynecol. 1996;174(3):812–7.

46. Johnson JM, Lange IR: Biophysical profile scoring in the management of the diabetic pregnancy. Obstet Gynecol. 1988;72:841–5.

47. Reece EA, Sivan E, Francis G, Homko CJ. Pregnancy outcomes among women with and without diabetic microvascular disease versus non-diabetic controls. Am J Perinatol. 1998;15:549.

48. O'Reilly-Green C, Divon MY. Sonographic and clinical diagnosis of macrosomia. Clin Obstet Gynecol. 2000;43:309–315.

49. Jazayeri A, Heffron JA, Phillips R, Spellacy WN. Macrosomia prediction using ultrasound fetal abdominal circumference of 35 cm or more. Obstet Gynecol. 1999;93:523–6.

50. Miller RF, Johnson EB, Devine P. Sonographic "fetal symmetry" predicts shoulder dystocia. Am J Obstet Gynecol. 2007;193:S45.

51. Ben-Haroush A, Yogev Y, Rosenn B, Hod M, Langer O. The postprandial glucose profile in the diabetic pregnancy. Am J Obstet Gynecol. 2004;191:576.

52. Gestational Diabetes. ACOG Pract Bull No. 30. American College of Obstetricians and Gynecologists. Obstet Gynecol. 2001;98:525–38.

53. American Diabetes Association: Gestational diabetes mellitus. Diabetes Care. 2004; 27(Suppl 1):S88–S90.

54. HAPO Study Cooperative Research Group. Hyperglycemia and adverse pregnancy outcomes.N Engl J Med. 2008;358(19):1991–2002.

55. Crowther C, Hiller J, Moss J, et al. Effect of treatment of gestational diabetes mellitus on pregnancy outcomes. N Engl J Med. 2005;352(24):2477–86.

56. Whitelaw B, Gayle C. Gestational diabetes Obstetrics, Gynaecology and Reproductive Medicine. 2010;21:2–41.

57. Nelson A. Intermediate-term glucose tolerance in women with a history of gestational diabetes: Natural history and potential associations with breastfeeding and contraception. Am J Obstet Gynecol. 2008;198(6):699 e1–e7.

58. Gunderson E, et al. Duration of lactation and incidence of the metabolic syndrome in women of reproductive age according to gestational diabetes mellitus status: A 20-year prospective study in CARDIA (Coronary Artery Risk Development in Young Adults). Diabetes Care. 2010;59(2):495–504.

59. Steube A. Breastfeeding and diabetes – benefits and special needs. Diabetes Voice. 2007;52(1):26–9.

60. Ferrara A, Ehrlich SF. Strategies for diabetes prevention before and after pregnancy in women with GDM.Curr Diabetes Rev. 2011 Mar;7(2):75–83.

61. Nice clinical guideline 37. Routine postnatal care of women and their babies July 2006.

62. Kjos SL. Optimal contraception for the diabetic woman. In: Textbook of Diabetes and Pregnancy. Hod M. 2003;589–96.

63. Summary of expert consensus : Diabetes and Metabolism. 2010;36:695–9.

64. Visser J, Snel M, Van Vliet HAAM. Hormonal versus non-hormonal contraceptives in women with diabetes mellitus type 1 and 2. Cochrane Database of Systematic Reviews 2006, Issue 4. Art. No.: CD003990. DOI: 10.1002/14651858.CD003990.pub3.

65. Schaefer-Graf UM: Association of breast-feeding and early childhood overweight in children from mothers with gestational diabetes. Diabetes Care. 2006;29:1105–7.

66. Gobl CS, Bozkurt L, Prikoszovich T, Winzer C, et al. Early possible risk factors for overt diabetes after gestational diabetes mellitus. Obstet Gynecol. 2011;118:71–8.

67. Verier-Mine O. Outcomes in women with a history of gestational diabetes.

68. Screening and prevention of type 2 diabetes. Literature review. Diabetes& Metabolism. 2010;36:595–616.

69. ACOG Committee on Obstetric Practice. Postpartum screening for abnormal glucose tolerance in women who had gestational diabetes mellitus. Obstet Gynecol. 2009;113(6):1419–21.

70. Division of Nutrition PA, and Obesity, Centers for Disease Control and Prevention. 2008 Physical Activity Guidelines for Healthy Pregnant or Postpartum Women. 2008. Available from: ://www.cdc gov/physicalactivity/everyone/guidelines/pregnancy. html. Accessed 2010.

71. Kieffer E. Health behaviors in women with a history of gestational diabetes mellitus in the Behavioral Risk Factor Surveillance System. Diabetes Care. 2006;29(8):1788–93.

Tuberculosis in Pregnancy

Rucha S Dagaonkar, Zarir Udwadia

Tuberculosis, that 'Captain of all men of death' (John Bunyon) has never known barriers of caste or class. Some of the famous women struck with 'consumption' include Kamala Nehru, Dr Anandibai Joshi, Eleanor Roosevelt, and the Bronte sisters, to name a few. Today tuberculosis is a leading cause of maternal mortality in the BRIC (Brazil, Russia, India and China) countries and in Sub-Saharan Africa. Although tuberculosis continues to have a major impact in the developing world, in the developed world it remains an important concern in view of HIV infection, immigration and the emergence of an aging population with its attendant non-communicable diseases. These last have been recognized as risk factors for the development of TB disease.

Epidemiology in the Female Population[1-3]

Tuberculosis (TB) is among the three leading causes of death in women in the reproductive age group, with 320,000 women dying from TB in 2010. More women of child-bearing age are killed by TB than all causes of maternal mortality combined. TB-infected women in the reproductive age group are also more susceptible to the development of active disease as compared to men of the same age group. TB has been linked to about a fourth of HIV-related deaths in women. The disease also has a considerable sociocultural impact that contributes to delay in diagnosis, inadequate treatment and even abandonment of the patient by her family.

TB infection and TB Disease in Pregnancy

About 30% of immunocompetent adults develop TB-infection after exposure, and they have a 10% lifetime risk of development of active TB. Patients with HIV infection have a 70% chance of acquiring TB infection upon exposure to the bacillus and furthermore, have a 10% annual risk of the development of active TB disease.[4] The classical environmental factors found to increase chances of TB infection include: overcrowding, poor ventilation, poor nutrition, and repeated close contact with an infective patient. Homelessness, alcoholism, immunosuppression (pathological and iatrogenic) and presence of certain non-communicable diseases (diabetes mellitus, metabolic syndrome, and tobacco-dependence) have also been associated with an increased risk of TB infection and disease.[5]

The exact predisposition produced by pregnancy towards the development of TB infection and TB disease, is not known. However, in a study of 286 patients in Tanzania,[6] it was found that the prevalence of latent tuberculosis infection (LTBI) was higher in pregnant women than in the general population. This suggests an increased risk of TB infection during pregnancy.

A British study[7] that included nationwide pregnancy data spanning over 12 years has found that the crude TB rate for (pregnancy and postpartum) was 15.4 per 100,000 person-years, and for non-pregnant patients, was 9.1 per 100,000 person-years, which was a significant difference. Interestingly, the postpartum TB risk was significantly higher than outside pregnancy. But the risk during pregnancy was not increased as compared to TB risk outside pregnancy.

Factors Predisposing to Development of Active TB

The HIV co-infection is the most potent factor for development of active TB. In a recent study[9] from Kwa-Zulu, Natal it has been found that TB-HIV coinfected pregnant women are 32 times more likely to die than are those without HIV infection.

Non-communicable diseases[5] have also been found to contribute to the development of active TB. Diabetes mellitus increases the relative risk of TB to 3.3, possibly because of adverse effects on cell-mediated immunity. Delayed sputum-culture conversion has also been observed in diabetics with TB and postulated to be a factor in the development of drug-resistance.

Alcohol consumption of > 40 day has been found to confer three-fold increased risk for development of TB, and also reduced adherence to treatment, which may contribute to development of drug resistance. Tobacco smoking also increases the risk of TB 2 to 3 times.

Etiology

The causative agent 10–13 of tuberculosis is the bacillus *Mycobacterium tuberculosis* (genus *Mycobacterium*, family *Mycobacteriaceae*, order *Actinomycetales*). The TB bacilli are slender rod-shaped organisms that are non-sporing and non-motile, and not encapsulated. They resist decolorization with both sulfuric acid and absolute alcohol. Hence, they are known as acid and alcohol fast bacilli (AAFB) or as acid fast bacilli (AFB).

The most common mode of development of TB-infection is through inhalation of the bacilli in the form of droplet nuclei exhaled by infective patients. Other modes of infection such as direct inoculation of infective secretions into the skin are also known to occur.

Pathology

After inhalation of infective droplet nuclei, TB infection leads to formation of the 'primary complex' in the lungs that includes the site of infection (primary focus) and the draining lymph nodes. This is known as the 'Ghon's complex'. Upon inhalation, the bacilli are engulfed by the alveolar macrophages wherein they are either killed or they remain dormant. Dormant bacilli are cordoned within granulomas formed by epithelioid giant cells. The bacilli that cannot be thus contained cause a bacillemia and reach the draining lymph nodes. Here, further granuloma formation occurs. Thus, the pulmonary parenchymal site of infection and the draining lymph nodes together form the Ghon's complex. Extra-pulmonary sites get seeded with TB bacteria at the time of the bacillemia. Primary pulmonary tuberculosis commonly occurs in childhood, and the infection is generally well-contained within the primary complex.

Genital infection occurs via the hematogenous route. Endometrial TB is a common cause of infertility. If pregnancy occurs, then endometrial TB is also a cause of congenital tuberculosis via the transplacental route. Tuberculosis has not been found to cause reduced placental blood flow during pregnancy.[14]

Caseating epithelioid cell granulomas are the pathological hallmark of TB and these granulomas may also show AFB.

Clinical Features

The cardinal symptoms of pulmonary tuberculosis include: cough, sputum production, fever, and weight loss. Programmatic guidelines say that any patient with cough lasting for two weeks or more should be investigated for the possibility of tuberculosis.

Tuberculosis can present with virtually any set of clinical features. Important among these are the syndrome of 'pyrexia of unknown origin', fever and vomiting in a patient of TB-meningitis, chronic lower backache in the patient with TB-spine and hypoxia in the patient with miliary tuberculosis.

Clinical Features in the Pregnant Patient

Pulmonary tuberculosis (PTB) is a very common clinical presentation of tuberculosis in pregnancy, although the disease can frequently be extra-pulmonary.[8] The symptoms include cough, usually of greater than two weeks' duration, associated with expectoration. Hemoptysis may be present. There may be associated low grade fever with an evening rise in temperature. Weight loss caused by TB may be masked because of the weight gain seen in normal pregnancy. Hence, lack of expected weight gain should be looked out for.

Dyspnea, another feature of normal pregnancy may also be seen in PTB, as also in miliary tuberculosis and with tuberculous pleural effusions.

Lower backache associated with constitutional symptoms may be seen in TB of the spine.

Vomiting, which may occur as a part of normal pregnancy, usually subsides by the end of the first trimester. However, projectile vomiting in the setting of fever, loss of appetite, weight loss and neck stiffness should raise the suspicion of TB meningitis. A case of meningeal TB during early pregnancy, misdiagnosed as hyperemesis gravidarum has been reported.[15]

Abdominal pain is an obvious cause of concern in the pregnant patient. The symptoms of abdominal tuberculosis include abdominal pain, loss of appetite and fever. Intestinal obstruction may occur. Tuberculous peritonitis though rarely reported, has been known to occur during pregnancy.[16]

Tuberculosis is also associated with a broad spectrum of hematological manifestations. Important among these is anemia of chronic disease. This may add to the nutritional anemia seen in pregnancy, and contribute to such symptoms as fatigue, breathlessness and tachycardia, which may be mistakenly attributed to those produced by pregnancy. Thrombocytopenia may be seen with disseminated tuberculosis.

In a small study of 27[17] patients with TB in pregnancy, it was found that cough (74%), weight loss (41%), fever (30%), were the predominant symptoms. About a fifth of pregnant TB patients may be asymptomatic.[8]

In a study[18] of 471 patients,[17] it was found that although pulmonary involvement was predominant, extra-pulmonary involvement was quite common (nearly 9%). The commonly affected extra-pulmonary sites in that study were: lymph nodes, skeleton and kidneys. Today, HIV infection is an important problem during pregnancy and is overall the most potent risk factor for the development of active tuberculosis. HIV co-infection also confounds the laboratory and radiological features of tuberculosis. Patients with low CD4 and T cell counts (less than 200 cells/cumm) often have sputum smear negative (but culture-positive) PTB. They are four times[9] more likely to develop extra-pulmonary tuberculosis. The radiological features in HIV co-infected patients may also be nonspecific, thus, making the diagnosis a challenge.

Overall, the clinical picture of TB during pregnancy resembles that seen in non-pregnant patients, especially with PTB. In endemic areas and in patients with risk factors for TB disease, a high index of suspicion should be maintained, for both pulmonary and extra-pulmonary TB.

TB and Female Factor Infertility[19,20]

Endometrial/fallopian tube TB (genital tuberculosis; GTB) infection is an important cause of female factor infertility in endemic areas. This form of disease may only be discovered at the time of investigations for infertility. Empiric anti-TB treatment (ATT) has been reported to result in favorable outcomes in certain such cases. However, the accuracy of these findings has been questioned, and empiric ATT is not a treatment option for infertility. The obvious concerns here are ATT drug toxicity and emergence of drug resistance with unwarranted use of these medications. When GTB is suspected as a cause of infertility, a fertility expert and a TB specialist must both be consulted (personal communication).

Tests like PCR have a very poor specificity for genital tuberculosis as the risk of environmental contamination is high. At the authors' institute, which has a WHO accredited Intermediate Reference Laboratory for TB diagnosis, samples, such as endometrial tissue, are not accepted for TB PCR. We strongly discourage the use of TB PCR on endometrial samples to diagnose TB.

Clinical Interaction of TB and Pregnancy

A 1953[21] study looked at the natural history of tuberculosis in pregnancy. Sanatorium therapy was given to 250 pregnant women with tuberculosis. No chemotherapy was given, as was acceptable at that time. They were followed up during pregnancy and for one year thereafter. It was found that the proportion of patients with clinical improvement was similar to that of those with disease progression. The majority of patients remained stable throughout the period of observation, including those with advanced pulmonary TB. The maximum risk seemed to exist in the immediate postpartum months. The authors of this study recommended the implementation of measures such as forceps delivery in order to reduce the duration of labor. A study of 1565[22] preterm and full-term deliveries conducted in New York was published in 1975. Ten percent of the patients had active tuberculosis during or prior to pregnancy. There was no significant difference between the birth-weight of infants with tuberculous mothers and those born to non-tuberculous ones.

However, more recent data from the WHO database paints a different picture. Adverse maternal and fetal outcomes are being reported with TB in pregnancy. Of particular importance among these are: pre-eclampsia, vaginal bleeding, low birth-weight, prematurity, perinatal and fetal death. In a study of 33[23] pregnant patients with extra-pulmonary tuberculosis, it was found that TB lymphadenitis did not have an adverse effect on pregnancy outcome. However, TB at other sites was associated with higher rates of hospitalization, and the infants of such patients had low Apgar scores and birth weights. The cause of hospitalization in most cases in this study was either directly related to the TB, or its sequelae (for example, ankle effusion in skeletal TB, deep venous thrombosis in TB spine with paraplegia).

Effect on the Fetus[24-30]

Transplacental transmission of TB infection to the fetus remains a concern. Other modes of mother to child transmission (MTCT) of TB include aspiration of infected amniotic fluid during childbirth, and later on, via the inhaled route. The rate MTCT of TB has been noted to be 15% in the three weeks after birth. Congenital TB is rare and may be diagnosed using the Cantwell's criteria. In a study comparing 79 pregnancies complicated by maternal PTB, with normal pregnancies, the following adverse perinatal outcomes were reported: significantly lower birth weight, 2-fold increase in risk of prematurity, 6-fold increase in perinatal deaths, and increased risk of small for gestational age neonates. The authors also found that adverse outcomes were associated with late diagnosis of PTB, irregular treatment and advanced stage of the disease. Maternal TB (especially with HIV coinfection) is also a risk factor for childhood TB (Table 13.1).

Latent TB Infection in Pregnancy

A study from Pune,[29] India has found that maternal tuberculosis increases the risk of transmission of HIV infection from mother to child even in the postpartum period. The relative risk of death in infants of HIV positive mothers with active

TABLE 13.1 Summary of adverse obstetric and fetal outcomes with maternal tuberculosis

Adverse outcomes reported with TB during pregnancy
Low birth weight
Prematurity
Fetal growth retardation
Congenital tuberculosis in the neonate
Fetal death
Antenatal hospitalizations
Perinatal death
Increased rate of mother to child transmission of HIV

TB was increased 2.2–3.4-fold. The study recommended that isoniazid preventive therapy should be considered in the Indian scenario in mothers with HIV infection. However, the precise diagnosis of latent TB infection in pregnancy, especially in HIV co-infected patients is an issue currently under study.

The standard test for LTBI diagnosis is the Tuberculin Skin Test (TST), and is safe in pregnancy. The newer tests like the Interferon Gamma Release Assays (IGRAs), are less invasive, but more expensive. While IGRAs have been found to show consistent results in patients with strong test-positivity at baseline, their concordance with the TST has been variable, and they have not yet replaced the TST as a standard test for LTBI diagnosis.[31]

As per the CDC[32] guidelines, LTBI in pregnancy should be treated immediately, (after exclusion of active TB disease), if the patient is HIV infected or has had recent contact with an infective TB patient. If the patient is not immediately at risk for development of active disease, the INH preventive therapy (IPT) may be deferred until after delivery, keeping in mind the increased risk of INH hepatotoxicity in the immediate postpartum period. The standard regimen for IPT is tablet isoniazid 300 mg orally daily for 9 months. Pyridoxine supplementation is essential, both during pregnancy and lactation. Breastfeeding is permitted in lactating women, but pyridoxine supplementation for both mother and child are recommended by the CDC. However, not enough isoniazid is excreted via the breast milk, to treat LTBI in the infant.

However, in countries with a high incidence of LTBI, like India, there are no recommendations for IPT. The benefit of this treatment remains unproven in these cases. At the author's institute, it is not a practice to routinely treat LTBI in pregnant patients.

Diagnosis

The diagnosis of active disease depends on the clinical features, HIV status and local epidemiology of tuberculosis in a given region. The cardinal clinical features have been already discussed. A clinical algorithm commonly followed for the diagnosis of tuberculosis consists of evaluation of the patient with a suggestive clinical presentation, using a sputum smear examination for AFB, and a chest radiograph.

If the chest radiograph is suggestive of TB, or if the sputum smear is AFB positive, anti-TB treatment is initiated. If these are negative the patient may either receive empiric TB treatment, or be investigated for other causes for their symptoms. In a study of 799 HIV infected pregnant women, it was found that screening them for tuberculosis by checking for the classical symptoms (cough, fever, night sweats or weight loss) had a negative predictive value of 99.3%. Chest radiography and the TST did not prove to be very useful.[33]

The diagnosis of TB can present considerable difficulty in the pregnant patient owing to overlap in clinical features. A median diagnostic delay of 7 weeks has been found in one study. A chest radiograph with an abdominal shield may be safely performed in pregnancy and the patient should be given this benefit, if TB is suspected.

Microbiology

The diagnosis of pulmonary tuberculosis is by sputum culture for *Mycobacterium tuberculosis*. If the patient is unable to produce sputum, it may be induced using saline nebulization. Bronchoscopy may be required in patients who are unable to expectorate sputum and in whom microbiological diagnosis is essential. This includes MDR-suspects and patients at risk for various other infections (i.e. immunosuppressed or HIV infected patients). Guidelines[34] for performing bronchoscopy in the pregnant patient are available. Extra-pulmonary TB is often challenging to diagnose and invasive tissue sampling of lymph nodes and deep seated abscesses may be required.

The gold standard for diagnosis of tuberculosis is the demonstration of the *Mycobacterium tuberculosis* complex in culture, of body fluids or tissue samples. TB culture is commonly performed using solid media (Lowenstein-Jensen medium). Liquid media systems (TB-MGIT) reduce the turn-around time and allow for faster performance of drug sensitivity testing (DST).

Molecular Methods

Molecular methods of detection of *Mycobacterium tuberculosis* have emerged as an exciting new development in TB diagnostics, having the potential to be point-of-care diagnostic modalities, and provide simultaneous diagnosis of drug resistance. The two molecular methods that have made their way into practice guidelines are: the Line Probe Assay (LPA; Hain test) and the GeneXpert MTB/RIF (a Real Time Polymerase Chain Reaction test; RT-PCR).[35,36]

Treatment of Tuberculosis

General Principles

Combination therapy is a must as drug resistance occurs with monotherapy. Development of active TB often occurs in the setting of poor nutritional status and defective immunity; hence, nutritional support and treatment of any underlying immunosuppression are extremely important for success of chemotherapy. Because of the increased pill burden (or use of inject able drugs), and prolonged duration of the ATT regimen, there is a chance of lack of patient compliance. Directly Observed Therapy (DOT) has hence found wide application in the setting of National TB Control Programs (NTP). Ensuring compliance is a key to successful TB treatment and to avoid development of drug resistance. For this, patients must be counseled comprehensively regarding the dosage, duration and adverse effects of ATT drugs and followed up.

Screening for HIV infection has been incorporated as a part of routine ante-natal care around the world. It has been suggested that screening for tuberculosis be also made a part of antenatal care, in order to improve case-finding, and ensure treatment of active TB as early as possible.

Whenever possible, sputum (or tissue samples) should be evaluated for TB culture in order to obtain a definitive diagnosis of TB, rule out infection with other agent, and to obtain drug-sensitivity testing. The samples should be tested as far as possible in laboratories accredited by the authorities for mycobacterial culture and DST. Chest radiography is an essential component for diagnosis of 'sputum smear negative PTB' and in the diagnosis of pleural effusions or mediastinal lymphadenopathy. A routine chest radiograph with an abdominal shield is safe, and must be done when tuberculosis is a possible diagnosis.

The central role of good nutrition should never be forgotten when treating the pregnant TB patient.

Chemotherapy

Standard ATT consists of a combination of the following four "first line" drugs: Rifampicin (R), Isoniazid (H), Ethambutol (E) and Pyrazinamide (Z). The term "drug sensitive TB" connotes infection with a strain that is in vitro sensitive to the four first line drugs. The term "multi-drug resistant TB (MDR TB)" indicates in vitro resistance to both R and H at least. The term "poly-drug resistance" indicates in vitro resistance to more than one drug, but sensitivity to either H or R, or to both. The following 'second line drugs' (SLD) are used to treat MDR TB: aminoglycosides (kanamycin, amikacin), capreomycin, fluoroquinolones (ofloxacin, levofloxacin, moxifloxacin), thioamides (ethionamide, prothionamide), cycloserine and PAS. Aminoglycosides and fluoroquinolones form the two key components of anti-MDR TB treatment. The term XDR TB connotes MDR TB with additional resistance to either of these two agents. The following drugs can be used in these cases: linezolid, amoxicillin-clavulanic acid, meropenem, clofazimine, clarithromycin.

It must be remembered that second line drugs and newer anti TB agents are less potent and much more toxic (and expensive) than the first line drugs. This is particularly important, in view of the sobering fact that drug resistance seems to be man-made, and totally-drug resistant tuberculosis (with reference to currently available drugs) is a looming danger.[37]

The dosages and the US-FDA pregnancy categories of each of the drugs have been tabulated below. The HREZ combination has been safely used in pregnancy,

TABLE 13.2 First line drugs used for anti-tuberculosis treatment

First Line Drugs/ Daily Dose	Adverse Effects	US FDA Pregnancy Category	Remarks
Rifampicin (R) 10 mg/kg Maximum : 600 mg PO OD	Hepatotoxicity, allergic reactions, thrombocytopenia, GI irritation, contraceptive failure, reddish orange discoloration of body fluids, contact lenses	C	Taken on empty stomach
Isoniazid (H) 5 mg/kg Maximum : 300 mg PO OD	Peripheral neuropathy, hepatotoxicity, GI irritation psychosis, allergic reactions, drug induced SLE	C	Pyridoxine supplementation essential in both mother and infant
Pyrazinamide (Z) 25 mg/kg Maximum : 2000 mg PO; up to 2 divided doses	Hepatotoxicity, joint pains, hyperuricemia	C	Dose adjustment essential with renal failure. Joint pains may be controlled with analgesics and drug may be safely continued
Ethambutol (E) 20 mg/kg Maximum : 1200 mg PO OD	Dose dependent oculo-toxicity, reduced peripheral vision.	C	Patients should be instructed to report any visual disturbance immediately
Streptomycin (S) 15 mg/ kg. Maximum 1 gm/ day IM	Nephrotoxicity, ototoxicity, vestibulotoxicity	D	Same as for kanamycin (Table 13.3)

and full dosages can be given as per weight. Table 13.2 showing the standard drugs as recommended by the WHO, for drug-sensitive tuberculosis:

The standard four drug regimen (HREZ) has been used safely during pregnancy and it should be continued. There is a recent murine model in which fetal transaminitis with ATT has been demonstrated. However at present, there is no contraindication to HREZ during pregnancy. An interesting case-control study from Hungary,[38] did not find an increased risk for congenital malformations with oral ATT; but this was a small study. The dosage schedule for PTB is: HREZ for the first 2 months (intensive phase; IP) followed by HR for the next 4 months (continuation phase; CP). Intermittent therapy is given in many national TB-control programs, but daily therapy can also be given. In areas with a high level of isoniazid monoresistance, HRE are given in the continuation phase. The treatment duration for bone and central nervous system (CNS) tuberculosis (i.e. cerebral, meningeal) is one year. The hepatic transaminase and bilirubin levels may be monitored as per American Thoracic Society Guidelines,[39] or if the patient has symptoms suggestive of hepatotoxicity. Changes in the regimen should only be made under the supervision of a TB specialist.

The WHO recommendations for treatment of MDR TB[40] have been published. Aminoglycosides and fluoroquinolones form the cornerstone of anti-MDR-TB therapy, and these must be supported by at least ethionamide, cycloserine,

TABLE 13.3 Second line drugs used for treatment of multi-drug resistant tuberculosis

Second Line Drugs	Common Adverse Effects	US FDA Pregnancy Category	Remarks
Kanamycin, Amikacin 15 mg/kg Maximum dose: 1 g/day. Kanamycin is given IM Amikacin may be given IV	Nephrotoxic, ototoxic, Vestibulotoxic. Can produce fetal ototoxicity. Pain at IM injection site	D	Dose adjustments in patients with reduced CrCl. Compatible with breast feeding. Potentiating of adverse effects with loop diuretics. Respiratory depression can occur if given with non-depolarizing muscle relaxants
Capreomycin 15 mg/kg IM	Nephrotoxic, ototoxic, Vestibulotoxic. Can produce fetal ototoxicity. Pain at IM injection site	C	Said to not have cross resistance with aminoglycosides
Ofloxacin : 400–600 mg/ day PO in divided doses Levofloxacin: 500–750 mg/ day PO OD Moxifloxacin: 400 mg PO OD	Nephrotoxicity, fetal cartilage malformations, dysglycemia, cardiac rhythm disturbance, GI upset, dizziness, hepatotoxicity (moxi-floxacin)	C	Compatible with breast-feeding. Dose adjustment required if CrCl < 30 ml/min. Moxifloxacin said to have lower potential for cross resistance with the other two. Ciprofloxacin is not recommended for use as ATT
Ethionamide 500–750 mg/ day in one or 2 divided doses PO Maximum 1 g/ day	Hypothyroidism, nausea, vomiting, stomatitis, occasionally psychotic manifestations, neuropathy, hepatitis, blurred vision	C	Not advisable with hepatic impairment, porphyria. Reduce dose with reduced CrCl. Pyridoxine supplementation advisable
Para-amino Salicylic Acid (PAS) 150–200 mg/ kg or 10–12 g/ day in divided doses. May dilute with water/orange juice	GI upset, hypothyroidism, occasionally increased prothrombin, crytsalluria	C; Congenital defects reported with use in 1st trimester	May increase isoniazid levels. Sodium PAS to be avoided with renal impairment. Caution with G6PD deficient patients
Cycloserine 500–750 mg/ day in 1 or 2 divided doses PO. Maximum 1 g/day	Neuropsychiatric disturbance, gum inflammation, visual disturbance, para-esthesias, suicidal ideation	C	Supplement vitamin B6 to infant. Additive CNS effects with isoniazid

pyrazinamide and ethambutol. Drugs like PAS, clofazimine, linezolid, amoxicillin-clavulanate, and meropenem may be used to form a combination of at least 4 effective drugs. The use of molecular methods for rapid diagnosis of MDR-TB has been advocated for MDR suspects and HIV infected patients.

The Indian MDRTB guidelines[41] have the following standardized treatment: kanamycin, ofloxacin, ethionamide, cycloserine, ethambutol and pyrazinamide for the intensive phase and omission of kanamycin and pyrazinamide for the continuation phase. Serial sputum cultures are used to decide upon the duration of the IP 6-9 months and CP (18–24 months). Birth control is advised, in female patients of child-bearing age and a pregnancy test is done before starting treatment. With patient consent, pregnancies of less than 20 weeks gestation are medically terminated and the standardized MDRTB therapy is given. If the patient wishes to continue the pregnancy, kanamycin is replaced with PAS. Ethionamide is omitted only during the first 12 weeks of pregnancy. Kanamycin may be restarted after delivery and continued until end of the intensive phase.

In the authors' experience, SLD including aminoglycosides have been safely used throughout the duration of pregnancy, with no adverse maternal or fetal outcomes. However, the mother must be counseled about the potential fetal toxicity of these agents and offered the choice of MTP, if she prefers. Recent studies have also documented a good safety profile of standard SLD during pregnancy, although unsatisfactory outcomes have also been reported.[42] Projected rates of spontaneous abortions and congenital malformations on ATT lie between 2 to 3%;[43] but accurate predictions cannot be made. A study [44] of 5 MDR TB patients, who became pregnant while on a standardized regimen (amikacin, ofloxacin, cycloserine, prothionamide) reported no adverse maternal outcomes or fetal malformations. A study of 38[45] pregnant patients with drug resistant TB (over 80% had MDR TB), each treated with an individualized regimen, that generally included an aminoglycoside, a fluoroquinolone and ethionamide as part of a 5 drug combination, was published recently. Around 60% of the patients were declared cured and the fetal outcomes were comparable to those in non-TB pregnancies. The authors recommended that medical termination of pregnancy should not be routinely offered to pregnant patients with MDR TB as second line agents may safely continue in pregnancy.

Surgical Treatment

Invasive procedures such as aspiration of effusions, drainage of abscesses, decompression of the spine, lysis of intra-abdominal adhesions and so forth are important for palliation and for obtaining tissue samples for culture. Radical measures such as lung resection (lobar resection or pneumonectomy) may be indicated in cases of localized disease with poor response to chemotherapy, or in case of a cavitary lesion causing hemoptysis. A case of therapeutic pneumoperitoneum[46] created to induce lung collapse in a post-partum patient has been reported. Measures like thoracoplasty and plombage were used in the past for TB. A multidisciplinary approach involving the obstetrician, TB specialist, surgeon and a pediatrician, is advisable.

Key Messages

- The gold standard for laboratory diagnosis of TB is demonstration of *Mycobacterium tuberculosis* in body fluids/tissue samples.
- Pregnancy can pose an increased risk for development of TB disease in the mother and can also confound the correct diagnosis.
- Standard first line ATT is safe throughout pregnancy. Multiple reports of safe use of SLD for MDR TB in pregnancy are available in the literature. Hence, MTP may be avoided in such cases after careful consideration of the clinical scenario.
- Active TB in pregnancy should definitely be treated. The treatment of LTBI (if at all indicated) may be deferred. HIV coinfection is an important consideration.
- Preventive measures such as standard antenatal care, nutrition and contraception all are vital in order to target TB as a cause of maternal mortality.
- A multidisciplinary approach for treatment of TB in pregnancy is recommended.

References

1. WHO 2011/2012 Tuberculosis Global Facts. Available at: http://www.who.int/tb/publications/2011/factsheet_tb_2011.pdf
2. WHO Tuberculosis Control. http://www.who.int/trade/distance_learning/gpgh/gpgh3/en/index5.html
3. WHO 2009 Women and Tuberculosis. Available at: http://www.stoptb.org/assets/documents/resources/factsheets/womenandtb.pdf
4. Sharma SK, Alladi Mohan, Tamilarasu Kadhiravan. HIV-TB co-infection: Epidemiology, diagnosis and management. Indian J Med Res. 2005;121:550–67.
5. Creswell J, Raviglione M, Ottmani S, Migliori GB, Uplekar M, Blanc L, et al. Tuberculosis and noncommunicable diseases: neglected links and missed opportunities. Eur Respir J 2011;37:1269–82. DOI: 10.1183/09031936.00084310
6. Sheriff FG, Manji KP, Manji MP, Chagani MM, Mpembeni RM, Jusabani AM, et al. Latent tuberculosis among pregnant mothers in a resource poor setting in Northern Tanzania: a cross-sectional study.BMC Infect Dis. 2010;10:52.
7. Zenner D, Kruijshaar ME, Andrews N, Abubakar. Risk of Tuberculosis in regnancy: A National, Primary Care-based Cohort and Self-controlled Case Series Study. Am J Respir Crit Care Med. 2012;185(7):779-84. Epub 2011.
8. Llewelyn M, Cropley I, Wilkinson RJ, Davidson RN. Tuberculosis diagnosed during pregnancy: a prospective study from London. Thorax. 2000;55:129–32.
9. Naidoo K, Naidoo K, Padayatchi N, Abdool Karim Q. HIV-associated tuberculosis. Clin Dev Immunol. 2011;2011. pii: 585919. Epub 2010 Sep 13.
10. Huard RC, Fabre M, de Haas P, Oliveira Lazzarini LC, van Soolingen D, Cousins D. Novel genetic polymorphisms that further delineate the phylogeny of the *Mycobacterium tuberculosis* complex. J Bacteriol, 2006;188:4271–87.
11. Brosch R, Gordon SV, Marmiesse M, Brodin P, Buchrieser C, Eiglmeier K. A new evolutionary scenario for the *Mycobacterium tuberculosis* complex. Proc Natl Acad Sci USA. 2002;99:3684–9.
12. van Soolingen D, de Haas PEW, Haagsma J, Eger T, Hermans PWM, Ritacco V. Use of various genetic markers in differentiation of *Mycobacterium bovis* strains from animals and humans and for studying epidemiology of bovine tuberculosis. J Clin Microbiol. 1994;32:2425–33.
13. Alexander KA, Laver PN, Michel AL, Williams M, van Helden PD, Warren RM, Novel *Mycobacterium tuberculosis* complex pathogen, *M. Mungi*. Emerg Infect Dis. 2010;16:1296–9.

14. Singh N, Bahadur A, Mittal S, Malhotra N, Bhatt A.Comparative analysis of endometrial blood flow on the day of hCG by 2D Doppler in two groups of women with or without genital tuberculosis undergoing IVF-ET in a developing country.Arch Gynecol Obstet. 2011;283(1):115-20. Epub 2010 Aug 6.
15. Kutlu T, Tugrul S, Aydin A, Oral O. Tuberculous meningitis in pregnancy presenting as hyperemesis gravidarum.J Matern Fetal Neonatal Med. 2007;20(4):357–9.
16. Sakorafas GH, Ntavatzikos A, Konstantiadou I, Karamitopoulou E, Kavatha D, Peros G. Peritoneal tuberculosis in pregnancy mimicking advanced ovarian cancer: a plea to avoid hasty, radical and irreversible surgical decisions. Int J Infect Dis. 2009;13(5):e270–2. Epub 2009 Jan 8.
17. Good JT Jr, Iseman MD, Davidson PT, Lakshminarayan S, Sahn SA. Tuberculosis in association with pregnancy. Am J Obstet Gynecol. 1981;140:492–8.
18. Hammer CS, Hirschman SZ. Infections in pregnancy. In:Cherry SH, Berkowitz RL, Kase NC, eds. Medical, Surgical and Gynecologic Complications of Pregnancy, 3rd ed. Baltimore:Williams and Wilkins. 1985:14–15.
19. Mondal SK, Dutta TK. A ten year clinicopathological study of female genital tuberculosis and impact on fertility.JNMA J Nepal Med Assoc. 2009;48(173):52–7.
20. Jindal UN, Verma S, Bala Y. Favorable infertility outcomes following anti-tubercular treatment prescribed on the sole basis of a positive polymerase chain reaction test for endometrial tuberculosis. Hum. Reprod. 2012 doi: 10.1093/humrep/des076.
21. Hedvall E. Pregnancy and tuberculosis. Acts Med Scand 1953;147:1–101.
22. Schaefer C, Zervoudalds IA, Tucks FF, David S, et al Pegnancy and pulmonary tuberculosis. Obstet Gynecol. 1975;46:706–15.
23. Jana N, Vasishta K, Saha SC, Ghosh K.Obstetrical outcomes among women with extrapulmonary tuberculosis.N Engl J Med. 1999;341(9):645–9.
24. Jana N, Vasishta K, Jindal SK, Khunnu B, Ghosh K. Perinatal outcome in pregnancies complicated by pulmonary tuberculosis.Int J Gynaecol Obstet. 1994;44(2):119–24.
25. Abalain ML, Petsaris O, Héry-Arnaud G, Marcorelles P, Couturaud F, Dobrzynski M, et al. Fatal congenital tuberculosis due to a Beijing strain in a premature neonate.J Med Microbiol. 2010;59(Pt 6):733–5. Epub 2010 Mar 4.
26. Peng W, Yang J, Liu E.Analysis of 170 cases of congenital TB reported in the literature between 1946 and 2009. Pediatr Pulmonol. 2011;46(12):1215–24. doi: 10.1002/ppul.21490. Epub 2011 May 27.
27. Lin HC, Lin HC, Chen SF. Increased risk of low birthweight and small for gestational age infants among women with tuberculosis. BJOG. 2010;117(5):585–90. Epub 2010 Feb 15.
28. Grange J, Adhikari M, Ahmed Y, Mwaba P, Dheda K, Hoelscher M, et al. Tuberculosis in association with HIV/AIDS emerges as a major nonobstetric cause of maternal mortality in Sub-Saharan Africa.Int J Gynaecol Obstet. 2010;108(3):181–3. Epub 2010 Jan 13.
29. Gupta A, Bhosale R, Kinikar A, Gupte N, Bharadwaj R, Kagal A, et al. Six Week Extended-Dose Nevirapine (SWEN) India Study TeamMaternal tuberculosis: a risk factor for mother-to-child transmission of human immunodeficiency virus. J Infect Dis. 2011;203(3):358–63.
30. Gupta A, Nayak U, Ram M, Bhosale R, Patil S, Basavraj A, et al. Byramjee Jeejeebhoy Medical College-Johns Hopkins University Study Group. Postpartum tuberculosis incidence and mortality among HIV-infected women and their infants in Pune, India, 2002-2005.Clin Infect Dis. 2007;45(2):241–9. Epub 2007 Jun 4.
31. Worjoloh A, Kato-Maeda M, Osmond D, Freyre R,Aziz N, Cohan D. Interferon gamma release assay compared with the tuberculin skin test for latent tuberculosis detection in pregnancy. Obstet Gynecol. 2011;118(6):1363–70.

32. Latent Tuberculosis Infection: A Guide for Primary Health Care Providers. Available at http://www.cdc.gov/tb/publications/LTBI/treatment.htm

33. Gupta A, Chandrasekhar A, Gupte N, Patil S, Bhosale R, Sambarey P, Ghorpade S, Nayak U, Garda L, Sastry J,Bharadwaj R, Bollinger RC; Byramjee Jeejeebhoy Medical College–Johns Hopkins University Study Group. Symptom screening among HIV-infected pregnant women is acceptable and has high negative predictive value for active tuberculosis. Clin Infect Dis. 2011;53(10):1015–8. Epub 2011 Sep 21.

34. Bahhady IJ, Ernst A.Risks of and recommendations for flexible bronchoscopy in pregnancy: a review.Chest, 2004;126(6):1974–81.

35. WHO factsheet for Tuberculosis Diagnostics Xpert MTB/RIF Test. Available at: http://www.who.int/tb/features_archive/factsheet_xpert_may2011update.pdf

36. Molecular Line Probe Assays For Rapid Screening of Patients at Risk of Multidrug-Resistant Tuberculosis (MDR-TB) Policy Statement. Available at: http://www.who.int/tb/features_archive/policy_statement.pdf

37. Udwadia ZF, Amale RA, Ajbani KK, Rodrigues C.Totally drug-resistant tuberculosis in India.Clin Infect Dis. 2012;54(4):579–81. Epub 2011 Dec 21.

38. Czeizel AE, Rockenbauer M, Olsen J, Sørensen HT. A population-based case-control study of the safety of oral anti-tuberculosis drug treatment during pregnancy. Int J Tuberc Lung Dis. 2001;5(6):564–8.

39. Jussi J Saukkonen, David L Cohn, Robert M Jasmer, Steven Schenker, John A Jereb, Charles M Nolan,et al. behalf of the ATS Hepatotoxicity of Antituberculosis Therapy Subcommittee. An Official ATS Statement: Hepatotoxicity of Antituberculosis Therapy. Am J Respir Crit Care Med, 2006;174:935-52. DOI: 10.1164/rccm.200510-1666ST

40. WHO Guidelines for the programmatic management of drug-resistant tuberculosis 2011 update. Available at :http://whqlibdoc.who.int/publications/2011/9789241501583_eng.pdf

41. DOTS-Plus Guidelines. Available at: http://health.bih.nic.in/Docs/Guidelines-DOTS-Plus.pdf

42. Oliveira HB, Mateus SH.Characterization of multidrug-resistant tuberculosis during pregnancy in Campinas, State of São Paulo, Brazil, from 1995 to 2007. Rev Soc Bras Med Trop. 2011;44(5):627–30.

43. Hageman, JR Congenital and perinatal tuberculosis: discussion of difficult issues in diagnosis and management. J Perinatol. 1998;18,389–93.

44. Tabarsi P, Moradi A, Baghaei P, Marjani M, Shamaei M. Mansouri N, . Chitsaz E, Farnia P, Mansouri D, Masjedi M, Velayati A. Standardised second-line treatment of multidrug-resistant tuberculosis during pregnancy. Int J Tuberc Lung Dis. 15(4):547–50. doi:10.5588/ijtld.10.0140

45. Palacios E, Dallman R, Muñoz M, Hurtado R, Chalco K, Guerra D, et al. Drug-resistant tuberculosis and pregnancy: treatment outcomes of 38 cases in Lima, Peru. Clin Infect Dis. 2009;48(10):1413–9.

46. Antoniou M, Chloros D, Spyratos D, Giouleka P, Sichletidis L.Therapeutic pneumoperitoneum in a patient with pulmonary tuberculosis and persistent fever. BMJ Case Rep. 2011;2011. pii: bcr0520102968. doi: 10.1136/bcr.05.2010.2968.

Plate 1

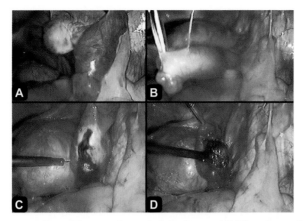

FIG. 4.2 Salpingostomy for a right ampullary tubal pregnancy. (A) Dilated ampullary portion with a tubal pregnancy; (B) A dilute vasopressin solution is injected in the anti-mesenteric part of the tube; (C) A linear incision is made with a monopolar needle cautery; (D) The tubal pregnancy is flushed out with a suction irrigator (hydro dissection)

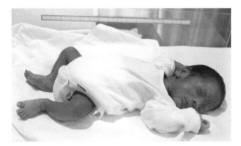

FIG. 6.1 Preterm baby delivered from a surrogate

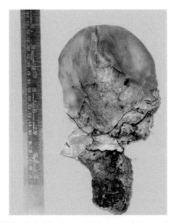

FIG. 6.2 Hysterectomy specimen of a term surrogate for placenta accretra

Index